Epidemiology in Nursing and Health Care

With contributions by

Karen Labuhn, R.N., Ph.D.
Assistant Professor
School of Nursing
University of Virginia
Charlottesville, Virginia

Linda Shortridge, R.N., M.N.
Assistant Professor
College of Nursing and Health
University of Cincinnati
Cincinnati, Ohio

Mary Ann Woodbury, R.N., M.P.H.
Epidemiologist/Biostatistician
Conoco, Inc.
Ponca City, Oklahoma

Epidemiology in Nursing and Health Care

Barbara Valanis, R.N., Dr. P.H.
Professor, College of Nursing and Health
Associate Professor, Department of Environmental Health,
Division of Epidemiology and Biostatistics
College of Medicine
University of Cincinnati
Cincinnati, Ohio

ACC APPLETON-CENTURY-CROFTS/Norwalk, Connecticut

0-8385-2225-4

90 91 92 93 94 / 10 9 8 7 6

Prentice-Hall of Australia, Pty. Ltd., Sydney
Prentice-Hall Canada, Inc.
Prentice-Hall Hispanoamericana, S.A., Mexico
Prentice-Hall of India Private Limited, New Delhi
Prentice-Hall International (UK) Limited, London
Prentice-Hall of Japan, Inc., Tokyo
Prentice-Hall of Southeast Asia (Pte.) Ltd., Singapore
Whitehall Books Ltd., Wellington, New Zealand
Editora Prentice-Hall do Brasil Ltda., Rio de Janeiro

Library of Congress Cataloging-in-Publication Data

Valanis, Barbara.
    Epidemiology in nursing and health care.

    Includes index.
    1. Epidemiology. 2. Nursing. I. Title. [DNLM:
1. Delivery of Health Care. 2. Epidemiologic Methods.
3. Epidemiology. 4. Nursing. WA 950 V136e]
RA652.V34 1986   614.4   86-1157
ISBN 0-8385-2225-4

Contents

v

Preface

This text is designed to provide an introduction to the concepts and methods of epidemiology and to issues in application of epidemiology to clinical practice, public health, and health administration. The author believes that epidemiology is an essential discipline for clinical and community health practice. The importance of this science for the clinician or public health practitioner is demonstrated by the inclusion of epidemiology courses in most medical school and nursing school curricula. Epidemiology provides ways of thinking about health and disease and tools for critical appraisal of the medical and nursing literature. It stimulates a questioning approach to practice which can reduce the probability that treatments or interventions, inadequately supported by research, will be introduced and accepted. Epidemiological thinking can also increase the probability that unusual and/or associated events will be promptly recognized.

Writing of this text was initiated when the author was teaching an epidemiology course in a baccalaureate nursing program and was unable to find a suitable text. Although numerous introductory texts were available, they were oriented toward readers interested in doing epidemiological research or in using epidemiology in community health. None dealt adequately with issues relevant to the clinician. Since the time this text was begun, several clinical epidemiology texts have been published, but they are aimed exclusively at physicians and limit the spectrum of applications and issues to medical practice. This text, while written primarily for nurses, both those who work in institutions and those in community health settings, is relevant for health administrators and for others in public health. Physicians may find it useful for review in preparing for examinations in preventive medicine.

The book is divided into three sections. The first six chapters cover the basic concepts and methods of epidemiology. Chapters seven through ten present data on the major causes of morbidity and mortality for four stages of the life cycle, pregnancy and infancy, childhood and adolescence, young and middle-aged adults, and older persons. The final five chapters discuss issues in the application of epidemiology to disease control and surveillance activities, screening programs, clinical decision-making, health planning and evaluation, and research into the etiology and natural history of disease.

The author hopes that, for some readers, the introduction to epidemiological thinking presented in this book will stimulate an interest in persuing further studies. For the majority of readers, she hopes that the strategies of epidemiology presented herein will add a new and rewarding dimension to their clinical and administrative practice.

Acknowledgments

This book has been influenced by many persons. The author's initial interest in epidemiology was stimulated by Zena Stein, who together with Mervyn Susser and Holger Hansen nourished and profoundly influenced the growth of that interest by their thinking and support. Without them, this book would never have been. The book might not have been started without Mary Curnen, who began writing an introductory text with me nearly 10 years ago. Although we abandoned that project, Mary insisted that in deciding on career goals I should not let go of my nursing background as a special link to epidemiology, and that decision contributed in large measure to this book. Ralph Buncher, by being supportive of my clinical orientation, providing me access to materials from his files, and his tacit expectation that I would indeed finish this book in good time, made an invaluable contribution. I would also like to thank my professional colleagues and students both in the College of Nursing and the College of Medicine at the University of Cincinnati who provided ideas, feedback, and moral support. My contributing authors, Karen Labuhn, Linda Shortridge, and Mary Ann Woodbury, I thank for their timely and excellent work.

Reading draft manuscripts for clarity, content, and format is a time-consuming task, devoid of glory, but invaluable to the author. Thus I wish to thank the reviewers, Elayne Kornblat, Carol Hogue, Diana Hackbarth, Shirley Thompson, and especially Linda Lee Daniel, whose overview comments were most helpful. Thanks also to Jean Cahall and Mary Ann Woodbury, who read the entire manuscript, providing detailed feedback on passages that were incomplete, unclear, irrelevant, or nonsensical. Kenneth Radack provided such feedback on the clinical decision-making chapter and profoundly influenced my thinking on the content. Brenda Riggins, with much patience and good humor, assisted enormously by typing and retyping a good number of these chapters. Thanks to all the other typists who helped with this task, often contending with deadlines and difficult-to-read hand-drafted manuscripts.

All my contacts with the publisher, Appleton-Century-Crofts, were helpful and pleasant. I wish in particular to thank Marion Kalstein-Welch and Brian Dietz for their helpful and skillful assistance. I would also like to thank all the staff who worked quietly behind the scenes to bring this project to completion.

Finally, and most importantly, I owe an emormous debt to my husband, Kirk Valanis, whose unfailing support and confidence gave me the courage to start and then later to complete this work, and to my daughter, Karin Mayleas, whose life most certainly would have been different if her mother had not been absorbed in this project. Thank you for understanding your mother's need to do this.

Epidemiology in Nursing and Health Care

Section I

Introduction and Methods

Epidemiology: What Is It About

Epidemiology is a term derived from the Greek language (epi = upon; demos = people; logos = science). It is a science concerned with health events in human populations. In practical terms, it is the study of how various states of health are distributed in the population and what environmental conditions, life-styles, or other circumstances are associated with the presence or absence of disease. Epidemiologists are essentially medical detectives concerned with the who, what, where, when, and how of disease causation. By searching to find who does and who does not get sick with a particular disease and determining where the illness is and is not found, under what particular circumstances, epidemiologists narrow down the suspected causal agents. When an agent is finally identified, public health officials can take steps to prevent or control the occurrence of the disease.

The process of investigating the disease generates other information that is useful to public health officials and to medical and nursing clinicians. Epidemiological investigations may provide measures of disease frequency that are useful in assessing the need for specific community health services, as for example, rates of occurrence of stroke in different age groups and the expected rate of disability among those having a stroke. These data permit estimation of both the probable number of hospital beds needed and the required staffing for home care and rehabilitation programs. Epidemiologists also generate information about the natural history of a disease—how disease occurs and progresses in the human host; they identify the various signs and symptoms of the condition and the usual patterns of presentation. They may identify physiological changes that, because they occur prior to presentation of clinical signs and symptoms of the diseases, are identifiable only through laboratory tests. Such tests can then be used for early case-finding so that, where effective treatment is available, it can be instituted to arrest the progression of the disease.

In the process of describing disease patterns, epidemiologists may identify new clinical syndromes, refine disease classifications, or identify factors that are associated with a high risk of developing a particular condition. Such information is useful to physicians in making differential diagnoses and deciding on the most effective treatment. Nurses use such information in physical assessments or in selecting groups for specific health education programs. When a specific causal agent is identified, programs to eliminate the agent from the environment or to protect the human population from the agent can be instituted. Because epidemiology provides these basic data needed for decision-making in public health, it is considered one of the basic sciences of public health, just as anatomy, physiology, biochemistry, and genetics constitute basic sciences for medicine and nursing.

DEVELOPMENT OF EPIDEMIOLOGICAL SCIENCE

For thousands of years people have been trying to explain what causes disease. Supernatural events are often used to explain the occurrence of illness. Hippocrates (460 to 377 BC) attempted to explain disease occurrence on a rational rather than a supernatural basis. In several books, *Airs, Waters and Places, Epidemics I,* and *Epidemics II,* he pointed out that disease is a mass phenomena, one that affects groups or populations as well as individuals. He differentiated between endemic disease, that which tends to be always present at a low level, and epidemic disease, occurrence of a given illness clearly in excess of the normal frequency. Further, he noted that environment and lifestyle are related to the occurrence of disease (Adams, 1886).

Even in biblical times, public health measures were instituted. These were based solely on observations about the occurrence of diseases in populations, since the causes were unknown. For example, the practice of isolating persons with a disease such as leprosy was based on the observation that the disease often developed in persons who came in contact with ill persons. Many religious laws or practices grew out of similar observations. The Jewish prohibition of eating pork may have developed from the observation that eating pork frequently resulted in illness (trichinosis). Incest laws are thought to have grown out of observations regarding the high occurrence of congenital malformations and other conditions associated with close consanguinity. Most of these measures were based on observations comparing people who got sick with those who did not, and most involved epidemics of disease. During each epidemic there was often a clear excess of disease that seemed to be associated with certain events.

In more recent history, James Lind suspected that scurvy might be related to the limited diet of sailors. In 1747, he conducted a small experiment in which small groups of ill sailors were given different supplements to their standard diet. Those receiving citrus fruits recovered while the others did not. Some years later, measure were taken to prevent the use of certain water supplies on the basis of the investigative observations of John Snow in England. His work in the 1850s led him to suspect contaminated water as the source of cholera outbreaks. The advent of quantitative measures of disease frequency, called rates, enabled him to determine that rates of cholera were much higher among those persons drinking the water than among those who did not. This was well before the actual isolation of the cholera vibrio by Koch in 1883.

/ The use of rates to measure the frequency of disease occurrence provided a scientific basis for the growth of systematic methods to study disease. These systematic methods, when applied to the investigation of disease patterns as they relate to the distribution of potential causal factors, form a basis for the science of epidemiology. Investigations based on these methods have, over the years, provided a substantial amount of data about human health and disease. This accumulation of data provides an epidemiological body of knowledge about what factors are associated with the occurrence and progression of diseases. The scope of this body of epidemiological knowledge is broadening with time. The earliest epidemiological investigations focused most frequently on infectious conditions, such as plague, cholera, or typhoid, rather than on noninfectious conditions (stroke, mental retardation), because much of the world was plagued with epidemics of infectious disease accompanied by high mortality. As a result, we now have considerable information about such illnesses.

Common nutritional diseases, such as scurvy and pellegra, were important focuses of epidemiological study early in the twentieth century. Chronic illnesses, such as heart disease and cancer, became major causes of mortality and morbidity as infectious and nutritional diseases were controlled. Thus, during the last half century, in particular, epidemiological investigation has expanded to include all diseases, communicable, noncommunicable, acute, or chronic, irrespective of whether their frequency shows short-term epidemic fluctuations. Further, epidemiology today is not limited to the study of diseases or patterns of ill health. It can also focus on other health-related characteristics of populations. Instances of this focus include studies of body weight in relation to height and of blood group subtypes in different population groups. By extending its scope to include mental and social conditions in addition to disease, epidemiology has helped behavioral scientists, social workers, community health planners and, in general, all those concerned with the health and well-being of human populations. It is truly multidisciplinary, providing information to the medical, social, and behavioral sciences, and drawing upon these sciences in its research. A strength of epidemiology as a science is its multidisciplinary approach to health problems, because the broader the scope of observation, the greater are the chances for uncovering the many factors that contribute to poor health. This recognition has led in recent years to a wider spectrum of professionals who participate in epidemiological research. Although the majority of epidemiologists in the past were physicians and nurses, today the field attracts sociologists, psychologists, anthropologists, environmentalists, and many others.

Thus far, we have considered epidemiological methods by which data are collected and the body of knowledge accumulated by the discipline. These represent two of the three characteristics generally considered to differentiate one scientific discipline from another. The third characteristic is the underlying theory that guides the collection of data. Stallones (1980) pointed out that the theory of a discipline is its most distinctive feature. He proposed the following as the central axiom upon which epidemiology is based:

> Axiom: Disease does not distribute randomly in human populations.
>
> Corollary 1: Nonrandom aggregations of human disease are manifested along axes of measurement of time, of space, of individual personal characteristics, and of certain community characteristics.
>
> Corollary 2: Variations in the frequency of human disease occur in response to variations in the intensity of exposure to etiologic agents or other more remote causes, or to variations in the susceptibility of individuals to the operation of those causes (p. 80).

This axiom recognizes that patterns of disease occurrence or other alterations of states of health in human communities are determined by forces that can be identified and measured and that modification of these forces is the most effective way to prevent disease. A definition of epidemiology should therefore reflect this theoretical basis for the discipline.

In recent years there has been considerable discussion among epidemiologists attempting to formulate a single best definition of modern epidemiology (Lillienfeld, 1978; Frerichs & Neutra, 1979; Evans, 1979; Rich, 1979). The following definition reflects the major components of the modern discipline: *Epidemiology is the study of the distribution of states of health and of the determinants of deviations from health in human populations*. The purposes of modern epidemiology are to (1) identify the etiology of deviations from health, (2) provide the data necessary to prevent or control disease through public health intervention, and (3) provide data necessary to maximize the timing and effectiveness of clinical interventions.

EPIDEMIOLOGY AND THE CLINICIAN

Although historically, epidemiological research has often grown out of clinical practice and observation, the focus of epidemiology differs from that of clinical practice. Clinical practice focuses on the health of the individual. The focus of epidemiology is the health of the group to which the individual belongs, whether this group is large or small, representative of a "natural" population (family, school, community, nation) or of a more heterogeneous "aggregate" (club, party). The *clinical* description of a disease differs from its *epidemiological* description in so far as the former relates to an *individual patient* whereas the latter describes a *group of individuals* similarly affected. Here the epidemiologist has to single out, in terms of probabilities, averages, and means, those characteristics that are significantly more common in the diseased population.

Practicing clinicians make use of epidemiological information in their art of diagnosis; they also contribute to epidemiological knowledge of disease through careful observation, examination, and laboratory workup of their patients. Accurate case definition is essential to the epidemiologist. Although the unit of observation in epidemiology is basically a population group, measures of disease frequency are based on the appropriate diagnosis of a disease in each individual patient. By relating clinical signs and symptoms of current patients with those of similar cases previously encountered, either in their own experience or as reported in literature, clinicians and epidemiologists may identify a clustering of similar cases and thus identify and classify new diseases. The recent identification of acquired immune deficiency syndrome (AIDS) as a new illness, restricted to certain population groups, required awareness on the part of clinicians that they were seeing the same unusual symptoms in multiple patients within a short time period and the awareness that all these patients had some common characteristics. In this instance, the early cases were among homosexuals. Since that time, other population groups, such as hemophiliacs and drug addicts, have also been observed to have a high rate of this condition (MMWR, 1985). Patterns of symptoms often cluster in a particular age group, geographical area, or time period. Recognition of such patterns is the first step in learning what causes a particular disease.

A recent example of this epidemological thinking is the investigation of Legionnaire's disease. A unique set of symptoms, resulting in high mortality rates, were recognized primarily among attendees of the American Legion Convention in Philadelphia. Later, while reviewing case records from several previous small epidemics of unknown origin, epidemiologists discovered that these epidemics were of the same conditions as those seen among the Legionnaires. Comparison of the circumstances surrounding each outbreak led to the hypothesis that the organism may have been disseminated through air conditioning systems (Frazer & McDade, 1979). Another instance of epidemiological thinking occurred when several physicians discovered that each of them had recently treated a patient with an unusual cell type (adenocarcinoma) of vaginal cancer. A further unusual factor was that each of the cases occurred in teenaged girls, an unusual age for vaginal cancer. These observations led to a search of hospital records to determine whether further cases could be located, and a study to learn what might be common to all the cases followed. The common factor appeared to be fetal exposure to diethylstilbesterol (DES), a drug that at one time was given to women during pregnancy to reduce the occurrence of spontaneous abortion. This case illustrates the importance of complete recording of information on the onset of symptoms and of laboratory data by hospital personnel.

Nurses working on an inpatient medical unit of a large urban hospital thought they were seeing an unusually high occurrence of bladder infections among patients with indwelling catheters. When they checked unit records they found that during the most recent 3 months, the rate of new infections was three times that of the previous 3 months. Approximately 3 months before, a new brand of catheter had been purchased to replace the more expensive brand used on the unit. Further examination of nursing notes revealed that the frequency with which the new, less expensive catheters became displaced and had to be reinserted was much higher than with the previous brand. The nurses thus recommended to the hosptial administrator that the more expensive brand be reinstated as the cost in added personnel time, illness, and use of multiple catheters per patient was far greater than the few cents saved per catheter with the new brand. Following a return to the original brand, reinsertion rates and rates of bladder infection returned to the previous low level. This example of epidemiological thinking illustrates the importance of being aware of the usual frequency with which events occur, and the need for adequate records with which to validate one's observation that the observed frequency of an event did indeed change.

In general, epidemiological studies rely heavily on health data that are recorded for purposes other than epidemiological investigation. Thus physicians, nurses, and other health personnel are essential in providing the required data. Further, because these clinical personnel are regularly in contact with patients, they are in a superb position to note patterns of disease occurrence and progression and to raise questions about anything unusual. Understanding epidemiological methods can lead to "thinking epidemiologically" and increases the likelihood of appropriate observation. Thus, most medical schools and nursing schools offer some training in epidemiology.

Clinical personnel frequently make use of epidemiological data in the course of their practice. As previously mentioned, physicians use knowledge of the patterns of disease occurrence to make differential diagnosis. Nursing assessments utilize knowledge of distribution of symptoms in relation to age to determine whether a particular symptom needs follow-up or intervention. A blood pressure of 140/90 is probably no cause for alarm in an 80-year-old, but most likely requires intervention in a 25-year-old. Additionally, epidemiological input is useful to clinical personnel in determining the optimum therapy, the dosage of medication, and the duration of treatment. For example, through the systematic observation of a considerable number of children who have undergone surgery at different ages for repair of congenital heart disease, it is now possible to select the most appropriate age for this intervention.

Early detection of disease may contribute to improved prognosis. Identification of risk factors for breast cancer, for example, permits the identification of high-risk women who need more frequent screening to identify a cancer before metastasis and for cautious use of drugs, such as reserpine, which some studies have shown to enhance cancer risk. Furthermore, these high-risk women should be taught how to do self-breast examinations so they can monitor themselves between physical examinations for any occurence of a lump.

COMPONENTS OF EPIDEMIOLOGY

The term epidemiology has come to refer both to the particular methods applied in studies of disease causation and to the body of knowledge that arises from such investigations. The collection of epidemiological knowledge is usually termed substantive epidemiology, although some authors may refer to it as descriptive epidemiology. To avoid confusion for the reader, the author of this book has chosen to reserve the term descriptive epidemiology for the first phase of epidemiological research. The term substantive epidemiology is used to refer to the cumulative body of knowledge generated through epidemiological research. This comprises the epidemiological descriptions of various diseases and states of health, including their natural history, patterns of occurrence, and factors associated with high risk of developing the condition (risk factors).

USES OF EPIDEMIOLOGY

Different systems for classifying uses of epidemiology have been devised. The author has used a system that classifies uses into seven categories:

Investigation of Disease Etiology and Determination of the Natural History of Disease. Because the purpose of epidemiological investigation is to delineate the etiology of disease, thus providing the data needed for control or eradication, etiological studies represent a major use of epidemiological methods. These studies produce information on the natural history of the disease. Natural history refers to the processes normally leading to disease occurrence, prior to any intervention, and to the course and outcome of the disease process. It includes the description of the disease process from the first forces creating the disease stimulus in the environment or elsewhere, through the time of host–agent interaction, and to the resulting response in humans, including illness, recovery, permanent disability, or death. In order to prevent disease, the cause(s) of the disease must be identified and the means by which causal agents are transmitted to the human host must be understood. In contrast to epidemiological studies, which emphasize the prepathogenic or early pathogenic stages of disease in total population groups, research carried out by clinicians, whether by physicians, nurses, or other groups, is largely concerned with patient responses to treatment (physiological and psychological) during the later stages of the natural history. Clinical research is usually based only on the study of patients who have sought treatment for symptoms of illness.

Although there are epidemiological studies based solely on populations of hospitalized cases, the evolution of a complete body of knowledge about the natural history of a disease demands the study of a spectrum of ascertainable cases in a population, including those cases too mild to have sought or require medical treatment. Without this spectrum of disease severity, it is impossible to understand the natural history. Thus, epidemiological research studies often produce a different picture of the disease than do studies derived only from data on hospitalized patients. As an example, recent data show that half or more of the deaths of middle-aged men from coronary heart disease occur in the initial days of the first clinical attack of coronary thrombosis. Because a substantial portion of these deaths occur in the first hours before the patient reaches the hospital, these cases are never part of clinical research. In addition, there are many cases of "silent" myocardial infarction (MI) that are generally unknown to the clinician (Russek and Zohman, 1951). These data provide important information, however, that can be used for planning early intervention directed toward identification and treatment of the "silent MI" group through early treatment of high-risk individuals. In addition, the data on the high early mortality associated with clinical attacks suggest the need for mobile life squads trained in cardiopulmonary resuscitation with readily available equipment.

Identification of Risks. Risk refers to the probability of an unfavorable event. In epidemiology, the term generally refers to the likelihood that people who are without a disease, but who come in contact with certian factors thought to increase disease risk, will acquire the disease. Factors associated with an increased risk of acquiring disease are called risk factors. These factors may be part of the physical environment, such as toxins, infectious organisms, radiation, or part of the social environment, such as stressful life events, divorce or death of a spouse. They may also be behavioral, like smoking and lack of exercise, or inherited, like hemoglobin S, which increases risk for infection.

In general, the risk to an individual of developing a particular disease can be estimated only on the basis of the experience of whole populations of individuals. Once this experience is known, the relevant risks can be calculated for persons who are similar to those in that population. Further, population data on disease occurrence can provide data for estimating the effect of a public health intervention on disease rates. Epidemiological methods are used to collect the appropriate data and to estimate these risks.

Risk to an individual of developing a disease due to a particular exposure is derived by comparing the occurrence of disease in a population exposed to the causal agent to the occurrence of disease in a nonexposed population. This measure, called a *relative risk ratio,* estimates how much the risk of acquiring a disease increases with exposure to a particular causal agent or known risk factor. Thus, a relative risk ratio of 5 implies that the risk of acquiring that disease is five times greater for someone exposed to an etiological agent than for someone not exposed. Relative risk ratios are a useful tool for identifying factors that represent increased risk for development of a disease. Diabetes, obesity, hypertension, and smoking are considered risk factors for cardiovascular disease because populations with these characteristics show several times the rate of that disease as do populations without those conditions or behaviors. Once these risk factors are identified, public health programs can be instituted to change high-risk behaviors, such as smoking, and to identify high-risk individuals through comprehensive screening programs that ensure medical treatment to reduce risk. In addition, nurses and other clinicians can counsel high-risk individuals regarding methods to reduce their risk by adopting healthier life-styles. Relative risk ratios are discussed in more detail in the chapters on epidemiological methods and measures.

An estimate of the effect on disease occurrence of public health intervention to eliminate exposure to a causal agent is provided by a measure called *attributable risk.* This measure subtracts the rate of disease occurrence (incidence) in the nonexposed population from the rate of disease occurrence (incidence) in the exposed population. If a nonsmoking population develops cardiovascular disease at a rate of 350 per 100,000 and a smoking population develops cardiovascular disease at a rate of 685 per 100,000, then 335 cases per 100,000 population are attributable to cigarette smoking and should be preventable if cigarettes were banned.

Identification of Syndromes and Classification of Disease. This use of epidemiology relates directly to clinical medicine. Broad descriptive clinical and pathological categories often include very different elements. Variations in their statistical distribution and in the ways in which diseases progress or behave in a population (natural history) may make it possible to distinguish elements of one disease from another. Previously, all vascular diseases were classified together. As epidemiological data accumulated, it became clear that cerebrovascular disease and cardiovascular disease were distinct conditions, although both shared the characteristic narrowing or occlusion of a blood vessel as a preceding mechanism. Populations with high rates of cerebrovascular disease, such as the Japanese, had low rates of cardiovascular disease whereas populations with high rates of cardiovascular disease had lower rates of cerebrovascular disease (Morris, 1975).

Clustering of signs, symptoms, and similarities of natural history allows the identification of syndromes. Rubella syndrome was identified as a collection of malformations and functional problems common to offspring of mothers infected with rubella during pregnancy, particularly during the first trimester (Gregg, 1941). A more recent example is the identification of toxic shock syndrome as a definable group of symptoms characterized by fever of greater than 102°F, rash, desquamation of skin, particularly on the extremities, hypotension, and involvement of three or more of the following organ systems: gastrointestinal, muscular, mucous membrane, renal, hepatic, hematologic, central nervous system and negative results shown on the tests in Table 1–1 (MMWR, 1980).

Differential Diagnoses and Planning Clinical Treatment.
Descriptive data, such as age and sex distribution of disease incidence, aid the clinician in understanding the condition and in sorting through multiple possible diagnoses that present with the same or similar symptoms. Such data also facilitate the planning of treatment. Recognizing the association of age with prognosis for long-term survival in breast cancer, for example, will likely influence treatment and may also influence follow-up programs. Breast cancers diagnosed premenopausally tend to be more lethal than postmenopausal breast cancer, and thus require more aggressive treatment and closer follow-up. Mumps may be a mild self-limiting disease in childhood, but in adult men it can lead to infertility. Public health intervention to reduce susceptibility or to prevent exposure of men who did not acquire that infection during childhood is therefore crucial.

TABLE 1–1. TOXIC SHOCK SYNDROME CASE DEFINITION

1. Fever (temperature $\geqslant$38.9°C [102°F]).
2. Rash (diffuse macularerythroderma).
3. Desquamation,1–2 weeks after onset of illness, particularly of palms and soles.
4. Hypotension (systolic blood pressure $\leqslant$90 mm Hg for adults or <5th percentile by age for children <16 years of age, or orthostatic syncope).
5. Involvement of 3 or more of the following organ systems:
   a. Gastrointestinal (vomiting or diarrhea at onset of illness).
   b. Muscular (severe myalgia or creatine phosphokinase level $\geqslant 2 \times$ULN[a]).
   c. Mucous membrane (vaginal, oropharyngeal, or conjunctival hyperemia).
   d. Renal (BUN[b] or Cr[c] $\geqslant 2 \times$ULN or $\geqslant$5 white blood cells per high-power field–in the absence of a urinary tract infection).
   e. Hepatic (total bilirubin, SGOT[d], or SGPT[e] $\geqslant 2 \times$ULN).
   f. Hematologic (platelets $\leqslant$100,000/mm³).
   g. Central nervous system (disorientation or alterations in consciousness without focal neurologic signs when fever and hypotension are absent).
6. Negative results on the following tests, if obtained:
   a. Blood, throat, or cerebrospinal fluid cultures.
   b. Serologic tests for Rocky Mountain spotted fever, leptospirosis, or measles.

[a]Twice upper limits of normal for laboratory.
[b]Blood urea nitrogen level.
[c]Creatinine level.
[d]Serum glutamic oxaloacetic transaminase level.
[d]Serum glutamic pyruvic transaminase level.
(From Follow-up on toxic shock syndrome. *Morbidity and Mortality Weekly Reports, 29*, 442.)

Surveillance of the Health Status of Populations. Surveillance means keeping watch over. Epidemiological descriptions of diseases provide data on who is at high risk of contracting a disease, in which geographical locations it is more likely to occur, and when in time it is most frequently observed. This information alerts health workers to situations that should be monitored for early indication of a disease outbreak so that early detection programs may be set up and intervention promptly instituted. As an example, influenza rates tend to increase during late fall and early winter. Specific types of influenza are likely to recur in 2- to 3-year or 4- to 6-year cycles (Benenson, 1980). Groups at high risk of becoming seriously ill and dying of influenza are infants, young children, and the elderly. By monitoring the population for the initial increase in cases of influenza, through reports of deaths due to influenza, an increase in cases seen at emergency rooms, or an increased rate of absence from schools or work due to respiratory illness, public health officials can identify the signs of an outbreak early and can take steps to immunize susceptible populations at high-risk of complications to prevent occurrence of the illness in these individuals.

In an additional example, the descriptive epidemiology of measles indicates that it occurs most frequently among school-age children, that rates vary by season with highest rates in the fall, and that there are long-term cycles with increased rates every other year in large communities and at less frequent intervals in smaller communities, where outbreaks tend to be more severe. Measles is transmitted from person to person by close contact; therefore, it tends to occur in locations where children congregate (Benenson, 1975). Armed with this information, the school nurse can be alert to signs and symptoms of measles during the fall and can follow up on absences to determine if measles caused the absence. Numerous absences may indicate a need to review the immunization status of the school population. Although most schools, in theory, require up-to-date immunizations for students to be admitted, all too often monitoring does not occur and follow-up programs must be instituted to obtain immunizations for the susceptible children.

Monitoring of newly diagnosed cancer cases or of birth defects can alert officials to clusters of cases that may suggest clues as to their causes. The occurrence of several cases of adenocarcinoma of the vagina of young girls was noted by physicians in Boston. They realized that the occurrence of several cases in a short period of time in this age group was a highly unusual event. Their follow-up investigation identified as the probable causal agent DES, a drug given to the mothers of these patients during their pregnancies (Herbst & Scully, 1972).

Community Diagnosis and Planning of Health Services. Epidemiology provides the facts about community health. It describes the nature and relative size of the health problems to be dealt with, as well as how they are distributed in terms of geographical location, age group, socioeconomic group, and so on. This kind of information is the basis for planning the number and types of services required to meet the needs of a particular community. A neighborhood with a high proportion of elderly individuals is likely to have high rates of cardiovascular disease, cancer, and other chronic, debilitating diseases. Particularly if it is a low income neighborhood, elderly residents may lack the financial resources to travel to a distant source of medical care. Thus, health planners need to consider either setting up a satellite clinic in the neighborhood, providing transportation or home services, or both. Maternal–child health services can be planned to meet the needs of a community with a young population and a high birth rate. Family planning facilities, well-child centers, which include immunization services and health education programs aimed at prevention of disease through promotion of good health habits, may be appropriate.

Evaluation of Health Services. Because many health services are initiated as an effort to treat a community problem identified by epidemiological data, these same data, used as a monitoring device, are useful in the evaluation of these services. For example, one means of evaluating the effectiveness of a maternal–child health center established to reduce the rates of morbidity and mortality among mothers and children is to follow closely the morbidity and mortality rates and see if they drop and remain low after the health center begins operation. Specifics of how epidemiology can be used to plan and evaluate health services are discussed in Chapter 15.

REFERENCES

Adams, F. *The genuine works of Hippocrates.* (trans. from the Greek) New York: William Word, 1886.

Benenson, A. S. (Ed.). *Control of communicable disease in man* (13th ed.). New York: American Public Health Association, 1980.

Evans, A. S. Letter to the editor. *American Journal of Epidemiology,* 1979, *109,*379–382.

Frazer, D. W., & McDade, J. E. Legionellosis. *Scientific American,* 1979, *241,* 82–99.

Frericks, R. R., & Neutra, R. Letter to the editor. *American Journal of Epidemiology,* 1978, *108,* 74–75.

Greg, N. M. Congenital cataract following German Measles in the mother. *Trans Opthalmol Soc Aust,* 1941, *3,* 35.

Herbst, A. L., Kurman, R. J., & Scully, R. E. Vaginal and cervical abnormalities after exposure to stilbesterol in utero. *Obstetrics and Gynecology,* 1972, *40,* 287–298.

Koch, R. *Investigations into the etiology of traumatic infective diseases.* (W. Watson Cheyne, trans.) London: The New Sydenham Society, 1880.

Lilienfeld, E. D. Definitions of epidemiology. *American Journal of Epidemiology,* 1978, *107,* 87–90.

Lind, J. *A treatise of the scurvy.* Edinburgh: Kincaird and Donaldson, 1753. Reprinted in C. P. Steward & D. Guthrie, (Eds.), *Lind's treatise on scurvy.* Edinburgh: University Press, 1953.

MMWR. Follow-up on toxic shock syndrome. *Morbidity and Mortality Weekly Reports* (CDC), September 19, 1980, *29*(37), 441–445.

MMWR. Update—Acquired Immunodeficiency Syndrome—United States. *Morbidity and Mortality Weekly Reports* (CDC), May 10, 1985, *34*(18), 245–248.

Morris, J. N. *Uses of epidemiology.* New York: Churchill and Livingston, 1975.

Rich, H. Letter to the editor. *American Journal of Epidemiology,* 1979, *109,* 102.

Russek, H. I., & Zohman, B. L. Chances for survival in acute myocardial infection. *JAMA,* 1951, *156,*765.

Stallones, R. A. *Annual Review of Public Health,* 1980, *1,* 69–82.

Snow, J. *On the mode of communication of cholera* (2nd ed.). London: Churchill, 1855. Reprinted in *Snow on cholera.* New York: Commonwealth Fund, 1936.

2

Some Useful Concepts in Epidemiology

A number of concepts are essential to the principles and methods of epidemiology. Understanding these concepts enables the clinical practitioner or the public health professional to interpret the epidemiological literature and to apply this information in their practice. Three crucial concepts are discussed in this chapter: natural history of disese, levels of prevention, and causality. Some other concepts relevant to epidemiology are included under the discussion of the three major concepts. Presentation of additional concepts, such as that of an epidemic, has been postponed to other chapters where auxiliary information that contributes to understanding of the concept is presented.

NATURAL HISTORY OF DISEASE

Natural history of disease is the process by which diseases occur and progress in the human host. This process involves the interaction of three different kinds of factors: the causative agent(s), a susceptible host (human), and the environment. As long as a state of equilibrium exists between host, agent, and environment, a state of health is maintained. A disequilibrium, such as an increase in the amount of the agent resulting from a change in environmental conditions, increases the likelihood that a susceptible host will be exposed. An increase in host susceptibility because of lack of sleep, malnutrition, excessive stress, aging, or a variety of other factors also increases the risk of disease. Changes in the environment contribute to changes in host susceptibility as well as to the conditions for viability of the agent.

The Agent

An *agent* is a factor whose presence causes a disease or one whose absence causes disease. An example of the former is Salmonella, which causes salmonellosis; an example of the latter is lack of vitamin D, which leads to rickets. Categories of causative agents include physical, chemical, nutrient, biological, genetic, and psychological agents. Physical agents include mechanical forces or frictions that may produce injury or atmospheric conditions such as extremes of temperature and excessive radiation. Chemical agents are those that affect human physiology through chemical action. These agents include substances that may occur as dusts, gases, vapors, fumes, or liquids. Nutrient agents are chemical in nature, but refer specifically to basic components of the diet. Agents transmitted from parent to child through the genes are genetic agents. Psychological agents are those stressful social circumstances in the environment that affect physiology by psychosomatic means. The category of biological agents includes all living organisms, including insects, worms, protozoa, fungi, bacteria, rickettsia, and viruses. This class of agents is infectious in nature.

Certain characteristics of agents affect their ability to produce disease in the host. For infectious agents, the characteristics are infectivity, pathogenicity, and virulence. These characteristics are measured by the infection or attack rate, pathogenicity rate, and case fatality rate, respectively. These rates provide a means of population surveillance, allowing public health officials to assess the nature of the problem they are dealing with and to plan appropriate intervention. Characteristics of infectious agents are discussed further in Chapter 5.

Important characteristics of noninfectious agents include concentration and toxicity for chemical agents, size, shape, and intensity for physical agents, chronicity or suddenness for psychological agents, and homo- or heterozygocity of genetic material for genetic agents. These are discussed in relation to non-infectious diseases in Chapter 6.

The Environment

Environment refers to all external conditions and influences affecting the life of living things. Physical, biological, and socio-economic environments provide reservoirs where agents can reside and/or reproduce and modes of transmission for transporting agents from the reservoir to a human host. The *physical environment* includes the geological structure of an area and the availability of resources, such as water and flora, that influence the number and variety of animal reservoirs and certain insects that function as vectors to carry an agent from the reservoir to the host. Weather, climate, and season are important influences in the physical environment.

The *socioeconomic environment* contributes to the types of infectious agents in a locality because social and economic conditions relate both to the extent of environmental sanitation practices, such as disposal of garbage and excreta, and to the availability of medical facilities for immunization and medical care. The socioeconomic environment may also influence the noninfectious agents. More psychological stressors may be found in poorer socioeconomic environments than in better ones. Poor socioeconomic neighborhoods are more likely to be located near industrial plants, which may produce dangerous chemicals or emit physical particles of agents such as asbestos or coal tar.

Finally, there is the *biologic environment,* which includes living plants and animals that may serve as either the reservoir or the vector for transmission of an infectious agent. Brucellosis is a disease in which animals, particularly cattle, swine, sheep, goats, horses, and reindeer, serve as reservoirs for human infection. The disease is transmitted from these animals to humans by contact with tissues, blood, urine, vaginal discharges, aborted fetuses, or placentas, and by ingestion of milk or dairy products from infected animals. Pasteurization of milk is an effective control measure for the general population. Special animal inspection and disposal procedures and education of farmers, animal handlers, and slaughter house workers help to control the spread of the disease among these groups (Benenson, 1980). In the case of plague, wild rodents are the usual reservoir, although infective fleas serve as the mode of transmission of the disease to humans (Benenson, 1980).

The Host

A *host* is the individual human in whom an agent produces disease. Disease can occur only in a host who is susceptible. Lack of susceptibility may be due to immunity or to inherent resistance. Immunity relates to lack of susceptibility to infectious agents whereas inherent resistance is broader, including lack of susceptibility to all types of agents. Immunity is the resistance on the part of a host to a specific infectious agent. Immunity can be humoral (antibodies in the blood) or cellular (specific to each type of cell). The role of immunity varies with the type of infectious agent. Immunity can be passive or active. Passive immunity is attained either naturally (maternal transfer of antibodies to the fetus) or artifically by inoculation of specific protective antibodies (immune serum globulin for prevention of infectious hepatitis or diphtheria antitoxin for diphtheria prevention). Passive immunity is temporary; in the newborn it usually lasts 6 months, during which time the infant is only protected against infections experienced by the mother and for which she has made antibodies. By contrast, active immunity is long lasting and may protect an individual for life. It is attained naturally by infection, with or without clinical manifestations, or artifically by the inoculation of vaccine obtained from fractions of products of the infectious agent or of the agent, itself, in killed, modified, or variant form. The principal of active immunity is used in many of the major vaccination programs such as for diphtheria and polio. It was also the basis for the successful worldwide program to eradicate smallpox through an international vaccination and surveillance program.

In contrast to immunity, the term inherent resistance refers to the ability to resist disease independently of antibodies or of specifically developed tissue response. It commonly rests in anatomical or physiological characteristics of the host; it may be genetic or acquired, permanent or temporary. The concept of inherent resistance is useful in understanding host resistance both to infectious agents as well as to other types of agents. Factors such as general health status or nutrition, for example, may affect resistance to disease. Someone in good health who maintains good nutrition and a regular schedule of rest and exercise may be exposed to the common cold virus and resist infection even though the person is not immune to the organism. Similarly, this same individual, if exposed to psychological stress, may resist ulcers better than would someone in poorer general health.

The Disease Process

Occurrence of disease in a human host is not a single event at one point in time. Rather it is a process occurring over a period of time—the natural history of the disease.

The natural history may be divided into two periods, prepathogenesis and pathogenesis. Each of these periods is further subdivided into two stages. Stages in prepathogenesis are susceptibility and adaptation. Stages in pathogenesis are early pathogenesis and clinical disease (Fig. 2–1). Clinical disease is defined as disease that is detectible because of symptoms experienced by the patient or signs apparent to a clinician during a physical examination. Pathological changes detectible only by laboratory or other tests are considered preclinical in the model. Thus, tests that can detect disease earlier than it would normally be detected through presence of physical signs and symptoms, i.e., screening tests, detect disease during the stage of early pathogenesis.

These stages and the events that occur at each stage can be used as a basis for determining intervention measures. Table 2–1 outlines the stages of the natural history for any disease and identifies points of intervention.

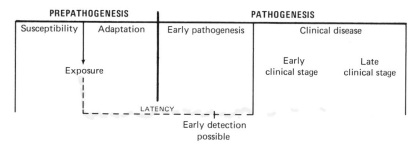

Figure 2–1. The natural history of disease.

TABLE 2–1. NATURAL HISTORY OF DISEASE AND APPLICATION OF PREVENTIVE MEASURES

Period	Stage	Events	Level of Application of Preventive Measures	Specific Interventions
Prepathogenesis	Susceptibility	1. Interrelations of various host, agent, and environmental factors bring host and agent(s) together	Primary prevention	Health promotion (health education, nutrition counseling, adequate housing, personal hygiene, etc.)
		2. Disease-provoking stimulus is produced in the known host		Specific protection (immunizations, sanitation, removing occupational and environmental hazards, use of specific nutrients, etc.)
	Adaptation	1. Adaptive processes are initiated		

Pathogenesis				Level of Prevention	Action
Presymptomatic disease	A. Early pathogenesis	1.	Interaction of host and stimulus continues after failure of adaptive response		
		2.	Stimulus or agent becomes established (if infectious agent, increases by multiplication)		
		3.	Beginning tissue and physiological changes		
	B. Discernible early lesions	1.	Clinical recognition of disease is possible through laboratory or other tests that detect early physiological changes	Secondary prevention	Early diagnosis and prompt treatment (screening, case-finding, selective examination)
		2.	Patient develops early symptoms that go unrecognized		
Clinical disease		1.	Acute illness	Tertiary prevention	Disability limitation (treatment to arrest disease process)
		2.	Disability		Rehabilitation retraining for maximum use of remaining capacities, facilitating reentry to the family unit and to the workplace
		3.	Defect		
		4.	Chronic state		
		5.	Death		

(Adapted from Leavell, H. R. & Clark, D. W.. *Preventive medicine for the doctor in his community.* New York: McGraw-Hill, 1958.)

In the first stage, *susceptibility,* disease has not yet developed, although the groundwork has been laid through presence of factors that favor its occurrence. For example, poor eating habits and fatigue resulting from lack of sleep, which are often present among college students during exam week, represent risk factors that favor the occurrence of the common cold. If exposure to an agent occurs at this time, a response will occur. Initial responses reflect the normal adaptation response of the cell or functional system (e.g., the immune system). If these adaptation responses are successful, then no disease occurs and the process is arrested in the adaptation stage.

The next stage in the natural history is the stage of *presymptomatic disease,* sometimes called *early pathogenesis.* At this stage, the individual has no symptoms indicating the presence of illness. Adaptation, however, has been unsuccessful and pathogenic changes have begun. These changes, which may be detectable by sophisticated laboratory tests, are called subclinical because they are below the level of the *clinical horizon,* an imaginary line dividing the point where there are detectable signs and symptoms from that where there are not. Premalignant changes or early malignant tissue changes in the cervix, for example, may be detected by a Papanicolaou (Pap) smear long before a woman experiences symptoms and before signs are visible to an obstetrician on visual examination.

Stage four in the natural history is *clinical disease.* By this stage, sufficient anatomical or functional changes have occurred to produce recognizable signs and symptoms. This stage includes a range of disease severity from early clinical disease to that so advanced that death is inevitable. Possible outcomes, once a patient has entered this stage, may be complete recovery, residual defect that produces some degree of disability, or death. In an attempt to further understand this stage, clinicians and researchers have developed classification schemes for varying degrees of disease severity, including the staging systems used for malignancies, and the functional and therapeutic classifications used for cardiac disease.

Exposure of the host to an agent occurs during the stage of susceptibility. In the case of infectious agents, exposure is followed by an *incubation period,* a time when the organism multiples to sufficient numbers to produce a host reaction and clinical symptoms. This time period is relatively short, usually hours to months. For diseases caused by noninfectious agents, however, this time period from exposure to onset of symptoms, called the *induction period* or *latency period,* may be years to decades. Accidents resulting from a severe psychological stressor may occur shortly after initial exposure to the stressor. Ulcers, as a consequence of psychological stress, may require years of exposure. One of the shorter known latency periods for cancer is the 5-year latency period for leukemia in children exposed to radiation. Lung cancer resulting from asbestos exposure may have a latency period of 40 years between exposure and detection of the disease. Exceptions to these general rules about time from exposure to onset of symptoms for noninfectious agents do occur. For example, some chemical agents cause almost instantaneous, acute episodes of poisoning. The end of the incubation or induction period is the point of disease detection, whether by screening or by appearance of clinical signs and symptoms, although the time of clinically observable illness has conventionally been used.

Another difference between diseases caused by infectious agents and those caused by noninfectious agents or by still unidentified agents is the likelihood for the former to be conditions of a chronic nature. Most, but not all, diseases with infectious causes are of relatively short duration. The patient is usually ill for a period ranging from a few days to several months and generally recovers without any residual disability, or, if the illness was severe, may die from the illness. The patient who has recovered rarely requires long-term follow-up, although there are exceptions. Tuberculosis and rheumatic heart disease, which results from a staphylococcal infection, are diseases caused by infectious agents that are chronic in nature. The herpes virus may produce a single acute infection or may become chronic with repeated outbreaks of the infection following periods of remission. In the case of noninfectious agents, there is often residual disability requiring prolonged medical treatment and rehabilitation programs. Patients with cardiovascular disease, for example, are likely to require ongoing supervision with prescribed medications, control of diet, and indefinite modifications of life-style.

LEVELS OF PREVENTION

The natural history of a disease provides the basis for planning intervention. Because a disease evolves over time and pathological change becomes less reversible as the disease process continues, the ultimate aim of intervention programs is to halt or reverse the process of pathological change as early as possible, thus preventing further damage. Three levels of intervention, based on the three stages of disease natural history, have proved useful (Table 2–1). Because the goal of intervention at each of the three levels is to prevent the pathogenic process from evolving further, the three levels are called primary, secondary, and tertiary prevention.

Primary prevention is aimed at intervening before pathological changes have begun, during the natural history stage of susceptibility. Primary prevention seeks to keep the agent away from contact with the host, or to eliminate or reduce host susceptibility. These aims are accomplished through two types of activities, general health promotion and specific protection. General health promotion includes all activities that optimize the environment and favor healthy living. Thus efforts to improve the physical environment, whether that of outdoors, home, school, or work would be included. Health education aimed at educating the population about good nutrition, hygiene, the need for rest and recreation, preparation for retirement, or the harmful effects of smoking or drug use is a form of general health promotion. Specific protection refers to measures aimed at protecting individuals against specific agents. These measures include immunization against specific disease, such as diphtheria or polio, and removal of harmful agents from the environment, as with sewage treatment, pasteurization of milk, or chlorination of water. Since 1900, the effects of primary prevention can be seen in the dramatic reduction in mortality from infectious diseases, which is largely a result of environmental manipulation and immunization programs (Fig. 2–2). This reduction in infectious disease mortality, particularly among infants, young children, young women, and the elderly, has led to a larger total population and to the advent of chronic disease as a major public health concern. As fewer people die of infectious disease, more live to older ages where chronic diseases are common. Also, industrialization and changes in life-style have increased exposure to potential causal agents of noninfectious disease. These epidemiological transitions are discussed at length in Chapter 4.

Secondary prevention seeks to detect disease early, treat promptly, and cure disease at its earliest stage, or, when cure is not possible, to slow its progression, prevent complications, and

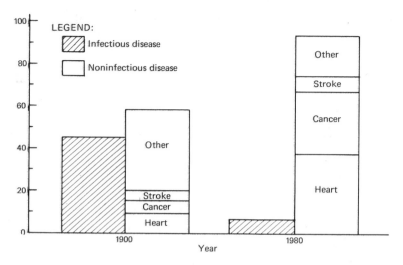

Figure 2–2. Proportional distribution of deaths from infectious and major noninfectious diseases, United States, 1900 and 1982.

limit disability. Secondary prevention is thus focused primarily on the stage of presymptomatic disease or on the very early stage of clinical disease. Screening is the most common form of secondary prevention. Many screening tests can detect early physiological indicators of disease before the individual has any symptom of illness. Examples include the Pap smear for cervical cancer, hearing tests for hearing impairment, the skin test for tuberculosis and the phenylalanine test for phenylketonuria (PKU) in infants. Such screening programs have become very popular in recent years as improved technology has led to a proliferation of available test procedures. Detection and treatment of conditions at the stage allowed by screening tests provide benefits ranging from prevention of mental retardation in children with PKU by maintaining a special diet until adulthood, through preservation of life for cancer patients whose disease is detected while in the early stage, where it is curable. In the case of communicable diseases, early detection and treatment benefits not only those who are detected and treated; the screening programs provide primary prevention for other persons in proximity to affected individuals because they will no longer be exposing others to the infectious agent. For example, the VDRL can screen for venereal disease and identify infected individuals who are treatable. Once treated they cannot transmit the disease to others. Further discussion of epidemiological issues in the planning, implementation, and evaluation of screening programs is presented in Chapter 13.

Tertiary prevention includes limitation of disability and rehabilitation of those persons for whom residual damage already exists. Activities are focused on the middle to later phases of clinical disease, when irreversible pathological damage produces disability. Exercise therapy to preserve muscle tone, restore motion, and prevent contractures in stroke patients is a form of tertiary prevention, because it limits disability and begins the process of rehabilitation by maximizing the individual's residual capacities. Psychosocial and vocational services are usually part of a rehabilitation program as well.

Comparison of Prevention for Infectious and Noninfectious Diseases

Primary prevention for the control of communicable disease utilizes measures aimed at preventing the spread of the infectious agent from those environments that harbor it to individuals who are susceptible and who may be exposed, and at increasing host resistance. The former can be achieved by modifying or eliminating the environment in which the infectious agent lives, by interfering with the means of transmission to the human host, or by increasing host immunity. Immunization programs and general health maintenance efforts are used to increase host immunity. Control is facilitated by the maintenance of surveillance programs to quickly identify new cases and to follow up with isolation methods to prevent exposure of susceptibles, or by instituting specific treatments to limit the period of communicability and progression of pathology (secondary prevention). Tertiary prevention plays a smaller role in infectious disease programs than in noninfectious programs because infectious disease less often results in permanent disability.

In the case of infectious diseases, illness can be prevented if the agent is destroyed or otherwise removed from the environment, or if specific protection is instituted through vaccination programs. These programs are effective because the infectious agent is necessary to produce the disease. For chronic conditions caused by noninfectious agents, however, there is usually no single necessary agent. Emphysema, for example, may result from smoking, from air pollution, from genetic susceptibility, or from a variety of other agents. Each and every agent must be eliminated to assure control of disease incidence. For this reason, measures aimed at specific protection through removal of hazardous substances from the workplace or other environment, often will reduce occurrence of the disease associated with exposure, but will not eliminate it. Isocyanates, for example, have been implicated as a cause of asthma. Because they are only one of many causes, however, elimination of workplace agents, although it may dramatically reduce the occurrence of attacks among the worker population, will not eliminate the disease entirely, even among those workers.

Synergistic effects of two or more agents are frequently seen in instances of causation by noninfectious agents. For example, nonsmoking workers exposed to asbestos have an increase of about eight times in the risk of dying from lung cancer when compared to nonsmoking, nonexposed individuals. Workers who smoke and are exposed to asbestos, however, are estimated to have 92 times the risk of the nonsmoking, nonexposed individuals (Kleinfeld, Messite, & Koozman, 1967). This is of concern because control efforts often must settle for minimizing rather than eliminating exposure to workplace agents. The synergistic effect of other agents could mean that substantial risk remains even with low level exposures. It was hoped that if exposures to harmful environmetnal agents could be kept low, then the latency period before onset of symptoms would be so long that the average individual would not develop problems until old age. Because synergism may shorten latency periods, producing illness in the prime of life even at low exposure levels, the reduction of behavioral risks such as smoking is crucial.

Because of these factors, efforts aimed at primary prevention of chronic, noninfectious conditions such as heart disease must focus, for example, on maternal diet during pregnancy, diet of the child during early life, regular exercise, and education programs regarding the hazards of smoking. Although success cannot be guaranteed, prospects for success are greatest if intervention occurs early in life, before physiological risk factors such as obesity and elevated cholesterol levels are permitted to develop. Because these physiological states involve cellular changes that are steps in the development of disease, risk factor reduction is already secondary prevention.

CAUSALITY

A Statistical Approach to Causality

As commonly used, the term *cause* is understood to mean a stimulus that produces an effect or outcome. In epidemiology also, cause deals with the production of an effect or outcome. Because epidemiologists must investigate causality by assessment of statistical associations, the operational definition of cause is a factor whose frequency varies with that of the health condition of interest. An increase or decrease in the amount or frequency of the causal agent produces a parallel increase or decrease in the frequency of the health condition.

A cause can be any of a large number of characteristics relating to time, place, person, or events. A health condition is likely to have multiple causes. Because an epidemiologist must rely on statistical measures of association to investigate causal relationships between a stimulus and an outcome, it is important to understand ways in which events or circumstances may be related in statistical terms.

The first question to be addressed is whether a statistical relationship exists between two factors. Stated another way, the first step in investigating statistical relationships between two factors or events is to determine whether any relationship (association) that does exist can be expected to occur by chance alone or whether the two factors occur together with a frequency greater than would be expected by chance. This is determined by applying one of a variety of statistical tests for independence or association, such as the chi square test or a correlation coefficient. If such a test is statistically significant, then the two factors are not independent—they do have a statistical relationship that is not explained by chance alone.

A table compares rates of developing complications following mastectomy in women with and without anxious personalities. A chi square test is statistically significant at $p<.05$. At least 95 times out of 100, one would not expect to find such differences in complication rates between the two personality types by chance alone. The two factors—personality and complication rates—are not independent. The presence of a statistically significant association does not mean, however, that personality type causes complications. Determination of a statistically significant association is only the first step in assessing whether a relationship is causal. If there is a strong statistical association between two factors or events, however, it may suggest the possibility of a causal association.

It is important to stress that statistical associations are determined for categories or groups and not for individual instances. In the previous example, although groups of women with anxious personalities are more likely to have complications following mastectomy than are women not undergoing mastectomy, it is not possible to say that any individual with an anxious personality will have complications, although, if the association is causal, an individual with an anxious personality will be more likely to have complications than an individual without.

Once it has been determined that two factors are not independent, i.e., that they have a statistically significant association, the next step is to determine whether the relationship is causal. Statistically significant (nonindependent) factors may be causally or noncausally related. A *noncausal relationship* can be statistically significant because the hypothetical causal factor varies systematically with the actual causal variable. When uncontrolled, its effect cannot be distinguished from that of a causal variable with which it is highly correlated. Paternal age, for example, shows a statistically significant relationship with infant birth weight. This association occurs because paternal age is highly correlated with maternal age, the actual causal variable; most husbands and wives are close in age, so the two vary together. In this instance, it is difficult to derive any logical biological explanation for why a father's age should affect the birth weight of a child, so a researcher finding this association would suggest that it is not causal and would search for an explanation for the association. It is possible in the process of epidemiological investigation to identify such factors or variables through appropriate analysis. However, it is important for clinical practitioners to bear in mind when reading the epidemiological literature that in the early stages of epidemiological investigation of a problem, published reports may not yet have identified such noncausal relationships. Guidelines to facilitate the process of interpreting the epidemiological literature in regard to the validity of causal evidence will be presented later in this chapter.

Causal relationships may be of two types, direct and indirect. It is important for epidemiologists to distinguish between direct and indirect relationships in order to provide complete information on the natural history of a disease.

Direct causal associations are those in which a factor causes a disease with no other factor intervening.

Causal factor ——————→ Outcome

An example of a direct cause would be the tubercule bacillus or any other infectious organism.

Tubercule bacillus ——————→ Tuberculosis

Apparent directness depends on the limitations of current knowledge; what is considered a direct association may be identified as indirect when information arising from further studies of causal mechanism reveals a new, more direct cause for the association. A historical example is the association of certain water sources with the outbreaks of cholera observed by Dr. John Snow in England in 1853 (Snow, 1855). Subsequent intervention to ban the identified sources of water reduced greatly the incidence of cholera. We now know that it was not the water itself, but rather the cholera vibrio that was the direct cause of the cholera epidemics.

For public health practitioners interested in reducing or eliminating onset of disease, the distinction between direct and indirect cause is often not crucial, as the available information may be a sufficient basis for initiating intervention. For clinicians who more often deal with patients with signs or symptoms of disease already present, however, the distinction is more crucial. We shall illustrate this point with the example of toxic shock syndrome (TSS). The direct cause of this condition is the staphylococcal organism. Tampons are an indirect (contributing) cause. Public health officials could intervene even before the staphylococcal organism was identified as the direct cause. Education programs were aimed at eliminating use of tampons or changing the way tampons were used to reduce the risk of developing toxic shock; specifically, it was suggested that women avoid the super absorbent tampons, change the tampons frequently using good hygienic practices, and avoid leaving the tampons in at night (MMWR, 1980). Clinicians, on the other hand, needed to know that the organism was the cause of the symptoms in order to treat patients appropriately. Knowledge of the role of tampons, however, is also useful to clinicians who need to counsel toxic shock patients regarding the risks of resuming tampon use.

In *indirect causal associations,* a third variable, an intervening variable, occupies an intermediate stage between the cause and effect. If, in the model below, A is causally related to D (A is the cause and D the effect), but only through the interposition of one or several linked factors such as B and C, the association between A and D is one of an indirect causal relationship.

$$A \longrightarrow B \longrightarrow C \longrightarrow D$$

One example is the relationship of cigarette smoke to chronic bronchitis. Breathing air polluted by cigarette or other smoke (A) causes damage to the respiratory epithelium (B); this damage increases the susceptibility of the epithelium to infection (C); this results in chronic bronchitis (D). In this example, knowledge about B and C is not essential to primary prevention of chronic bronchitis; eliminating the inhalation of cigarette smoke may greatly reduce the frequency of occurrence of chronic bronchitis. For purposes of secondary and tertiary prevention, however, understanding B and C is important. Awareness of the role of epithelial damage on the development of chronic bronchitis offers an opportunity to test for early epithelial changes in high-risk individuals. Although it may not be possible to reverse the damage, counseling these individuals as to their risk for bronchitis and the role of smoking may at least encourage them to reduce their use of cigarettes. Furthermore, individuals with epithelial damage are more susceptible to infection. They should be advised to avoid close contact with individuals known to have acute respiratory infections and to seek early treatment to avoid further damage in the event that they develop an infection.

In the previous example of toxic shock syndrome, tampons are an indirect cause of the disease. The direct cause is staphylococcal organisms in the vagina. The tampons are a contributing cause in that they create an ideal environment for proliferation of the organism (MMWR, 1980). From the standpoint of primary prevention, the disease could be prevented by eliminating tampon use or changing the way in which they are used. Theoretically, it could also be prevented by treating women who are vaginal carriers of staphylococcal organisms with antibiotics, but this is less practical because of the expense and difficulty of identifying carriers and the possibility that the organism will recur again following treatment. From the standpoint of treatment (tertiary prevention), however, knowing that staphylococci is the direct cause is useful because the physician can treat the disease with antibiotics to eliminate the source of the infection.

The Concept of Multiple Cause

Thus far, for simplicity of presentation, we have discussed causality as if each disease had a single cause, although we have implied in the section on levels of prevention, that this is not the case. Historically, since early epidemiology focused on outbreaks of diseases with infectious origins, the idea of single cause was quite workable for control of the disease. Cholera outbreaks could be controlled by eliminating the source of the cholera vibrio. Diphtheria could be eliminated through vaccination programs. Scarlet fever could be kept from spreading by imposing a quarantine on all exposed individuals. These measures were effective because infectious agents were necessary to produce the disease. Therefore, elimination or isolation of the agent and elimination of host susceptibility through vaccination were effective measures.

With the advent of chronic diseases of noninfectious origin as major causes of morbidity and mortality, however, modern epidemiology has been forced to move from the single cause conceptualization of causality to one that recognizes the presence of multiple causes in any biological phenomenon. The concept of multiple cause is applicable both to infectious and noninfectious causes. The staphylococci, for instance, was identified as *the* cause of toxic shock syndrome because this organism must be present for the disease to occur. This does not mean necessarily that it will always cause a clinically recognizable disease. There are circumstances when the organism is present and no disease occurs. The host has to be susceptible to the organism; susceptibility reflects previous exposure to the organism, immune response, and so on. If the host is not susceptible, no disease occurs. The environment is also important because the likelihood of exposure to the organism may vary greatly in different geographical areas; if temperature and moisture conditions are not ideal for proliferation of the organism, exposure is less likely. With diseases caused by noninfectious agents, the single cause model is of limited usefulness because there is no single factor or agent that must be present to cause the disease. For example, even though smoking is recognized as a major cause of lung cancer, nonsmokers and individuals who have never been exposed to the cigarette smoke of others do get lung cancer. Clearly, there must be other substances that cause the disease. Nonsmokers exposed to asbestos may develop lung cancer. Furthermore, smokers who are exposed to substances such as asbestos are more likely to develop lung cancer than are those smokers not exposed to asbestos. Exposure to multiple causal factors may have an additive or multiplicative effect.

In a different example, automobile accidents may result from numerous factors such as speeding, faulty equipment, heavy traffic, poor visibility, driver inexperience, or drinking and driving. Any of these factors could cause an accident. All are amenable to intervention, as through public education, better engineering design, better vehicle maintenance. Several of these factors together increase the risk of an accident. Such interrelationships between a multitude of factors, some known and some unknown, but all bearing ultimately on the cause of the disease, constitute the *web of causation*. It is, fortunately, not necessary to understand completely the intricacy of relationships between factors to institute adequate preventive measures.

Using our earlier definition of cause, numerous factors such as smoking, obesity, blood cholesterol level, and stress are causes of heart attack. The more of these factors present in an individual, the greater the risk of infarction. Because presence of these factors increases the risk for contracting a disease, we call them risk factors. Although we may not understand how these factors work or how they interact with each other, we can intervene and reduce the risk of heart attack by persuading individuals to give up smoking, to lose weight, or to change their diet to reduce cholesterol.

The ultimate determination of the causality of an observed association is reached through an epidemiological experiment.

For practical purposes, a factor is considered causal when reducing the amount or frequency of the suspected cause reduces the frequency of the effect, in this case, the illness of interest. If treating hypertensives to keep their blood pressure low reduces the frequency of stroke compared to the frequency of stroke in an equivalent, untreated group of hypertensives, hypertension would be considered a cause of stroke. Such experimental evidence of causality gives us an operational definition of a cause. A factor is a cause when a reduction in the frequency of the factor produces a reduction in the frequency of occurrence of the related disease.

Criteria for Evaluating Causality in the Literature

Studies reported in the literature may show conflicting results. An epidemiological experiment is not always feasible or desirable. In these instances, criteria based on available epidemiological data are needed for making decisions regarding intervention. Five criteria often accepted for assessing causality in such instances were used in the 1964 Surgeon General's Report (DHEW, 1964) for assessing the causal relationship between smoking and a variety of health outcomes. The five criteria are (1) correctness of temporality; (2) strength of the association; (3) specificity of the association; (4) consistency of the association; and (5) biological plausibility.

Correctness of temporality requires evidence that exposure to the causal factor did, in fact, occur prior to initiation of the disease process. For diseases such as cancer, definitive proof that the exposure occurred prior to the first cell transformations may be difficult to obtain, because there is a long period of latency during which cell replication and growth continues. It may be as long as 20 to 40 years after the initial exposure to a causal agent before the tumor is diagnosed. Suppose someone with lung cancer has been smoking for 10 years. Did smoking initiate the disease process or did it speed up tumor growth that was already initiated by another agent? The answer cannot be definitely established. But it is much more likely that smoking is causal if a patient smoked for 10 years prior to diagnosis than if he smoked for only 18 months. Clearly, however, if exposure can be shown to have not occurred before the disease, the relationship cannot be causal despite a strong statistical association.

Strength of the association is usually measured by a statistic called the relative risk ratio or alternatively, the odds ratio. In general, the larger the ratio, the stronger is the association and the greater is the likelihood that the association is causal. Some studies report correlation coefficients instead. Another aspect of strength of the association is dose-effect. The strength of association should be stronger at higher doses, or levels, of exposure.

Specificity of the association refers to the uniqueness of the relationship. The terms necessary and sufficient can be used to clarify this concept. If the disease can occur without the presence of a particular agent, the agent is not necessary. Lung cancer can occur in nonsmokers; toxic shock, however, cannot occur without exposure to the staphylococci. Sufficient refers to whether the agent is always able to produce the outcome. Although asbestos fibers are necesary to produce asbestosis, the fibers may not be sufficient; it is possible to be exposed to asbestos and not develop asbestosis. Exposure to flame is always sufficient to produce a burn, although severity may vary. Fire is not necessary to produce a burn, however, because burns may result from chemical exposures as well. A highly specific, therefore, unique association exists when an agent is both necessary for disease occurrence and sufficient, by itself, to produce the disease. Such a specific relationship would be causal. The closer an agent comes to meeting these criteria, the greater is the likelihood of causality. As discussed in the next section, however, meeting both the necessary and sufficient criteria simultaneously is incompatible with the concept of multiple causes.

Consistency of the association refers to the findings of various epidemiological studies. There may be conflicting results among reported studies on the association of a specific agent with a specific disease. Some studies may find no association. Others may find a positive association. The strength of the association may vary widely in the studies reporting a positive association. Barring major flaws in study designs, consistent findings of a positive association would be expected if the association is causal.

Biological plausibility, sometimes called coherence, implies the presence of a reasonable biological mechanism to explain the physiological process by which an agent could produce the specific disease of interest. Documentation of biological plausibility is dependent on other scientific disciplines such as physiology, microbiology, toxicology, and pharmacology. Causality demands a reasonable biological explanation for the observed association. Exposure of laboratory animals to an agent should, if an appropriate animal system is used, produce effects similar to those seen in humans.

REFERENCES

Benenson, A. S. (Ed.). *Control of communicable disease in man* (13th ed.). New York: American Public Health Association, 1980.

Kleinfeld, M., Messite, J., & Koozman, O. Mortality experience in a group of asbestos workers. *Archives of Environmental Health,* 1967, *15,* 176–180.

MMWR. Follow-up on toxic shock syndrome. *Morbidity and Mortality Weekly Reports* (CDC), 1980, *29*(37), 441–445.

Snow, J. *On the mode of communication of cholera* (2nd ed.). London: Churchill, 1855. Reproduced in *Snow on cholera.* New York: Commonwealth Fund, 1936.

U.S. Department of Health, Education, and Welfare. *Smoking and health: Report of the Advisory Committee to the Surgeon General of the Public Health Service* (PHS Publication No. 1103). Washington, D.C.: U.S. Government Printing Office, 1964.

Epidemiological Methods

SEQUENCE OF EPIDEMIOLOGICAL INVESTIGATION

Epidemiological investigations generally proceed in an orderly fashion, beginning with the observation and recording of existing patterns of occurrence for the condition under study. These observations, recorded as disease rates, are compared for various categories of person, place, and time characteristics. From these recorded observations, one generates a description of which specific characteristics are associated with high versus low frequency of disease occurrence. This first phase of investigation, called *descriptive epidemiology*, suggests hypotheses concerning etiology.

Description

To illustrate this sequence, suppose that investigators are interested in trying to learn what causes breast cancer. The first step is to obtain the rates of breast cancer for groups of people with different characteristics, in different geographical locations, and at various points in time. Although epidemiologists would prefer to have the rates of newly occurring cases, *incidence rates*, these are not generally available without a special survey or a source of regularly recorded cases such as a disease registry. Therefore, *mortality rates*, the rates of death from the disease, are generally used in early stages of the investigation. When rates of breast cancer mortality are examined, it is observed that breast cancer is rare among men and more frequent among whites than nonwhites, among single women than married women, and among those in higher socioeconomic groups than those in lower socioeconomic groups. Breast cancer occurs with increasing frequency in successively older age groups and shows a decreasing frequency as number of liveborn children increases and as age at first full-term pregnancy decreases. Rates of breast cancer also vary by geographical area. These rates are higher in the developed, western countries than in less developed countries. Rates are lowest in Asian countries such as Japan. Breast cancer mortality was increasing steadily in the early 1900's, but these rates have leveled off during the past 50 years or so, reflecting improvements in early detection and treatment. Now, there is little change in incidence rates for whites, but there continues to be a rise for nonwhites. This information constitutes an epidemiological description of breast cancer.

Analysis

Hypotheses suggested by the descriptive epidemiology of a condition are tested in the second investigative phase, *analytical epidemiology*. Because these analytical studies are based on observational data, a suspicion must be entertained that the observed association of a suspected causal factor with occurrence of a particular disease may be due to other factors. For instance, one factor could be genetic self-selection of individuals for use of harmful substances. There could also be confounding variables, factors which cause change in the frequency of disease and vary systematically with the hypothetical cause under study. When uncontrolled, the effects of confounding variables cannot be distinguished from those of the hypothetical causal variable. Confounding variables may be identified at a later stage of investigation. Suppose that a researcher noted that rates of spontaneous abortion increased with the number of pregnancies. Having more babies might not be a causative factor; the number of pregnancies is related to age of the mother. If physiological aging leads to a decreased capacity for carrying a pregnancy to term, then age would be confounding the original association between parity and spontaneous abortion rates. The physiological aging process actually contributed to the inability to successfully complete a pregnancy but, when the effect was not controlled, parity appeared to be a causal factor. In this example, parity is non-causally related to risk of spontaneous abortion. Because of this problem, multiple analytical studies on the same hypotheses are usually required to sort out these relationships.

Analytical studies may be done on either an ecological level or a relational level. Ecological studies compare large aggregates of people, usually of a defined geographical area, with another such large population. For example, cancer rates may be compared for the population of towns with polluted drinking water and that of towns with pure drinking water to assess whether water pollution is associated with elevated rates of cancer. Or, per capita data on fat consumption may be compared for countries with high and low rates of colon cancer in order to investigate a hypothesized causal role of fat consumption in the development of colon cancer. Such studies, although a useful first step in the analytical phase of investigation, are subject to the *ecological fallacy*. There is a fallacy in assuming that relationships observed among groups can be assumed for individuals. Although there may be a striking relationship between high cancer rates and polluted drinking water in the populations studied, there is not necessarily the same relationship observed on the individual level. Imagine, for example, that the majority of residents of the town with polluted water who developed cancer were men who worked in another town, where they were exposed to carcinogens in the workplace. They actually drank less of the polluted water than did the individuals remaining in the town.

Relational studies, on the other hand, do relate exposure and disease in the same individuals. The presence or absence of exposure is determined for each individual and the presence or absence of disease is assessed for each individual. The frequency of joint presence of disease and exposure is then assessed for this group of persons.

Four basic types of studies are commonly used: 1) cross-sectional studies; 2) case-control studies; 3) cohort studies; and 4) historical cohort studies. These designs may be used both in ecological studies based on aggregate data for entire populations and in relational studies where specific information on exposure and outcome for each individual is available. Other names used synonymously with these terms, along with the design of each type of study, are listed in Table 3–1. These designs differ in

TABLE 3–1. COMPARISON OF ECOLOGICAL AND RELATIONAL STUDY DESIGNS FOR OBSERVATIONAL STUDIES

Level of Study	Types of Studies	Other Common Terms for Study Design	Basic Design
Ecological	Cross-sectional	Correlational Ecological correlational Ecological survey	Rates of disease frequency for places are correlated with frequency of factors in those places at various points in time
	Case-control	Retrospective	Places with high rates of a disease are compared with places with low rates for levels of factors thought to be related to causing that disease
	Cohort	Prospective Longitudinal	Future rates of disease occurrence are compared for places with current environmental exposures and places known not to have such exposures
	Historical cohort	Retrospective–Prospective Nonconcurrent cohort	Rates of disease occurrence are compared for places with known past exposure to an environmental factor and places known not to have such exposures. Tracking of rates begins at the time of exposure and continues to the present

Relational	Cross-sectional	Correlational Prevalence study Prevalence survey Survey study	Current rates of exposure among individuals are correlated with current rates of disease frequency among these same individuals
	Case-control	Retrospective Case-comparison	Frequency of prior exposure to the study factor is compared for individuals with the study disease and a group of individuals without the disease, who are similar in regard to other characteristics
	Cohort	Prospective Longitudinal Prospective population	A group of individuals known to be exposed to a factor and a group of similar individuals not exposed are followed into the future and their respective incidence of the disease of interest is compared
	Historical cohort	Retrospective–prospective Nonconcurrent cohort Retrospective cohort Retrospective mortality Retrospective incidence	A group of individuals known to have been exposed to a factor at a time in the past are compared with a group of individuals not exposed and their rates of disease incidence or mortality compared from the time of exposure to the present

(From Valanis, B. The epidemiological model and community health nursing. In M. Stanhope & J. Lancaster, *Community health nursing: Process and practice for promoting health*. St. Louis: C. V. Mosby, 1984. p. 162.)

time frame, and therefore in selection of study groups, in
required numbers of subjects, in potential sources of data that
can be used, and in methods of analysis. The time framework for
these studies is illustrated in Figure 3–1.

Cross-sectional studies, also called prevalence surveys,
simultaneously ascertain the status of subjects on both the exposure factor and the disease of interest. Consider a study that
investigates the relationship of depression (the study factor) to
the occurrence of gastric ulcers (disease outcome), by simultaneously obtaining for a selected population measures of depression, using depression scales, and diagnosis of presence or absence of gastric ulcer, by physical examinations, history, and
tests. This cross-sectional study cannot establish the causal
nature of a relationship between depression and gastric ulcers
because the design does not allow the investigator to account for
the time sequence of events. It is impossible to know whether

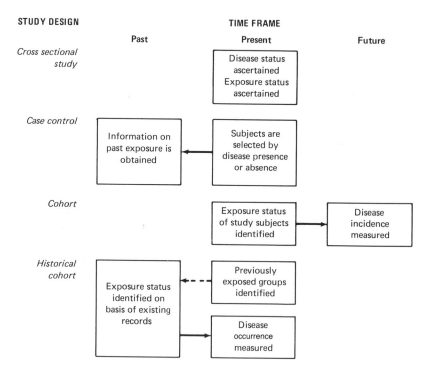

Figure 3–1. The time frame of four epidemiological study
designs.

depression occured prior to onset of ulcers, ulcers prior to the onset of depression, or whether the two occured together. This is a major limitation of all cross-sectional studies.

Case-control studies begin by identifying a group of cases who have the disease of interest and a comparable group of subjects without the disease, called a control group. Attempts are then made to determine the frequency of exposure to the study factor for each group. A recent case-control study investigated demographic characteristics of mothers, complications related to pregnancy and labor, the method of delivery, and newborn illnesses and injuries as risk factors for neonatal sepsis (Soman et al., 1985). In this study, cases were all 113 instances of sepsis identified on birth certificates in Washington state in 1980 to 1981. Controls were a sample of 347 births randomly selected from the 1981 Washington state birth certificates. Once cases and controls were selected, information as to presence or absence of each risk factor was obtained from each child's birth certificate. Relative frequencies of each factor of interest were compared for cases and controls using the odds ratio, which represents the odds in favor of having the disease with the factor present and with the factor absent, respectively.

Some general rules apply to case-control studies. Because of potential problems in establishing exposure status of subjects, the same sources of data on exposure should be available for the cases and controls; this reduces bias caused by better ascertainment of exposure for one group than for the other. When selecting controls, it is important that controls have the same chance as cases of being exposed to the study factor. This point is elaborated later in this chapter. Finally, a clear, unambiguous definition of a case is needed to facilitate selection of cases for the study. Optimally, cases should consist of all newly diagnosed (incident) cases with the specified characteristics during a specified period of time in a defined population. Incident cases are preferred to prevalent cases since use of prevalent cases can introduce bias that is caused by loss of patients who have a short disease course because of recovery or death. This is particularly a problem when the factor being investigated is also related to the probability of dying or recovering.

Cohort designs, whether prospective or historical in type, begin by classifying the study subjects according to their exposure status. Prospective cohort studies follow subjects into the future, monitoring the incidence of the disease of interest for all subjects. The disease incidence or mortality rates for various levels of exposure (e.g., high, medium, low, or no exposure) are then compared. If a relationship between exposure and disease occurrence is causal, one would expect to see a significantly higher rate of the disease in those exposed compared to those not exposed. This is measured by the relative risk ratio discussed later in this chapter. One would also expect to observe a dose-effect, i.e., an increase in disease incidence related to the level or dose of exposure. Perhaps the best known cohort study is the Framingham Study investigation of the factors associated with the risk of coronary heart disease (Dawber, 1980). This study, begun in 1949, has continued to the present. A representative sample of 5209 men and women aged 30 to 59 selected from the total population of Framingham, Massachusetts were examined by physical examination. The 5127 individuals determined to be free of coronary heart disease and therefore at risk of developing coronary heart disease (CHD) were reexamined every other year for evidence of CHD during the 30+ years of the study. Within the total study cohort of 5209, subjects were classified as to presence or absence of specific exposure factors of interest, e.g., diabetes, blood pressure, activity, blood cholesterol, and smoking, and incidence of CHD compared for the subgroups. Much of what we know about risk for CHD has emerged from this study and new data continues to be forthcoming. One of the most recent reports examined risk of sudden death among subjects with prior CHD and those with no prior CHD (Schatzkin, Cupples, Heeren, Morelock, and Kannel, 1984).

Historical cohort studies differ from prospective cohort studies in that both the exposure and the onset of disease have already occurred. Such studies require the availability of records that permit classification of individuals on the initial exposure and a way of reconstructing the disease history. This study design is frequently used in occupational studies. If one wished to study exposure to benzene in relation to incidence of bladder cancer, a historical cohort study would most likely be the design of choice. Because bladder cancer has a relatively low incidence, a large cohort would need to be followed many years into the future to generate enough cases of bladder cancer for statistical analysis. To further complicate matters, regulation of benzene exposures by OSHA has led to lower levels of exposure among workers in recent years. If there is a causal relationship between benzene exposure and bladder cancer, the incidence (or mortality rates) would be lower in groups with low exposure than in groups with high exposure. Thus, a prospective study of current workers would require an even larger sample size. Associated costs and the length of time before any answers would be available make such a study impractical.

If cohorts of workers with a wide variety of exposure doses that occurred in the past can be identified through available records, then a historical cohort study can be conducted. Suppose a sufficiently large cohort of workers with exposures to benzene between 1950 and 1960 can be identified. All such workers meeting specified eligibility criteria would be entered into the study and tracked until the present to establish their vital status—dead or alive—and if dead, the date, place, and cause of death. This would be done through use of social security records, motor vehicle license records, union records, or any other available source of data. A comparison (control) group of unexposed workers could be similarly identified and followed. Most often, historical cohort studies use general population age and time-specific mortality rates rather than incidence as a basis for comparison because of availability of mortality data. Using life-table methods, an expected number of deaths is calculated for the cohort of exposed workers based on the experience of the general population. The observed number of deaths in the cohort is then compared to this expected number. This ratio is known as a standard mortality ratio (SMR). Alternatively, a ratio based on proportional rates, the proportional mortality ratio, is sometimes used.

In both types of cohort studies accurate classification of exposure and disease outcome is essential. This is more easily achieved in the prospective study since the historical design relies on recorded data. Loss to follow-up is a potential problem in both these designs. Efforts must be directed at minimizing such losses and evaluating whether any systematic bias is introduced into the study by those subjects who have dropped out.

Ecological studies are generally based on aggregate data collected for other purposes. Data routinely collected by official agencies on water quality or air quality of a particular locality, for example, may be used as a measure of the level of exposure of a population to particular pollutants. These data are then examined in relation to rates of the disease of interest (usually mortality rates) for the resident population of that same locality. Because these data are already available, such studies are relatively inexpensive and quick to do. These studies often are done early in the process of epidemiological investigation and may be useful in hypothesis generation as well as in stage I hypothesis testing. Cross-sectional ecological case-control and historical cohort designs are useful in hypothesis testing. Ecological cohort studies, although theoretically possible, are rarely used in practice.

Relational studies require data, for each individual in the study population, on the presence or absence of exposure and on the level and time period when the exposure was present. In addition, information from each individual as to the presence or absence of the disease is required. Time of onset of the disease is also important information. In addition, relational studies try to obtain individual information regarding other factors that are already known to relate to the disease process or factors that may lead to false inferences if not controlled in study design or analysis. For example, in studies on pregnancy where the outcome of interest may be maternal health status or fetal health, the age of the mother will be important regardless of which exposure factor is the object of investigation. It is necessary to control for effects of age because it is known to have a strong impact on pregnancy outcomes, and if the exposure factor under study varies with age, it would appear to be causally related if age were not controlled. In other instances, age may interact with another exposure to produce a synergistic effect of that exposure.

Cross-sectional and case-control studies are generally used as first steps in the analytical phase of relational investigation because they can be done quickly, require small samples, and are relatively inexpensive. Historical cohort and (prospective) cohort studies generally require large samples, longer times to complete, and are expensive. On the other hand, they yield measures of incidence or risk; no incidence can be derived from the cross-sectional or case-control studies and any risk measures must be obtained by indirect means.

Experimentation

When sufficient evidence has accumulated from analytical studies suggesting that a specific factor is causally related to the occurrence of a particular disease, the experimental phase of epidemiological investigation is begun. This phase employs a study design called a randomized controlled trial. In contrast to the observational studies previously discussed, the investigator, not the individual, determines who is exposed or not exposed to each experimental condition and controls the nature of each experimental condition. Because it would be unethical to expose human subjects to an agent thought to be harmful, in most epidemiological experiments the study sample is chosen from individuals already exposed to the causal agent under study. The suspected causal factor is then taken away from one study group and their disease experience is compared with that of the group who remains exposed to the suspected factor. For example, if hypertension is thought to be a causal agent for stroke, patients with hypertension may be randomly assigned to a treatment group that is given medication to reduce blood pressure, whereas the remaining subjects receive either no treatment or diet treatment only. The two groups are then compared for the incidence of stroke. Thus, experimental studies have a similar design to that of a prospective cohort study. Because in experimental studies the investigator has control over who is or is not exposed, as well as over the experimental conditions, the problems of causal inference inherent to the analytical studies are not generally present. As a result, data from experimental studies are typically used to prove causal relationships.

Criteria for Evaluation of Published Studies

Certain methodological criteria must be met if results of a study are to be considered valid. When reading research reports in the literature, you should assess whether the following minimal criteria have been met.

1. Background and Study Hypothesis. Sufficient information on why the particular issue is being investigated should be presented to convince the reader that there is a need for the study. The background information should provide some indication of which factors are already known to be associated with the occurrence of the particular disease, because these factors need to be controlled in the design and/or analysis of the study. Hypotheses to be tested should be clearly spelled out since they ought to provide the basis for developing an appropriate study design.

2. Equivalence of Subjects in the Two Study Groups. All

studies require a control group. This is a group of persons with
whom the study group of interest can be compared in regard to
frequency of the factor of interest. In case-control studies, all
subjects are selected on the basis of presence or absence of the
disease whereas in any form of cohort study they are selected on
the basis of pesence or absence of exposure. In both instances it
is important that the comparison group be similar to the study
group (cases of the disease in case-control studies; exposed subjects in cohort studies) for factors other than the study factor.
For example, the groups should be of similar socioeconomic status, and similar race and sex. The same holds true for ecological
studies; there must be equivalence in the two populations being
compared. For case-control studies, such equivalence is important to insure that cases and controls have had an equal chance
of being exposed to the study factor. If they have not had an
equal chance, then a bias is introduced. For example, in a case-
control study to investigate the relationship of reserpine use to
occurrence of breast cancer, cases and controls should have
equal chances of receiving medical care, since the opportunity to
have reserpine prescribed is dependent on regular medical care.
If cases had more opportunity for medical care than the controls
(e.g. if the two groups were of different socioeconomic status),
then the study would find that reserpine use was more common
among breast cancer cases than among controls. This would be
due to bias in the study design rather than to a true excess
among cases. Similarly, in a cohort study (either historic or prospective), it is crucial that both the study group exposed to the
study factor and the nonexposed control group should have
equal probability of exposure to other factors that could be
related to development of the disease outcome of interest. For
example, in a study of the relationship of regular exercise versus no exercise to incidence of chronic obstructive pulmonary
disease, both the group exposed to regular exercise and those
not exposed to exercise should have similar frequencies of smoking. If one group has a higher percentage of smokers than the
other, the effect of smoking on lung function of that group will
make if difficult to evaluate the role of amount of exercise when
comparing the two groups. If smoking status is known, then
smokers in the regular exercise group could be compared with
smokers in the no-exercise group. However, if specific information on smoking is unavailable, the effect cannot be evaluated.

3. Similar Availability of Information on Study Factors for the Two Study Groups. If the data required for the study are not likely to be equally available and complete for both groups from the same source, then there is the likelihood that whichever group has a better source of information will show an excess of the factor under study (exposure for case-control studies; presence of disease for cohort studies).

4. Accurate Measurement of Study Factors. Important considerations are reliability and validity of measurement (discussed later in this chapter). These measurement issues relate both to the criteria for defining what constitutes a "case" of the disease under study and to the measurement of exposures and control factors.

5. Sample Size and Power. Presentation of the study design should address the issue of how the size of the study sample was determined and the statistical power of this sample size to answer the research question. Particularly in studies which did not find the hypothesized relationship between an exposure and a disease, it is impossible to know whether no relationship exists or whether the negative finding was due to inadequate sample size.

6. Analysis. The analytical techniques should be appropriate to the design of the study. A prospective study, for example, should use incidence rates and relative risk measures to capitalize on the strengths of the prospective design, rather than setting up the data for analysis as if it were retrospective in design. Although this seems obvious, there are studies in the literature where this was not done. Furthermore, confidence limits for risk ratios and other relevant tests should be provided. Presentation of data without such information makes interpretation of results difficult. Finally, the analysis should control for the potential confounding variables that were not controlled by the study design.

7. Discussion. Quality research will compare and contrast the results of their study to the findings of previous studies. Reasons for possible discrepancies in findings should be suggested, including a candid analysis of factors inherent in the design of the current study.

Sources of Data

Epidemiological investigations use data from a variety of existing sources, such as census data routinely collected by the government or medical record data maintained by hospitals. In other instances, the data may be generated for a specific study through surveys that include interviews and physical examinations.

Epidemiologists require four types of data:

1. Population statistics for denominators of rates
2. Frequency of health events (morbidity and mortality data)
3. Exposure for hypothesized causal factors or events
4. Linkage data that permit researchers to track individual study subjects over time

Data from a population census carried out every 10 years in many countries are the main source of population statistics. Census data include a count of the total population and a variety of information about geographical, economic, and personal demographic characteristics of individuals and households. Some of these data provide the denominator for routine health statistics.

Data on frequency of health events are of two types—mortality data and morbidity data. Mortality statistics are generally based on the numbers and causes of death listed on death certificates because, in most of the world, registration of deaths is required by law. As a result, these data provide a fairly complete record of the number of deaths. Accuracy of the reported cause of death varies from place to place, but these data are probably adequate indicators of the mortality count for major causes of death. International comparison of mortality has been facilitated by general use of the International Statistical Classification of Diseases, Injuries, and Causes of Death (ICD).

Deaths are one type of *vital statistic*. Vital statistics is a term used for the data collected from ongoing registration of "vital" events relating to births, deaths, and marriages. They include births and adoptions; deaths and fetal deaths; marriages, divorces, legal separations and annulments. Certification of births, deaths, and fetal deaths are the vital events of most use in epidemiological research. Birth certificates, for example, provide information for the numerator and for the denominator of various rates measuring health aspects of childbirth and infancy. Although in the United States certificates are filed locally, each state and certain large cities hold legal responsibility for registration and reporting of vital events. A standard format for certificates is recommended by the National Center for Health Statistics (NCHS) in conjunction with its Cooperative Health Statistics System (CHSS). While most states adopt these standard forms, the amount of available information varies since each state may determine the format and context of its own certificate. In order to facilitate epidemiological research based on mortality data, the NCHS established the National Death Index (NDI) in 1979. This central, computerized index is compiled by NCHS from tapes provided by the various state vital statistics offices. The NDI allows epidemiologists to trace people who have died through one central source rather than having to contact individual states.

Morbidity data, as a rule, are not routinely recorded and, therefore, are less accurate than mortality statistics. The two major sources of morbidity data probably are hospital records and notification systems, such as the reporting of some 37 infectious diseases decreed as reportable in most states. Another type of notification system is the reporting required by disease registries, such as cancer registries and birth defects registries. The U.S. Centers for Disease Control Systematically collect data on abortions, congenital anomalies, nosocomial infections and other conditions with preventable components. Special surveys may be conducted when data is not otherwise available. The National Health Survey, established by Congress in 1956, is conducted by NCHS and provides a continual source of information about the health status and needs of the entire country. Components of this Survey include The Health Interview Survey (includes approximately 40,000 households per year) and the Health and Nutrition Examination Survey. Additional NCHS surveys include the National Hospital Discharge Survey, the National Nursing Home Survey, and the National Family Growth Survey.

Summary statistics for a community are frequently available from organizations that routinely use them for health planning purposes. These organizations include health departments, regional planning agencies, hospitals, and a variety of governmental agencies. The rates most frequently used as indices of community health are listed in Table 3–2.

TABLE 3–2. RATES MOST FREQUENTLY USED AS INDICES OF COMMUNITY HEALTH

numerator = death or illness New cases
denominator = the population.
TOTAL population

	Usual population factor

General mortality rates

Crude death rate $= \dfrac{\text{No. deaths in a year}}{\text{Average (midyear) population}}$ *July 1st.* — per 100,000 population

Cause-specific death rate $= \dfrac{\text{No. deaths from a stated cause in a year}}{\text{Average (midyear) population}}$ — per 100,000 population

Age–specific death rate $= \dfrac{\text{No. deaths among persons in given age group in a year}}{\text{Average (midyear) population in specified age group}}$ — per 100,000 population

Proportional mortality rate $= \dfrac{\text{No. deaths from specific cause in specified time period}}{\text{Total deaths in same time period}}$ — percent of deaths

Case-fatality rate $= \dfrac{\text{No. deaths due to specified disease}}{\text{No. cases of specified disease}}$ — per 100 cases

Rates assessing morbidity

Incidence $= \dfrac{\text{No. of new cases of disease in place, from time 1 to time 2}}{\text{No. persons in place, midpoint of time period}}$ — per 100,000 population

Point prevalence $= \dfrac{\text{No. of existing cases in place, at time}}{\text{No. persons in place, at time}}$ — per 100,000 population

Maternal and infant rates

Maternal (puerperal) mortality rate $= \dfrac{\text{No. deaths from puerperal causes in a year}}{\text{No. of live births in same year}}$ — per 100,000 live births

Infant mortality rate $= \dfrac{\text{No. deaths in children less than 1 year of age during 1 year}}{\text{No. of live births in same year}}$ — per 1,000 live births

Neonatal mortality rate $= \dfrac{\text{No. deaths in a year of children under 28 days of age}}{\text{No. of live births in same year}}$ — per 1,000 live births

Fetal death rate $= \dfrac{\text{No. fetal deaths during year}}{\text{No. of live births and fetal deaths in same year}}$ — per 1,000 live births

Perinatal mortality rate $= \dfrac{\text{No. fetal deaths 28 weeks or more and infant deaths under 7 days of age during year}}{\text{No. of live births and fetal deaths 28 weeks or more gestation in same year}}$ — per 1,000 live births

Data on frequency of hypothesized causal factors is sometimes available from existing sources such as hospital records. This source might include data on factors such as drugs used, smoking history, reproductive history, previous diseases, or occupation. Unfortunately, completeness and accuracy of these records may vary widely. Records kept by employers and unions may be a source of information on toxic exposures experienced by workers. In other cases, the investigator must resort to special surveys using interviews or questionnaires to obtain information on exposure to hypothesized causal agents.

Sources of data that measure frequency of exposure or frequency of health events vary considerably in their accuracy. Clearly, if the information used to measure events is not accurate, erroneous conclusions may result from the study. Therefore, epidemiologists must be concerned with how accurately they can measure the events they are attempting to study.

The final type of data required by epidemiologists allows an investigator to follow a subject through time. Consider the example of a historical cohort study with the purpose of determining whether a group of workers exposed to benzene in 1945 has a higher rate of cancer of the urinary tract than do workers not exposed to benzene. In order to answer the research question, workers will be followed until 1984 or death, whichever comes first. Death certificates will be required to determine the cause of death of the deceased workers. The National Death Index mentioned previously will help here. For those still alive, physical examinations will be done. Many workers may have moved since 1945, so some means of locating them is required. Sources of data such as social security records, state motor vehicle records, and town registries must be used.

ISSUES OF MEASUREMENT

Two major aspects of measurement are the *reliability* of the measuring procedure or source of data, and the *validity* of the measurement. *Reliability* is the repeatability of a measurement. Factors that affect repeatability include variations in the attribute being measured, variability in a measuring instrument, and variations between measuring instruments or raters. Blood pressure, for example, is an attribute that varies in an individual. Stress and activity will each result in short-term changes in blood pressure. Furthermore, an instrument such as a sphygmomanometer used to measure blood pressure requires frequent recalibration to be sure that variation in measurement is minimal. Two nurses using the same sphygmomanometer to take the blood pressure of the same patient, one immediately after the other, may obtain different readings. All these factors contribute to a low reliability of blood pressure measurement. To maximize reliability of measurement, the conditions of measurement must be standardized. In this example, measures for all patients should be done under similar conditions, with well calibrated instruments used by a few nurses who have been trained to do the procedure in the same way.

Validity refers to the accuracy of the measurement. Stated another way, validity is how well the measurement represents reality. A measure must be reliable in order to be valid, but reliability alone does not produce validity. A measure may be precise but not accurate. For example, the tuberculin test may be used as a screening test for tuberculosis. Even if the reliability of the test administration and test reading is maximized, the test is not a totally accurate or valid test for tuberculosis. Although individuals with tuberculosis should test positive (a true positive reading and not a false negative reading), a reading may be positive for reasons other than presence of tuberculosis, such as having been previously vaccinated with BCG. Thus, a high rate of false positives may be observed. A positive sputum culture for tuberculosis is generally a more valid test for the presence of tuberculosis as long as reliability of testing is maximized. Even in this instance, validity is not 100 percent because false negative readings may occur if the specimen was inadequate or was improperly handled. Figure 3–2 illustrates reliability and validity using the concept of a target. Target A

Figure 3–2. A visual approach to the concepts of reliability and validity.

Target A
Reliable, but not valid

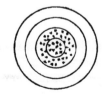

Target B
Less reliable, but valid

indicates a highly reliable, but invalid measure because the center of the target is the actual value. Target B shows a less reliable, but still reasonably valid measure. Were the reliability to decrease, then the validity would also decrease.

CONCEPT OF RATES

In epidemiology, a count or frequency of health events is of limited interest by itself. However, when frequency is used as the numerator of a fraction that expresses a proportion with specification of a relevant time frame, it is of great value and is called a rate. The reporting, for example, of three cases of infectious hepatitis without indicating if they occurred among 1000 students in a school (3/1000 = 0.3 percent) or among 20 in a dormitory (3/20 = 15 percent) is of little practical value to the epidemiologist or to public health practitioners, except for the fact that the number of cases of this disease may be useful to estimate the need for additional medical services. The rates, however, can be compared to rates for other times or places to assess trends and identify excesses of disease occurrence, or to evaluate progress in control efforts. For example, public health officials have recently observed that the rates of lung cancer deaths among women have been increasing rapidly since 1965 (Figure 3–3). It has been estimated that if these rates continue to rise at the present rate, lung cancer will overtake breast cancer as the leading cause of cancer mortality for women by 1985. Smokers who use oral contraceptives have higher rates of death from heart disease. In an attempt to reduce these preventable deaths, public health officials have instituted anti-smoking campaigns primarily directed at young women of reproductive age.

In another example, high rates of measles were observed among high school students by school nurses in Cook County, Illinois in 1976. Measles are unusual among this age group as highest rates have occurred among primary school children. When these cases were reported to the county health department, an investigation was begun. After investigating the exposure and immunization histories of these cases, it was learned that they were among the earliest groups vaccinated after the measles vaccine first became available. The students had been vaccinated before reaching 6 months of age. Since there was

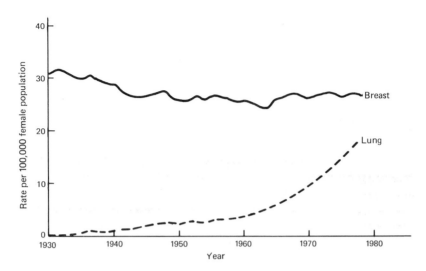

Figure 3–3. Age-adjusted death rates of women from breast and lung cancer, United States, 1930–1980. *(From Valanis, B. The epidemiological model in community health nursing. In M. Stanhope & J. Lancaster (Eds.),* Community health nursing: Process and practice for promoting health. *St. Louis: C. V. Mosby, 1984, p. 157.)*

residual maternal antibody still present in their blood, the vaccination did not stimulate active antibody production as intended. Thus, when maternal immunity waned, these persons were susceptible to the disease. As a result, such susceptible individuals were actively sought by county officials so they could be revaccinated before a new epidemic occurred (Kuter, 1977).

Both the increase in rates of lung cancer mortality in women and the increase in rates among the students in Cook County represent epidemics. *Epidemics* are defined as rates of disease significantly higher than the usual frequency. The usual frequency represents the *endemic* level. A third term, *pandemic*, is used to describe epidemics that include large areas of the world—a worldwide epidemic. Figure 3–4 illustrates the endemic fluctuation of rates. The peak in September represents an epidemic because it is clearly in excess of normal rates.

Rates are expressed by a numerator, a denominator, and by specification of person, place, and time. The numerator and denominator of rates may be *general* or *specific*. General rates refer to rates that include the total population whereas specific rates apply only to the population subgroup specified, e.g., all women, children under 17 years of age, or black males. Both

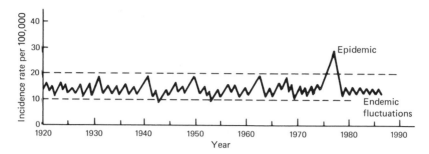

Figure 3–4. Schematic representation of endemic and epidemic rates. *(From Valanis, B. The epidemiological model in community health nursing. In M. Stanhope & J. Lancaster (Eds.)* Community health nursing: Process and practice for promoting health. *St. Louis: C. V. Mosby, 1984, p. 158.)*

numerator and denominator have to be similarly restricted by population characteristics (age, sex, and race), by place, and by time. When the denominator refers to a population that includes the numerator, the relative frequency is expressed as a *rate*. Stated another way, the events represented in the numerator arise from the population at risk in the denominator. For example:

$$\frac{\text{No. of new cases of uterine cancer in Cincinnati, Ohio, 1983}}{\text{No. of women in Cincinnati, Ohio, 1983}} \times 100{,}000$$

Because uterine cancer can only occur among women, only women are included in the denominator. The women in both the numerator and denominator are those living in Cincinnati, Ohio in 1983. The resulting rate is generally multiplied times some constant value, usually 100,000, in order that rates for different sized populations can be compared.

By contrast, although any fraction is encompassed by the general term ratio, in common usage *ratio* refers to a fraction where the numerator is not included in the denominator. The annual *fetal death rate* is the number of fetal deaths in a year related to the total number of annual births plus fetal deaths. The annual fetal death *ratio* is the number of fetal deaths in relation to the total number of live births only. Here the denominator does not include both the total population of affected and unaffected persons (live births and fetal deaths), but includes only the unaffected. A commonly used ratio is the sex ratio. The numerator is the number of men in a population; the denominator is the number of women in the population.

TYPES OF RATES

Death Rates (Mortality Rates)

Mortality rates may be crude—pertaining to the total population—or specific—pertaining to a population subgroup. The numerator of mortality rates includes all deaths that occurred in the population during a defined period of time, usually one year. Crude rates may include in the numerator all deaths from all causes, i.e., crude mortality rate for deaths in Ohio in 1983, or the numerator may be specific for a disease or condition, i.e., the crude mortality rate for pneumonia shown below. The numerator includes only deaths from pneumonia rather than including deaths from all causes. The denominator remains general, encompassing the entire population.

$$\frac{\text{No. of deaths from pneumonia in Ohio, 1983}}{\text{No. persons in population of Ohio, 1983}} \times 100{,}000$$

These crude rates provide one measure for the experience of the entire population. A crude rate of death from pneumonia, for example, includes deaths among men and women, and deaths among young and old. *Specific rates*, on the other hand, allow us to assess the experience of subgroups of a population. Sex-specific rates give us one rate for men, calculated as:

$$\frac{\text{No. of men dying from pneumonia in Cincinnati, 1983}}{\text{No. of men in total population of Cincinnati, 1983}} \times 100{,}000$$

If a similar rate is calculated for women, we can compare the rate for men with that of women. A similar procedure for specific age groups would allow us to compare the experience of younger persons with that of older persons. In this example, were we to look at actual age-specific rates, we would see that the rate of mortality from pneumonia is highest among the elderly.

Crude rates, which provide one rate for the experience of a total population, can present a problem if we wish to compare the population experience of one location with that of another because the distribution of characteristics within the population may vary. For example, suppose we wanted to compare population A and population B. As seen in Table 3–3, the age-specific rates of cardiovascular disease are the same in the two populations (see column 3). The crude rates (column 5) would lead us to believe that the experience of these populations is quite different, however. This occurs because population B has a large percentage of its members in the older age groups where rates of heart disease mortality are high, whereas population A has a heavier concentration of members in the younger age groups where rates of heart disease mortality are low. We might observe such a situation when comparing a state with a young population such as Alaska with a state such as Florida, which has a substantial elderly population.

A *"standardized"* or *age-adjusted* rate can be calculated to adjust for the difference in age distribution of populations. Essentially, age-adjusted rates allow one to answer the question, "suppose these populations have the same age distribution, how would their overall experience with this disease compare?" Calculation of these rates uses two pieces of basic information: 1) the actual age-specific rates for each population being compared and 2) a population distribution to which the specific rates are applied. The absolute number obtained will differ depending on the population distribution used. This number, although "fictitious" because of how it is calculated, nonetheless represents a valid way to compare the experiences of these two populations because it is not the absolute level but the relative position that is important. Therefore, it does not matter what population is chosen as the standard. For example, in Table 3–3, if we use the population distribution of population A in calculating the standardized rate for B, we obtain a rate of 22 for population B. Because the age-specific rates for the two populations are the same, this adjusted rate is the same as the crude rate for population A. If the distribution of population B is used for the calculation, we obtain a standardized rate of 31.7 for population A, the same as the crude rate of B. In both cases, we learn that population A and population B have the same rate of heart disease.

TABLE 3–3. COMPARISON OF DEATH RATES IN TWO POPULATIONS BY AGE SPECIFIC RATES, CRUDE RATES, AND ADJUSTED RATES

Age (years)	Population No.	%	Annual Age-Specific Death Rate per 1000	Annual No. of Deaths	Crude Death Rate per 1000	Adjusted Rate for B; A as Standard Population Age–Specific Rates — $\dfrac{Pop.\ B}{1000} \times Pop.\ A$ = Expected No. Deaths	Adjusted Rate — Adjusted Rate	Adjusted rate for A; B as Standard Population Age–Specific Rates — $\dfrac{Pop.\ A}{1000} \times Pop.\ B$ = Expected No. Deaths	Adjusted Rate
Population A									
<25	4000	40	2.0	8				$2.0 \times 1500 = 3$	
25–44	3000	30	4.0	12				$4.0 \times 3500 = 14$	
45–64	2000	20	50.0	100				$50.0 \times 4000 = 200$	
65+	1000	10	100.0	100				$100.0 \times 1000 = 100$	
All ages	10000	100		220	$\dfrac{220}{10000} = 22.0$			317	$\dfrac{317}{10000} = 31.7$
Population B									
<25	1500	15	2.0	3		$2.0 \times 4000 = 8$			
25–44	3500	35	4.0	14		$4.0 \times 3000 = 12$			
45–64	4000	40	50.0	200		$50.0 \times 2000 = 100$			
65+	1000	10	100.0	100		$100.0 \times 1000 = 100$			
All Ages	10000	100		317	$\dfrac{317}{10000} = 31.7$	220	$\dfrac{220}{10000} = 22.0$		

(From Valanis, B. The epidemiological model and community health nursing. In M. Stanhope & J. Lancaster (Eds.), *Community health nursing: Process and practice for promoting health*. St. Louis: C. V. Mosby, 1984.)

It should be remembered that these numbers are meaningful only as comparison and mean nothing alone. This leads us to the same conclusion we would have drawn by examining the age specific rates: these two populations have the same experience for heart disease mortality. You may ask—why not just compare the age-specific rates rather than going to so much trouble? This is a reasonable approach if you are trying to compare only two or three populations. However, if your aim is to compare rates for the 50 U.S. states, or 20 neighborhoods in a city, or for 50 different years, you might find the task of making sense of so many rates overwhelming. Use of a single standardized rate to represent the experience of each unit (state, neighborhood, year) makes the task manageable. In addition to standardization for age, rates can be standardized for differences in racial distribution, sex distribution, and for other characteristics associated with differences in specific rates that are distributed differently in the populations being compared.

Figure 3–5 illustrates the crude and age-adjusted death rates for the United States from 1930 to 1983. As discussed in Chapter 4, the average age of the United States has increased over the past 50 years as a result of increasing life spans and a declining birth rate. Because most of the major causes of death are chronic degenerative diseases and these diseases are most common among older persons, it is thus not surprising that the crude death rate for the years 1930 to 1983 does not show a substantial decline. Use of an age-adjusted rate, however, controls for the effect of the increasing age of the population. The age-adjusted rate in Figure 3–5, in sharp contrast to the crude rate, shows the dramatic decline in the death rate during the 53-year period.

Another kind of mortality rate compares the number of deaths from a particular illness, such as cancer, to deaths from all other causes. Such a rate, called a *proportional mortality rate*, is calculated:

$$\frac{\text{No. of cancer deaths in place in year}}{\substack{\text{No. of total deaths from all causes in place,}\\ \text{in year}}} \times 100 = \substack{\text{Percent of}\\ \text{deaths due}\\ \text{to cancer}}$$

This rate then tells us what percentage of all deaths are due to cancer. Other proportional mortality rates can be derived. The

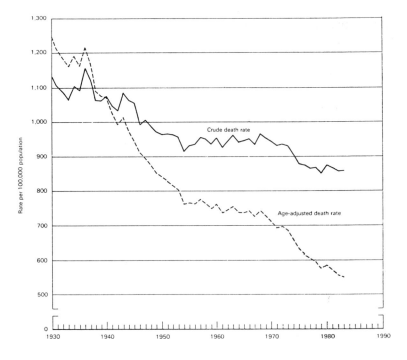

Figure 3–5. Crude and age-adjusted death rates: United States, 1930–1983. *(From NHS Monthly Vital Statistics Report.)*

denominator could be the total number of deaths from cancer if one were interested in what percent of all cancer deaths are due to breast cancer, in which case, the numerator would be the number of breast cancer deaths. In either instance, if the numerator is specific for certain age, sex, or race groups, the denominator has to be likewise restricted to these same groups. For instance, to calculate the proportional mortality rate for CHD in U.S. white males over 50 years of age in relation to all CHD deaths, the numerator would include all deaths in this restricted group of the general population; the denominator would be all CHD deaths in this segment of the population.

Morbidity Rates

The two most commonly used morbidity rates are incidence and prevalence. *Incidence rates* are a measure of all new cases arising in a population at risk during a defined period of time, usually 1 year.

$$\text{Incidence} = \frac{\text{No. of new cases in place during time of observation}}{\text{population in place at midpoint of time}} \times K$$

For the incidence rate shown above, the denominator uses the population size at the midpoint of the time period. This incidence rate, called a cumulative incidence, is the one commonly used for large general population estimates. As with rates discussed earlier, multiplication by a constant, K, facilitates comparing rates.

Other measures of incidence, such as incidence density, are modifications of the cumulative incidence rate. Incidence density is a measure often used in cohort studies where a defined group of persons is followed over time. To account for persons who die, who are lost to follow-up, or who have contracted the disease and are therefore not at risk for the whole time period of the study, a measure called person–years is used as the denominator of these incidence rates. A *person–year* represents one person at risk for 1 year. The numerator of the rate is the total number of cases accumulated over the study period.

$$\text{Incidence density} = \frac{\text{Total new cases accumulated during study period}}{\text{Person–years accumulated by study subjects}} \times K$$

This rate, yielded by dividing the numerator by the denominator, can subsequently be divided by the number of follow-up years to determine an average incidence density.

Incidence represents a measure of the risk for developing a particular disease. Thus, incidence rates are useful in studies of disease etiology; incidence rates for groups exposed to a putative etiologic agent are compared with incidence rates for groups not exposed. This measure, comparing the risk for two groups, is the relative risk ratio.

$$\text{Relative risk ratio} = \frac{\text{Incidence rate in exposed group}}{\text{Incidence rate in nonexposed group}}$$

A relative risk of 1.0 means that the risk is the same for both groups. A risk greater than 1.0 indicates excess risk in the exposed group. Statistical tests are used to determine whether any increase in risk is greater than would be expected by chance alone.

Incidence rates are useful for monitoring the occurrence of a disease in defined populations over time. Incidence rates are preferable to mortality rates for this purpose, because incidence reflects only diagnosed occurrence of the disease and not additional factors reflected by mortality rates, such as improvements in treatment leading to improved survival. Such monitoring of disease can alert public health personnel to the presence of new hazards in the environment. A sudden increase in a particular congenital malformation, for example, could indicate an environmental hazard that was recently introduced to that geographical area.

Special incidence rates, called attack rates, are frequently used in surveillance and control of infectious diseases. Attack rates are calculated when an identifiable population has been exposed to an infectious agent; the rate represents the incidence of illness among that exposed population. An example is the incidence of hepatitis B in a classroom of children exposed to a contageous classmate at a day-care center. Changes in attack rates may indicate a change in the immune status of a population, as with the Cook County measles epidemic discussed earlier, or may be an indication of a more virile strain of organism. These rates are discussed further in the chapter on communicable diseases.

Prevalence rates, when unspecified, usually refer to point prevalence. These *prevalence rates* are a measure of the existing number of cases present in a population at a given time. The numerator in a point prevalence rate can be likened to a snapshot of cases present when the picture is taken. The numerator of incidence rates, in contrast, is like a movie taken over a period of time.

$$\text{Point prevalence} = \frac{\text{No. of existing cases in place at point in time}}{\text{No. of persons in place at midpoint of year}}$$

In order to evaluate adequacy of existing services and to plan for future needs, public health officials require a measure of the case load requiring care. Prevalence is the measure generally used. Prevalence is not only a measure of current case load. Future prevalence can be projected by using incidence, recovery, and mortality rates to estimate changes in prevalence over time, because prevalence rates are a function of incidence and of the duration of the disease. A disease that is chronic in nature and that has low rates of mortality tends to increase the number of persons with the disease in the population if incidence remains the same. Death and recovery are the two most common factors that reduce the case load requiring care. A less common factor is substantial out-migration of individuals from the community.

The second type of prevalence rate is *period prevalence*. This rate is constructed from prevalence at a point in time, plus incidence cases and recurrences during a succeeding time period (e.g., 1 year).

$$\text{Period prevalence} = \frac{\text{No. of existing cases in place during period}}{\text{Average population of place during period}}$$

This rate is most useful for diseases that are episodic and for which exact date of onset is difficult to determine. It has been used most frequently in the mental health field. A variation of period prevalence, lifetime prevalence, is a measure of what proportion of a population has *ever* had a particular disease. This measure is also used primarily in psychiatric epidemiology.

Prevalence and incidence rates often give very different pictures of the disease status of a population. If two diseases have the same incidence rate but one of these is a chronic disease and the other an acute condition, they will have quite different prevalence rates. Assuming low case fatality rates for both, the chronic disease will show a high rate of prevalence whereas the acute condition will show a low rate of prevalence. In terms of provision of health services, the initial number of patients requiring treatment (reflected by the incidence rate) is the same for the two conditions. Need for long-term follow-up services (reflected by the prevalence rate) is quite different.

REFERENCES

Dawber, T. R. *The Framingham Study: The epidemiology of athero-sclerotic disease.* Cambridge, Mass.: Harvard University, 1980.

Kuter, B. *An Epidemiologic investigation of a measles epidemic in Cook County, Illinois.* Masters thesis, Columbia University, 1978.

Schatzkin, A., Cupples, L. A., Heeren, T., et al. Sudden death in the Framingham Heart Study. *American Journal of Epidemiology,* 1984, *120*(6), 888–899.

Soman, M., Green, B., & Daling, J. Risk factors for early neonatal sepsis. *American Journal of Epidemiology*, 1985, *121*(5), 712–719.

Epidemiological Transitions In Disease Patterns Over Time

This chapter focuses on historical changes in patterns of health and disease. The relationships of the health status of a population to demographic characteristics such as size, density, growth, and distribution is described. In addition, shifts in the health and demographic characteristics in relation to economic and social influences are discussed. Understanding the complex interdependence of the demographic characteristics and health status of populations is necessary for assessing and planning of health services because the health status of populations is not static, but constantly changing in response to population dynamics.

HISTORICAL POPULATION CHANGES

Archaeological evidence suggests that at the end of the last glaciation (10,000 BC) humans lived primarily as wanderers, gathering what food could be found. Populations were sparse and scattered. Through the years, as they wandered through changing environments and improved their means of food acquisition, population began to increase, reaching an estimated 10 million total world population by 8000 BC and rising to about 300 million by the advent of the Christian era largely because of the development of agriculture, which allowed groups to congregate in one place and to develop a more stable social system. This represented an annual growth rate of 0.06 percent across a period of 80 centuries. In comparison, modern rates of population growth are phenomenal (Table 4–1), rising from 0.29 percent between 1650 and 1750 to about 2.00 percent in the early 1960s (Broek and Webb, 1968). Since that time, population growth has slowed in most of the industrialized nations. In the period after 1960, population growth in Europe has been less than 1 percent annually, dropping to a low of 0.4 percent in 1980 to 1982 (Table 4–2). During this same time, rates have lowered to around 1 percent annually in other developed areas such as the United States, U.S.S.R., and Oceania (Australia, New Zealand, Papua New Guinea). Although there has been a slight slowing of the rate of increase in the less developed regions taken as a whole, the African population continues to increase at an annual rate approaching 3 percent (U.S. Bureau of the Census, 1983).

TABLE 4–1. WORLD POPULATION FROM 8000 BC TO PRESENT

Date	Population in Millions	Average Annual Increase		No. of Generations
		Millions	*Percent*	
8000BC	10			
1AD	300	0.036	0.06	266
1650	545	0.150	0.04	55
1750	728	1.8	0.29	
1800	906	3.5	0.44	
1850	1171	5.3	0.51	
1900	1608	8.7	0.64	13
1950[a]	2493	17.7	0.86	
1980[a]	4654	72.0	2.02	

[a]Amounts and rates of increase affected by improved collection of data
(Data 8000 BC to 1950 from Broek, J. Webb, J. *A geography of mankind.* New York: McGraw Hill, 1968, Table 18–1; 1980 data from *Statistical abstract of the United States, 1985.* Washington, D.C.: U.S. Government Printing Office, 1984.)

TABLE 4–2. WORLD POPULATION GROWTH BY CONTINENT, 1960 to 1982

Region	Midyear Population		Annual Rate of Growth (%)				
	1960	1980	60–65	65–70	70–75	75–80	80–82
Africa	277	499	2.5	2.6	2.7	2.8	2.9
Asia	1715	2738	2.0	2.5	2.3	1.9	1.8
Latin America	216	378	2.8	2.7	2.5	2.4	2.2
North America	199	257	1.5	1.1	1.1	1.0	1.0
Europe	425	488	0.9	0.7	0.6	0.4	0.4
U.S.S.R.	214	270	1.5	1.0	0.9	0.8	0.8
Oceania	16	23	2.1	2.1	1.9	1.3	1.4
World Total	3061	4654	1.9	2.1	2.0	1.8	1.7
more developed regions	945	1152	1.2	0.9	0.9	0.7	0.7
less developed regions	2116	3502	2.2	2.6	2.4	2.1	2.1

(Adapted from U.S. Bureau of Census, *Statistical Abstract of the United States, 1985* (105th ed.). Washington, D.C.: U.S. Government Printing Office,1984, Table 1515.)

FACTORS AFFECTING POPULATION SIZE AND COMPOSITION

Population growth, in general, is dependent on both the birth rates and the death rates. Migration is a third factor that may affect the population dynamics of a defined geographical area. Thus, an area with high birth rates, low death rates, and a balance between migration into and out of the area will show an increase in population. With a stable migration situation and death rates equal to or higher than birth rates, the population size will remain the same or decrease.

Early world population growth probably was attributable largely to increasing birth rates as mortality remained high. In more recent times, particularly during the last 100 years, death rates for all age groups have dropped dramatically in most of the world, resulting in a concurrent increase in life expectancy. When birth rates remain the same or increase simultaneously to a drop in death rates, a population explosion occurs. This is what we currently observe in Africa and, until the last 20 years, in Asia and Latin America.

Within countries, the rate of population growth is not the same for all subgroups of the population. In the United States, for example, between 1960 and 1980 the rate of growth for the white population was lower than that of the nonwhite populattion. Projections for the period between 1982 and 2025 estimate that the white population of the United States will increase 21.2 per cent, an annual average of 0.49 per cent. Estimates for the increase in the nonwhite population during the same time are 65.7 per cent, an annual average of 1.5 per cent (U.S. Bureau of the Census, 1983). Thus, if these rates of increase eventuate, the proportion of the U.S. population that is nonwhite will increase from the present 12.3 per cent to 16.9 per cent in 2025.

The U.S. nonwhite population is composed of numerous subgroups, including blacks, Hispanics, American Indians, Orientals, and others. The higher rate of growth observed during the past 20 years for nonwhites was a function of several factors; one of these was higher birth rates among the nonwhite population. Lifetime births expected by married women 18 to 34 years old are shown in Table 4–3 for 1967, 1975, and 1980. In 1975, for example, among blacks and Hispanics, the proportion of married women expecting to have four or more children was nearly twice that of married white women. A substantial immigration of Orientals including Thais, Vietnamese, Japanese, and Taiwanese and of Mexicans, Cubans, and other Hispanics during the 1970s has also contributed to a rapid increase in the proportion of the U.S. population that is nonwhite. In 1960, for example, the portion of the U.S. population either born in Asia

TABLE 4–3. LIFETIME BIRTHS EXPECTED BY MARRIED WOMEN 18 to 34 YEARS OLD—PERCENT DISTRIBUTION

Number of Births Expected	1967		1975			1980		
	White	Black	White	Black	Spanish Origin	White	Black	Spanish Origin
0	2.2	3.0	4.9	3.0	3.2	6.0	4.0	2.8
1	5.5	8.1	10.8	10.7	10.6	13.2	14.6	9.4
2	31.4	24.9	49.8	40.0	40.4	51.5	45.3	44.3
3	30.3	25.1	23.3	22.4	25.2	20.4	22.2	24.2
4+	30.6	39.0	11.1	24.0	20.5	8.8	14.2	19.4

(Adapted from U.S. Bureau of the Census, *Statistical Abstract of the United States, 1984* (105th ed.). Washington, D.C.: U.S. Government Printing Office, 1983, Table 92.)

or with at least one parent born in Asia was 3.4 percent. In 1970, the comparable figure was 5.2 percent. Similarly, in 1960, 6.8 percent of the U.S. population was born or had at least one parent born in Mexico, Cuba, or South or Central America. In 1970, the percentage increased to 11.5 percent. These changes reflect changes in immigration, as well as the higher birth rates.

CHANGES IN LIFE EXPECTANCY

In the Middle Ages, the average person had a short and uncertain life expectancy that varied somewhat by social class status. Aristocrats generally fared better than the common folk. Figure 4–1 shows typical survival curves for the people of York, England during the sixteenth century. Although early death was common among the townsfolk, with just over 10 percent living to age 40, close to half of the artistocracy lived to that age.

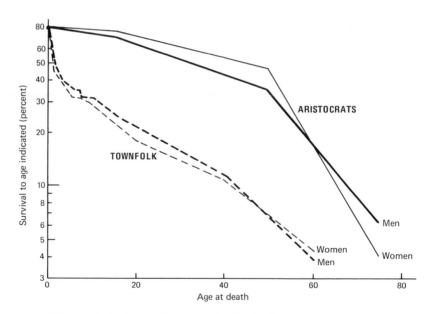

Figure 4–1. Survival curves for York, England townfolk and aristocrats in the sixteenth century. *(Adapted from Cowgill, U.M. The People of York: 1538–1812. Scientific American, 1970, 22, 104–112.)*

The average person was a constant prey of famine and disease, malign forces of nature, and the avarice and brutality of fellow countrymen. Widespread poverty was common. Methods of agriculture were crude and forces of nature such as floods, draught, unseasonable heat or cold, an unusual number of insect pests, or other natural hazards of farming, some of which today can be controlled by scientific means, might destroy a peasant's entire crop. As a result, famines, both local and widespread, were common occurrences. Epidemic diseases often accompanied famines, spreading like wildfire among a population already weakened by starvation. Even in good years epidemics were quite common. Poor sanitation and overcrowding facilitated the survival and spread of disease organisms. Poor nutrition increased death rates. Lack of hygiene led to high mortality from simple wound infection, postpartal infection, and infections of infancy.

In contrast to the Middle Ages, life expectancy today is long, 69.9 years for a white man born in the United States in 1979 and 77.6 years for a white woman born at the same time. Figure 4–2 shows the survival curves for white American women, between 1890 and 1978. Before the 1950s, survival was lower in the under-10-year age group because of high mortality among infants and young children 1 to 6 years of age. The same situation exists today in many Third World countries. High mortality in all age groups leads to a continual drop in the proportion of the population surviving at each successive age. In contrast, the survival curve for white American women in 1978 shows an almost constant proportion of the population surviving until age 50. Approximately 90 percent of the total U.S. population will survive to 55 years of age for those born in 1971 compared with approximately 55 percent of the population born in 1901. Half of the population born in 1901 died by age 65 whereas this median point for the population born in 1971 is about 77 years of age (U.S. Bureau of the Census, 1983).

As in York, England in the Middle Ages, we today observe differences in survival for various population subgroups. In the United States, for example, there are differences in survival at most ages by race, sex, and socioeconomic status. We have already presented in Chapter 1 the different mortality rates between blacks and whites; these are reflected in the differences in life expectancy—64.0 years for a black man born in 1970 compared to 70.6 years for a white man. Comparisons of life expect-

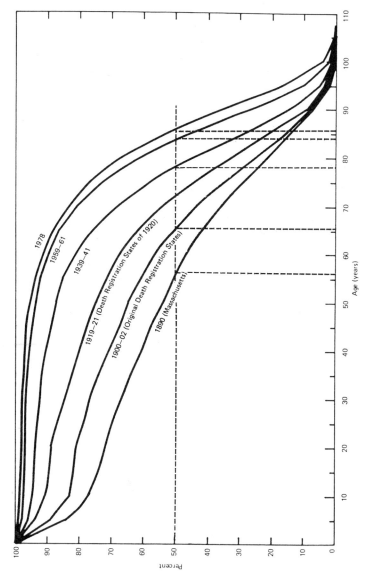

Figure 4–2. Percent surviving to each exact age of an initial cohort of white female births, according to various life tables for the United States: 1890 to 1978. Vertical dotted lines represent age of median survival. (*Adapted from U.S. Bureau of the Census. Current Population Reports Demographic and Socioeconomic aspects of aging in the United States, [Series P–23, no. 138]. Washington, D.C.: U.S. Printing Office, 1984, Figure 4–3.*)

ancy at different ages for whites and nonwhites, men and women are shown in Table 4–4. Women have a longer life expectancy than do men of either race.

Although life expectancies in Third world countries remain lower than in more industrialized nations, life expectancies have been rising quickly in recent years as death rates, particularly among infants and young children, have dropped. These changes have resulted from improvement in sanitation and living conditions and from the introduction of medical technology for prevention and control of disease. Emphasis on prevention and control of infectious disease through environmental hygiene, improved housing and nutrition, vaccination programs, and use of antibiotics for treatment of infection has been a primary factor in permitting populations to live longer.

The rate of transitions in life expectancy has occurred more rapidly in some places than in others. How quickly death rates in a country drop is dependent upon whether all these measures are introduced simultaneously, as in Cuba and China, or whether they were introduced gradually. The decrease in mortality in most western countries occurred gradually over 100 to 200 years because major improvements in sanitation and housing began more than a century ago, before the development of the medical technology of the twentieth century, such as vaccines and antibiotics. The transition in mortality and life expectancy was propelled by the social changes of the Industrial Revolution and accompanied by improved family and personal hygiene and improved nutrition. Countries that most recently

TABLE 4–4. AVERAGE LIFE EXPECTANCY IN YEARS BY RACE AND SEX FOR BIRTHS IN 1979

	Whites		Blacks	
Age	Men	Women	Men	Women
At Birth	70.6	78.2	64.0	72.7
20	52.3	59.5	46.4	54.8
40	33.9	40.2	29.6	36.2
50	25.1	31.0	22.1	27.8
65	14.2	18.7	13.3	17.2

(From U.S. Bureau of the Census, Statistical Abstract of the United States, 1984 (104th ed.). Washington, D.C.: U.S. Government Printing Office, 1983.)

began their prevention and control efforts have had access to these major technological advances. In most developing nations, the transition in disease mortality began around the 1940s and resulted largely from the introduction of medical technology simultaneous with a period of rapid social change. In most of these countries the transition in mortality rates is not complete (Omran, 1971).

Transitions in death rates produce several major effects on demographic patterns and social conditions. Figure 4–3 illustrates some of these using three patterns of mortality transition as identified by Omran (1971). Four effects are discussed below.

Change in Major Causes of Death. Because infectious diseases are more likely to affect the very young, controlling infectious disease has shifted the average age of death to an older

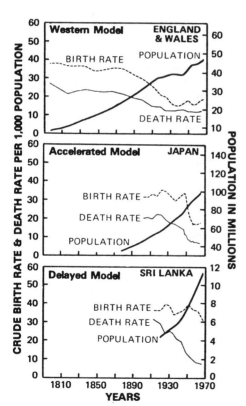

Figure 4–3. Epidemiological transition patterns for three different models of change. *(From Omran, A. R., The epidemiological transition; A theory of the epidemiology of population change.* Milbank Memorial Fund Quarterly, *1971, 49, 515.)*

age. Degenerative diseases, more common as causes of death in older persons, continue to emerge as major causes of death as age at death increases. Chronic diseases, such as heart disease are the most frequent causes of death from middle age onward. Table 4–5 shows the major causes of death in the United States in 1900 and 1982. Although infectious conditions topped the mortality lists in 1900, accounting for over one-third of deaths, coronary heart disease, cancer, and stroke are now the three major causes of death and account for more than 60 percent of all deaths.

TABLE 4–5. LEADING CAUSES OF DEATH IN 1900[a] AND IN 1982[b], UNITED STATES

	1900			1982	
Cause of Death	Deaths per 100,000 Persons	Percentage of all Deaths	Cause of Death	Deaths per 100,000 Persons	Percentage of all Deaths
All Causes	1719.1	100.0	All Causes	852.0	100.0
Influenza and pneumonia	202.2	11.8	Diseases of the heart	326.0	38.3
TB (all forms)	194.4	11.3	Malignant neoplasms	187.2	22.0
Gastritis	142.7	8.3	Cerebro-vascular diseases	68.0	8.0
Diseases of the heart	137.4	8.0	Accidents	40.6	4.8
Vascular lesions affecting the c.n. system	106.9	6.2	Chronic obstructive lung disease	25.8	3.0
Chronic nephritis	81.0	4.7	Influenza and pneumonia	21.1	2.5
All accidents	72.3	4.2	Diabetes mellitus	14.9	1.8
Malignant neoplasms	64.0	3.7	Suicide	12.2	1.4
Certain diseases of early infancy	62.6	3.6	Chronic liver disease and cirrhosis of liver	11.9	1.4
Diphtheria	40.3	2.3	Atheroselerosis	11.6	1.4
All other causes	615.3	35.9	All other causes	132.7	15.5

[a]Adapted from National Center for Health Statistics. *Progress in Health Services*, 1961, *10* (2).
[b]Adapted from Advance report, final mortality statistics, 1982. *Monthly Vital Statistics Report*, vol. 33, no. 9 (suppl.) DHHS Publication No. (PHS) 85–1120. Hyattsville, Md.: Public Health Service, 1984.

Similar shifts can be seen in countries that have more recently begun to reduce mortality from infectious disease. China, for example, following nearly 20 years of concentrated effort, has a proportion of deaths caused by heart disease, cancer, and stroke midway between the corresponding 1900 and 1978 figures for the United States.

X *Change in Age Distribution of the Population.* As epidemics of infectious diseases recede, fertility improves. In conjunction with improved child survival, there is an increased number of children who will grow to adulthood, moving in waves up through the population and changing the age distribution of the population. Figure 4–4 shows the population pyramids for the United States in 1900 and 1982. The 1900 pyramid is similar to that of the Middle Ages and of many developing countries, which are currently beginning the transition away from infec-

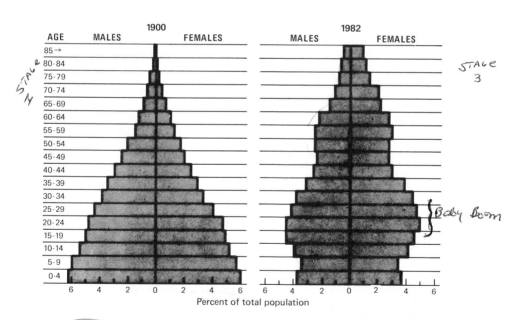

Figure 4–4. U.S. population pyramids, 1900 and 1982. *(Data from Bureau of the Census,* Historical statistics, colonial times to 1978, *Series A 23–25, and* Current population reports, *Series P–25, No. 929.)*

TABLE 4–6. INCIDENCE OF ACUTE CONDITIONS PER 100 PERSONS PER YEAR BY AGE, SEX AND CONDITION GROUP: UNITED STATES, JULY 1977 to JUNE 1978

Sex and Condition Group	All Ages	Under 6 Years	6–16 Years	17–44 Years	45 Years and Over
Men					
All acute conditions	206.0	385.6	273.0	197.3	115.5
Infective and parasitic diseases	22.6	64.9	33.3	18.0	8.4
Respiratory conditions	109.1	200.0	148.8	104.5	59.4
Digestive system conditions	9.4	11.5	12.6	9.1	7.0
Injuries	39.6	44.4	49.7	43.9	24.9
All other acute conditions	25.3	64.7	28.5	21.8	15.7
Women					
All acute conditions	231.1	377.4	284.7	245.7	146.0
Infective and parasitic diseases	25.7	57.7	36.6	24.9	12.6
Respiratory conditions	124.2	206.1	169.5	129.2	71.9
Digestive system conditions	10.5	16.8	11.6	10.9	7.7
Injuries	29.8	31.3	31.6	30.4	27.7
All other conditions	40.9	65.6	35.4	50.3	26.0

(Adapted from Ries, P. *Acute conditions: Incidence and associated disability* [DHEW Publication No. (PHS) 79–1560, series 10, no. 132]. Hyattsville, Md.: National Center for Health Statistics, 1979, P.5.)

tious diseases as major causes of death. It is characterized by a large number of persons in the younger age ranges and a rapid reduction in the proportion of the population in each successive age group, resulting in a very small number of individuals in the older ages. The pyramid for 1982 is fairly typical of countries that have completed the transition to a predominance of chronic, degenerative diseases. Here, we see a broadening of population in the middle and older age ranges and a substantial decrease in the very young ages, reflecting the lower birth rates that have resulted from the use of family planning techniques.

TABLE 4–7. DISTRIBUTION OF DEGREE OF ACTIVITY LIMITATION DUE TO CHRONIC CONDITION BY SEX AND AGE: UNITED STATES, 1978

Sex and Age	Total Population in Thousands	No Activity Limitation	Any Activity Limitation	Limitation Only in Major Activity[a]
		Percent Distribution		
Men				
All ages	103,174	85.7	14.3	10.8
Under 17 Years	30,096	95.8	4.2	2.2
17–44 years	42,951	90.0	9.1	5.5
45–64 years	20,734	75.7	24.3	19.7
65 years and over	9,393	51.8	48.2	43.2
Women				
All ages	110,655	85.9	14.1	10.3
Under 17 years	29,916	96.4	3.6	1.8
17–44 years	45,676	92.1	7.9	4.9
45–64 years	22,668	77.0	23.0	17.5
65 years and over	13,394	57.3	42.7	34.9

[a]Major Activity refers to ability to work, keep house, or engage in school or preschool activities. (From Givens, J. *Current estimates from the Health Interview Survey, United States, 1978.* [DHHS Publication No. (PHS) 80–1551] Hyattsville, Md.: National Center for Health Statistics, 1979.)

Change in the Sex Composition of the Population. Improvement in the survival of women during the childbearing years leads to a change in the sex composition of the population that becomes more marked as the population ages because men tend to become victims of degenerative diseases at younger ages than do women. The male to female ratio among children under age 14 in the United States in 1980 was 104.6. By ages 25 to 44, the ratio is 97.4 and it continues to drop. For persons aged 65 and older, the ratio is 67.6.

Change in the Major Causes of Morbidity. Although social changes were a major contributing factor in the transition from infectious to chronic diseases, improved health and longevity brought about further social changes and pressures. These include increased efficiency and productivity of the work force, increased economic expectation, the advent of the nuclear family, destruction in group cohesion, and problems of older citizens who face years of life with no productive employment, rising inflation, chronic health problems that may limit mobility, and a lack of family members in close geographical proximity to offer physical care and emotional support. Major causes of morbidity are often "man-made" diseases such as drug abuse, mental illness, accidents, and occupational-related diseases. These causes may be divided into acute and chronic illnesses. Rates of acute conditions and chronic illnesses vary by age, race, and sex. Table 4–6 shows incidence rates of common acute conditions by sex and age. Table 4–7 shows prevalence rates for major chronic conditions by sex and age.

Many of these conditions may be preventable. Those that are not preventable require medical and nursing intervention. In any event, awareness of which conditions are most common in each age and sex group and of the natural history of the conditions enables health professionals to function more effectively. The major causes of morbidity and mortality for the various age groups are discussed in Part 2 of this book in relation to measures for primary, secondary, and tertiary prevention.

REFERENCES

Broek, J., & Webb, J. *A geography of mankind.* New York, McGraw Hill, 1968.

Omram, A. R. The epidemiologic transition: A theory of the epidemiology of population change. *Milbank Memorial Fund Quarterly,* 1971, *49*, 509-516.

U.S. Bureau of the Census, *Statistical abstract of the United States, 1984* (105th ed.), Washington, D. C.: U.S. Government Printing Office, 1983.

5

Epidemiology of Diseases of Infectious Origin

Epidemiological investigation originated in response to outbreaks of infectious diseases. Study of the outbreaks of diseases, such as plague, cholera, and smallpox in Europe in the nineteenth century identified the etiology and mode of transmission of these diseases. Subsequently, measures were instituted for their control. Today, large explosive epidemics of communicable diseases are relatively rare and are confined mostly to the developing countries of the world in Africa, Asia, South and Central America. In these developing countries, controllable communicable diseases remain primary public health problems. Member states of the World Health Organization (WHO) from Africa and Asia, for example, list malaria and other parasitic diseases, tuberculosis, malnutrition, diarrheal diseases, leprosy, respiratory diseases other than tuberculosis, venereal diseases, measles, poliomyelitis, and tetanus (particularly neonatal tetanus) as their most important health problems.

Smaller outbreaks from a variety of infections may occur in limited geographical areas anywhere in the world. In the United States, public health officials are concerned at the present time with outbreaks of hepatitis, sexually transmitted diseases, salmonellosis, hospital-acquired infections, toxic shock syndrome, herpes, tuberculosis, influenza, and other respiratory infections. AIDS and listerosis are two infectious diseases that have recently made front page news. Thus, although the infectious diseases have decreased in frequency and prominence as major causes of morbidity and mortality, familiarity with infectious diseases and methods of control remains important. Some infectious conditions, e.g., venereally transmitted diseases, have actually increased in frequency in recent years. During the 1950s major public health efforts were devoted to public education programs and to case-finding and treatment programs for venereal disease. When rates of these diseases dropped, funds were diverted to other programs. Subsequently, importation of new antibiotic-resistant strains by veterans returning from abroad and changes in values and sexual behavior subsequent to introduction of the birth control pill in the 1960s contributed to an increase in these conditions, particularly gonorrhea, which began to decrease again only in the past few years. The most common notifiable infectious diseases are shown in Table 5–1.

As changes in the environment have modified the natural history of many diseases, man-made or artificial factors have changed the susceptibility of the human host to these infections. These factors have resulted from the broader use of immunosuppressive and cytotoxic drugs (i.e., in transplantation of organs, in cancer), from nutritional or metabolic deficiencies depressing host resistance (severity of measles in West Africa), and from the expanding use of antibiotics that modify the normal flora and make some areas of the body more vulnerable to pathogens.

This chapter discusses methods for control of infectious disease using the natural history model presented in Chapter 2. Specific examples of the use of the natural history of a disease in determining interventions for primary, secondary, and tertiary prevention are presented. This is followed by a discussion of methods for investigation of an outbreak.

MECHANISMS OF CAUSATION IN INFECTIOUS DISEASE

The cycle of disease transmission is a concept important to the prepathogenic and earliest pathogenic phase of the disease natural history. This cycle is illustrated in Figure 5–1. There are

TABLE 5–1. NUMBER AND RATE PER 100,000 POPULATION FOR NOTIFIABLE DISEASES IN THE UNITED STATES, 1983, WITH MORE THAN 500 REPORTED CASES

Disease	Number of Cases	Rate per 100,000
Amebiasis	6,658	2.95
Aseptic meningitis	12,696	5.49
Chancroid[a]	847	0.36
Chickenpox	177,462	99.65
Encephalitis (all forms)	1,795	0.76
Gonorrhea[a]	900,435	387.64
Hepatitis A	21,532	9.20
Hepatitis B	24,318	10.39
Hepatitis, Unspecified	7,149	3.09
Legionellosis[b]	852	0.43
Malaria	813	0.35
Measles (rubeola)	1.497	0.64
Meningococcal infections, total	2,736	1.17
Mumps	3.355	1.55
Pertussis	2,463	1.05
Rubella	970	0.41
Salmonellosis (excluding typhoid fever)	44,250	18.91
Shigellosis	19,719	8.43
Syphilis (primary, secondary)	32,698	14.08
Total—all stages	74,637	32.13
Toxic shock syndrome	502	0.24
Tuberculosis	23,846	10.19
Typhoid fever (cases)	507	0.22
Typhus fever, tick borne (Rocky Mountain spotted)	4,126	0.48

[a]Civilian cases only.
[b]Data recorded by date of report to state health department, rather than date of onset.
(Compiled from Annual summary, 1983. *Morbidity and Mortality Weekly Reports*, 1984, *32*(54), 114–115.)

three elements crucial to maintenance of the transmission cycle: the agent, a susceptible host, and the environment. Furthermore, requirements for maintenance of the transmission cycle include a reservoir, a portal of exit from the reservoir, a means of transport to the susceptible host (mode of transmission), and a portal of entry to the host. Each of these is discussed in the following sections.

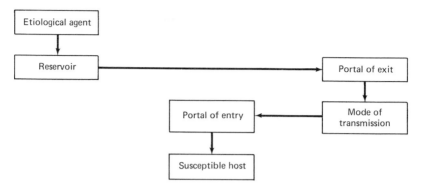

Figure 5–1. The cycle of infectious disease transmission.

The Agent

Infectious agents are invading, living parasites, either plant or animal, including metazoa, protozoa, fungi, bacteria, rickettsia, and virus. Table 5–2 lists some important diseases caused by each of these classes of infectious agents. These agents produce disease in a human host through one of three mechanisms:

1. Production of toxin
2. Invasion and infection
3. Infectious agents that produce immune response in host, thereby producing disease

An example of disease that results from the toxin produced by an infectious agent is staphylococcal food poisoning. The food contaminated with a staphylococci produces a medium in which the organism can multiply. The organism produces a toxin when the food is consumed, and the toxin produces illness. This is why symptoms of staphylococcal food poisoning appear soon after the food is consumed. In contrast, salmonella food poisoning does not produce symptoms until 12 to 24 hours after consumption of the food. Because the Salmonella produces disease through invasion and infection of the gastrointestinal mucosa, symptomatic response requires some time. Once recent disease of concern thought to be an example of the third method of disease production, i.e., through the immune response of the host, is acquired immune deficiency disease (AIDS). It is suspected that in

TABLE 5–2. DISEASES CAUSED BY VARIOUS TYPES OF INFECTIOUS AGENTS

Type of Agent	Disease	Specific Agent
Metazoa and protozoa	Hook worm	Filaria worm
	Acute amoebic dysentery	*Endamoeba histoytica*
Fungi	Histoplasmosis	*Histoplasma capsulation*
	Athletes foot	
Bacteria	Malaria	Plasmodian
	Strep throat, scarlet fever, rheumatic heart disease	Streptococci
	Syphilis	*Treponema pallidim*
	Tuberculosis	Mycobacteriam tuberculosis
	Plague	Yersinia pestus
Rickettsia	Legionaire's disease	L. pneumophilia
	Typhus (classical louse-borne)	Typhus exanthematicus
	Rocky Mountain spotted fever	Rickettsia rickettsi
Viruses	Common cold and other acute URIs	Rhinovirus, coronavirus
	Measles	Filterable virus
	Mumps	Paramyxovirus (measles)
	Chickenpox	Paramyxovirus (mumps)
	Polio	Herpes virus (varicella zoster)
	Encephalitis	Poliovirus
	Rabies	Alphavirus, flavivirus
	Yellow fever	Rhabdovirus
	Infectious hepatitis	Yellow fever virus
	Serum hepatitis	IH virus
		SH virus

response to a venereal infection the host's immune response leads to a form of autoimmune disease.

Host-related properties of an agent are infectivity, immunogenicity, pathogenicity, and virulence. *Infectivity* is the ability to lodge and multiply in a host, thus the ability to infect a host. The basic laboratory measure of infectivity is the number of infective particles needed to establish an infection. A more useful measure of this property for epidemiologists is the secondary attack rate. For contact transmitted infections, this is the frequency of infection occurrence among susceptible individuals within one incubation period of exposure. Infectivity can be detected through the presence of agent-specific antibodies produced by the host. The ability of an agent to induce such specific response in the host is called antigenicity or immunogenicity. Thus, when a serological survey of the exposed population can be conducted, an infection rate (IR) can be calculated:

$$IR = \frac{\text{No. of persons with antibody response}}{\text{Total no. exposed}}$$

Ideally persons with prior exposure, since they are not susceptible and have measurable antibody response, would be removed from both the numerator and the denominator, but unless baseline serological data on the specific population is available, this is not possible. Estimates of the percentage of the general population with antibody response can provide a guide.

The secondary attack rate and the infection rate permit us to order infectious diseases according to the relative infectivity of their causal agents. Table 5–3 shows the relative degree of infectivity for some common causal agents. Diseases that have high infectivity, such as measles or chickenpox, may be expected

TABLE 5–3. SOME WELL-KNOWN INFECTIOUS DISEASES ORDERED ACCORDING TO THREE HOST-RELATED PROPERTIES OF THEIR AGENTS

Relative Degree	Infectivity Basis: Secondary Attack Rate[a]	Pathogenicity Basis: Infected with Disease / Total Infected	Virulence Basis: Severe (e.g., Fatal) Cases / Total Cases
High	Smallpox Measles Chickenpox Poliomyelitis	Smallpox Rabies Measles Chickenpox Common cold	Rabies Smallpox Tuberculosis Leprosy
Intermediate	Rubella Mumps Common cold	Rubella Mumps	Poliomyelitis
Low	Tuberculosis	Poliomyelitis Tuberculosis	Measles
Very low	Leprosy (?)	Leprosy (?)	Rubella Chickenpox Common cold

[a]Limited to contact-transmitted diseases.
(From Fox, J., Hall, C., & Elveback, L. *Epidemiology: man and disease*. Toronto, Ontario: Collier-Macmillan, Canada, Ltd., 1970, p. 55.)

to spread quickly among a susceptible population. Leprosy, in contrast, appears to have low infectivity, requiring up to 30 years of close contact for successful transmission. However, this delay may also reflect a long period of incubation.

Pathogenicity is the ability of the agent to produce disease. Although an agent may successfully infect a host (lodge and multiply and produce an antibody response), it may not induce the signs or symptoms of disease. Whether the disease results from infection depends on such factors as the rapidity and extent to which the agent multiplies in the host, the extent of tissue damage resulting from agent multiplication, and whether or not the agent produces a toxin. In populations, pathogenicity of an agent is measured by the rate shown below:

$$\text{Pathogenicity} = \frac{\text{No. infected persons with clinical disease}}{\text{Total no. infected persons}}$$

The rate is specific to the relevant time frame for the current outbreak. The numerator is those persons with detectable signs and symptoms of disease, the denominator all those with antibodies to the disease organism.

Common childhood diseases, such as measles and chickenpox, are highly pathogenic; nearly all infected individuals show characteristic disease (Table 5–3). For polio, on the other hand, despite the severity of characteristic disease, infection produces typical paralytic polio only once in about 300 to 1000 times (Fox et al., 1970).

Virulence refers to the severity of the disease produced and is measured by the case fatality rate when death is the criterion for severity of disease.

$$\text{Case fatality rate} = \frac{\text{No. of fatal cases}}{\text{Total no. of cases}}$$

In other instances, criteria for severity may not be death, but rather, severe, permanent sequelae such as paralysis in the case of polio.

These measures provide a means of population surveillance, allowing public health officials to assess the nature of the problem they are facing in order to plan for intervention. Given limited fiscal resources, decisions must be made regarding which diseases should receive emphasis. An infectious disease caused by an agent of high infectivity, but low pathogenicity and virulence, is probably a poorer candidate for such resources than is one with low infectivity, but with high pathogenicity and/or virulence.

The Environment

Environment may be defined as all external conditions and influences affecting the life of an organism. Physical, biological, and socioeconomic environments provide reservoirs and modes of transmission for the agent. Physical environment includes the geological structure of an area and the availability of resources, such as water and flora, that influence the number and variety of animal reservoirs and arthropod vectors. Weather, climate, and season are important influences on these factors.

The socioeconomic environment contributes to the types of infectious agents in a location because social and economic conditions relate to the extent of environmental sanitation, pasteurization of milk, disposal of garbage and excreta, and the availability of medical facilities for immunization and medical care.

Finally, there is the biological environment, which includes other living plants and animals that may serve as either the reservoir or as the vector for transmission of an infectious agent. Because the agent is a living organism, it requires a place to live and to multiply. The habitat of the agent is called the reservoir. It may be any human, animal, arthropod, plant, soil, or inanimate matter that provides an environment for survival or reproduction. The reservoir is thus intimately related to the transmission cycle of the agent in nature. In the simplest cycle, the reservoir is the human body. For the majority of infectious diseases to which humans are subject, such as viral and bacterial respiratory infections, most staphylococcal and streptococcal infections, or venereal diseases, humans are both the host and the reservoir. Human reservoirs are individuals who have been infected. They may be acute clinical cases or they may be one of four types of carriers. When acute clinical cases are the reservoir and source of the infectious agent, disease control can be effected by isolating the individual until the period when he or she is infectious to other individuals has passed, thus preventing spread of the infection. This approach to control is effective only when the infectious period follows observable symptoms.

Such an approach is ineffective for controlling the spread of infection in diseases that have a stage in the natural history that includes an incubating carrier. This type of carrier is an individual who has been exposed to the disease organism prior to developing observable symptoms. By the time symptoms appear, the individual may have exposed many other persons to the infectious organism. This situation is present for many childhood infections, such as measles and chickenpox.

Other types of carriers are the inapparent carrier, the convalescent carrier, and the chronic carrier. The inapparent carrier is an infected individual whose infection remains subclinical; the carrier never develops observable symptoms but is shedding the organism and exposing others. The convalescent carrier is an infected individual who no longer has acute disease, but who remains infectious to others because of continued shedding of the organism. The infectious state may remain for weeks to months after symptoms are gone. Cholera and salmonella gastroenteritis are diseases that have a convalescent carrier state. Typhoid Mary is an infamous chronic-carrier type. Chronic carriers continue to harbor the viable organism indefinitely and remain infectious to others although they have no symptoms themselves. Chronic staphylococcal carriers among hospital workers, for example, can be a hazard to patients whose immune state is compromised.

Some agents are free-living in the environment, where, for example, soil and water serve as the reservoirs. The soil serves as reservoir for tetanus spores and for the rickettesia responsible for Legionnaire's disease. The cholera vibrio lives in organic matter found in water.

Animals are the reservoirs for other diseases of humans. Dogs, bats, and small wild animals are the reservoir for rabies; cows, pigs, and goats for brucellosis; and sheep for anthrax. An outbreak of the plague in California in the summer of 1980 was traced to its reservoir in ticks, which live on small wild animals in the mountains. In such instances the transmission cycle is complex, involving an intermediate host, the wild animal. In 1983, 40 cases of plague were reported and confirmed in the United States: 21 of these were among Indians whose lifestyle probably increases the likelihood of exposure (Barnes & Poland, 1985). A useful source of information about reservoirs and transmission cycles of specific infectious conditions in *Control of Communicable Disease in Man,* a handbook published by the American Public Health Association (Benenson, 1980).

The life cycle (transmission cycle) of an infectious agent is dependent on the reservoir where the agent resides and multiplies and on how it is transported from the reservoir to a susceptible human host. Such transport or transmission may be made by direct or indirect means. *Indirect transmission* is generally provided by a *vector,* which is some form of a living organism, or by a *vehicle,* which is an inanimate substance such as dust, water, or food. The malaria plasmodium, for example, lives and breeds in swamps from where it is transported by the mosquito to the human host. Airborne transmission by droplet nuclei also occurs between one infected person and another host. These particles remain suspended in air. This is a mode of transmission for influenza. *Direct transmission* is immediate transfer of an infectious agent from the reservoir, including another infected host, to an appropriate portal of entry in a susceptible host. This may involve direct contact between persons, such as kissing and sexual intercourse, or spread by droplets, as in sneezing and coughing, or direct exposure of susceptible tissues to such agents as bacterial spores lying on soil.

Portals of entry include the conjunctiva of the eye, the portal of entry for conjunctivitis; skin breaks as with hepatitis B; the gastrointestinal tract as with food poisoning, hepatitis A, or cholera; the respiratory tract as with influenza; the genitals as with venereal disease and toxic shock syndrome; and the urinary tract openings as with cystitis. These portals of entry serve also as portals of exit.

The cycle of disease transmission can be broken by eliminating the reservoir, by eliminating the means of transmission, or by eliminating both. In the case of malaria, control efforts have focused both on the elimination of the reservoir by draining swamps and other wet areas and on destroying the mosquito vector by aerial spraying with appropriate insecticides. The cycle of transmission by direct contact can be broken be eliminating the contact, as with use of condoms during sexual intercourse to prevent venereal disease. These examples represent primary prevention.

The Host

Disease can only occur in a susceptible host. Basic to the understanding of host resistance to disease is the concept of immunity. Immunity refers to the increased resistance on the part of a host to a specific infectious agent. Immunity can be humoral (antibodies in the blood) or cellular (specific to each type of cell). The role of each varies with the infectious agent and with the immune response of the host. Immunity can be passive or active. Passive immunity is attained either naturally (maternal transfer of antibodies to the fetus) or artificially by inoculation of specific protective antibodies (i.e., immune serum globulin for infectious hepatitis or diphtheria antitoxin for diphtheria prevention). Passive immunity is temporary; in the newborn it usually lasts 6 months, during which time the infant is protected only against infections experienced by the mother and for which she has made antibodies. By contrast, active immunity is long lasting and may protect an individual for life. It is attained naturally by infection, with or without clinical manifestations, or artificially by inoculation with vaccine obtained from fractions of products of the infectious agent, or from the agent itself in killed, modified, or variant form. The principle of active immunity is used in many major vaccination programs, such as those for diphtheria and polio. It was also the basis for the successful program to eradicate smallpox through an international case-finding, vaccination, and surveillance program. The dramatic change in incidence of rubella following introduction of a vaccine can be seen in Figure 5–2.

In contrast to immunity, the term *inherent resistance* refers to the ability to resist disease independently of antibodies or of specifically developed tissue response. It usually rests in anatomical or physiological characteristics of the host; it may be genetic or acquired, permanent or temporary. Factors such as general health status or nutrition may affect resistance to disease.

In the natural history cycle, the organism may or may not cause illness once it comes in contact with the human host. Assuming that a host is susceptible, infection will occur. Infection is defined as the entry and establishment of an infectious agent in a host. The minimum level of physiological reaction occurs when the agent propagates sufficiently to maintain its numbers without producing any identifiable sign of host reaction. This is termed colonization. If only subclinical infection (measurable through antibody tests but not clinically detectable) results, the host may never be identified as being infected. When clinical signs and symptoms are observed, infectious dis-

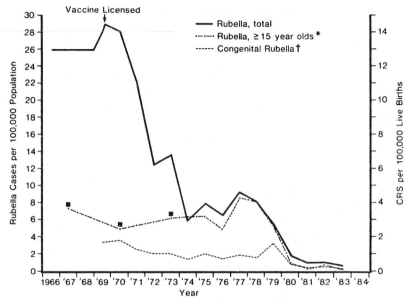

*Includes proration of unknown age cases in ≥ 15 year olds.

†Rate per 10⁵ births of confirmed and compatible cases of CRS by year of birth. Reporting for recent years is provisional, as cases may not be diagnosed until later in childhood.

■ Average annual United States estimate based on data from Illinois, Massachusetts, and New York City for the 3 year periods 1966–1968, 1969–1971, and 1972–1974. Age-specific data were not available for U.S. totals until 1975.

Figure 5–2. Incidence of reported rubella and of congenital rubella syndrome (CRS), United States, 1966–1983. *(From Annual summary 1983: Reported morbidity and mortality in the United States. Morbidity and Mortality Weekly Reports, 1984, 32(54), 49.)*

ease is present. Hosts at all three levels of infection may be capable of infecting others. As previously mentioned, the term carrier refers to infected persons without apparent clinical disease who represent a potential source of infection to others.

METHODS OF CONTROL

Because infectious diseases result from interactions among factors related to the host, the etiological agent, and the environment, methods of control are aimed at modification of these factors and their interactions. The particular factors involved vary from one disease to another. Therefore, specific interventions vary according to the epidemiology of the disease. A review of major approaches to control, however, provides a basis for planning control programs. Approaches to control of infectious disease involve the three levels of prevention discussed in Chapter 2: primary prevention, secondary prevention, and tertiary prevention. In general, measures for control of communicable disease are aimed at preventing the spread of the infectious agent from those environments that harbor it to individuals who are susceptible and who may be exposed. This can be achieved by modifying or eliminating the environment in which the infectious agent lives, thus inactivating the agents, by interfering with the means of transmission to the human host, or by increasing host immunity—all measures aimed at primary prevention. Control is facilitated by the maintainance of surveillance programs that quickly identify new cases and initiate isolation methods to prevent exposure of susceptibles or institute specific treatments to limit the period of communicability and progression of pathology (secondary prevention). Tertiary prevention plays a smaller role in infectious disease programs than in noninfectious programs because infectious diseases less often result in permanent disability. This is not to say that infectious agents never produce disability. Certainly such infectious conditions as tertiary syphilis or advanced stages of infectious endocarditis are associated with disability and require rehabilitative measures to optimize daily function.

We shall discuss control approaches within each level of prevention, then use specific diseases to illustrate an approach to control across the three levels. The presentation of a few specific examples, based on the epidemiology of a particular disease, illustrates how general approaches are applied to a particular case.

Primary Prevention

Table 5–4 lists three approaches to primary prevention of infectious diseases and the specific methods used in each of the three approaches, along with specific relevant activities. Primary prevention is aimed at intervening before the agent can become lodged in a host and begin to cause pathological changes. As shown in Table 5–4, this level of prevention seeks to keep the

TABLE 5–4. APPROACHES TO PRIMARY PREVENTION OF INFECTIOUS DISEASES

A. Breaking the chain of transmission of infection
1. Control of animals and other biological vectors of disease, e.g., arthropods, snails
2. Environmental control of air, dust, or dirt that may harbor infectious agents
3. Control of general sanitation—food, water, sewage
4. Personal measures for avoiding exposure or limiting spread of infectious diseases
   a. Good personal hygiene
   b. Proper food handling procedures
   c. Use of protective clothing or repellents to prevent insect bites
   d. Avoiding water, foods, animals, and insects likely to transmit disease
5. Use of aseptic technique in management of patients, their excretions and secretions (primary prevention for others)
6. Chemoprophylaxis before or after exposure to an infectious disease
7. Rapid case detection and specific chemotherapy to limit infectivity (secondary prevention for the patient, but primary prevention in terms of susceptibles in the environment)
8. Isolation of infectious cases and quarantine of their contacts
B. Inactivating the infectious agent
1. Use of physical methods
   a. Heat—pasteurization, adequate cooking of food, heat sterilization of infectious materials
   b. Cold—maintaining foods at low temperatures to inactivate organisms, e.g., parasites in meats, contaminants in other foods
   c. Radiation—ultraviolet light to inactivate infectious agents in air and on surfaces
2. Use of chemical methods
   a. Chlorinate water supplies and sewage affluents
   b. Disinfect infectious or potentially infectious material
C. Increasing host resistance
1. Use of immunobiologics—vaccines and toxoids for active immunization and immune globulins for passive immunization
2. Improvement in general health—proper nutrition, exercise, and so on

(Adapted from Last, J. (Ed.). *Communicable disease control in public health and preventive medicine.* New York: Appleton-Century-Crofts, 1980, p. 90.)

agent away from contact with the host by breaking the chain of transmission, by inactivating the agent, or by increasing host resistance.

The first three methods listed for breaking the chain of transmission are aimed at changing the environment. Environmental control programs such as chlorination of water supplies and sewage treatment plants that are aimed at the *reservoir* have had a major impact on the control of infectious diseases. In

Italy, Mussolini achieved the eradication of malaria in the vicinity of Rome by drying the "Marais Pontin" swamps, which were breeding the malaria parasite (Plasmodium). This was, unfortunately, done at the cost of an incredible number of lives as many of those who worked on this project soon died of malaria. Similarly, control of dust at construction sites can reduce spread of organisms whose reservoir is the dirt and whose *vehicle* is the dust.

Environmental measures to control infectious diseases may also be aimed at destroying the *vector* that transports the agent. This is the case for many viral encaphalitides that have mosquitoes as vectors. Here attempts have been made to abort urban epidemics by aerial spraying with suitable insecticide. This method, however, may disrupt the ecological balance for other living organisms; the effects of the insecticide should be specific, whenever possible, to the vector being eradicated.

The fourth method listed is a form of health promotion aimed at the human host. Encouraging "healthful behavior" to avoid potential harmful agents through good hygiene and use of protective clothing can break the chain of transmission.

Items 5 through 8 under breaking the chain of transmission, although involving cases of the disease, still constitute primary prevention because these measures are aimed at restricting the infection to the human reservoir and preventing the spread to other susceptible human hosts. Thus, although rapid case detection and early treatment may represent secondary prevention for the patient, they contribute to primary prevention for other susceptible hosts. Such control measures require surveillance programs to identify quickly new cases and to implement subsequently methods to keep infectious individuals away from susceptibles. The four methods most frequently used are isolation, quarantine, segregation, and personal surveillance.

Isolation usually refers to the separation of the infected persons during the period of communicability from others presumably uninfected. Patients with infectious diseases may be confined in isolation wards of a hospital or in the home. Table 5–5 shows the diseases for which isolation precautions are necessary. Persons who have been exposed to these patients prior to their isolation may be incubating the disease and be infectious to others although free of any signs or symptoms of illness. In the past it was common practice to quarantine those exposed individuals. *Complete quarantine* is defined as the limitation of

TABLE 5–5. CONDITIONS REQUIRING ISOLATION PRECAUTIONS[a]

Anthrax	Typhoid fever	Typhus
Dengue	*P. carinii* infection	Varicella
Diphtheria	Cholera	Viral hepatitis
Shigellosis	Neonatal diarrhea	Measles
Impetigo	Acute conjunctivitis	Mumps
Plague	Salmonellosis	Pertussis
Meningococcal	Poliomyelitis	Relapsing fever
meningitis	Rabies	Smallpox
Psittacosis	Scabies	Tuberculosis
Ringworm	Trachoma	Syphilis (primary)
Scarlet fever		

[a]The form of isolation (i.e., respiratory, stool, and so on) is determined by the epidemiology of each illness.
(From Marr, J. S. Epidemiologic considerations. In S. A. Berger (Ed.), *Clinical manual of infectious diseases.* Menlo Park, Calif.: Addison-Wesley, 1983, p. 342.)

freedom of movement of well persons exposed to a communicable disease, for a period of time no longer than the longest usual incubation period of the disease, in order to prevent direct contact with others not exposed. Complete quarantine, however, is rarely used today. More common is a *modified quarantine,* which selectively and partially limits movement of persons who may be susceptible to a disease and who are known to have been exposed. Nurses and women of childbearing age without a known history of German measles (rubella) or who do not demonstrate mandatory antibody levels would presumably be susceptible to German measles. If they have not been vaccinated and are planning a pregnancy, they should not work on pediatric wards with cases of this disease because maternal infection with rubella may cause severe damage to the fetus, particularly during the first trimester of pregnancy. In another example, individuals in contact with typhoid fever should be excluded from food handling until repeated cultures of the urine and feces have been negative for the typhoid bacillus. In some instances, immune persons have been exempted from provisions required of susceptible persons. For instance, following a case of whooping cough in a classroom, the nonimmune children may be excluded from school for 14 days after the exposure.

Segregation methods have been occasionally applied to facilitate the control of a communicable disease by the separation and observation of a group of individuals. Establishment of a sanitary boundary to protect uninfected from infected portions of a population would be an example. At times, certain areas of a city have been declared "off limits" to military personnel. In certain cases, *personal surveillance* methods may be used. This is the practice of close medical or other supervision of contacts in order to promote recognition of infection or illness but without restricting their movements. This is extremely useful in the field of venereal diseases. Sexual contacts of AIDS patients, for example, are closely monitored for symptoms of the disease. They are also discouraged from donating blood.

For susceptible persons such as hospital personnel and family members who must be exposed to infectious individuals in order to care for them, proper use of asceptic techniques in the management of the patient, secretions, and excretions can be protective. Proper management also includes appropriate disposal of contaminated materials to protect other personnel who may come in contact with these materials.

Inactivation of the agent is a second method of primary prevention. Such inactivation, whether by chemical or physical means, can be generally effective as in the use of fungicides to destroy potentially infectious agents at their sources. In other instances of intervention aimed at inactivating organisms, available methods must focus on inactivating the organism in a particular vehicle (for example, pasteurization of milk aimed at the agent for brucellosis). Although this method is effective at controlling the spread of the disease by consumption of milk, it is not an effective general control measure. Brucellosis can also be spread to handlers of infected animals such as farmers or butchers.

Primary prevention can influence inherent resistance of the host through health education programs and infant feeding programs, aimed at maximizing health status. Another approach to primary prevention aimed at the host is the immunization of susceptibles in the population. Immunization is done with vaccines obtained from fractions or products of the agent or from the agent itself in killed, modified, or variant form. *Vaccine* is a general term that applies to specific and actively immunizing agents, regardless of their origin, used against viral, rickettsial, or bacterial diseases. *Toxoids* are vaccines derived from denatured proteins that have lost their toxicity but retain much of their original antigenicity. The killed poliomyelitis virus vaccine (Salk) confers protection against the paralytic disease but not against infection; the live attenuated poliomyelitis vaccine

(Sabin) is thought to confer lifelong protection against subsequent infection by wild polio virus strains. Diphtheria toxoid, used in combination with tetanus toxoid and pertussis vaccine in a series of three intramuscular injections 4 to 6 weeks apart and DPT at 2 or 3 months of age is a routine procedure; a reinforcing or booster dose approximately one year after the third injection should be given. A list of the common vaccines used to prevent infectious disease in humans is given in Table 5–6.

TABLE 5–6. PRINCIPAL LICENSED BIOLOGICALS FOR HUMAN USE IN THE UNITED STATES, 1979

Disease	Inactivated Vaccine or Toxoid	Live Attenuated Vaccine	Immune Serum (animal)	Immune Serum Globulin (human)
Anthrax	x			
Botulism	x		x	
Cholera	x			
Diphtheria	x		x	
Hepatitis A				x
Hepatitis B				x
Influenza	x			
Measles		x		x
Meningococcal disease	x			
Mumps		x		(x)
Pertussis	x			(x)
Plague	x			
Pneumococcal disease	x			
Poliomyelitis	x	x		(x)
Rabies	x		(x)	x
Rh disease of newborns				x
Rocky Mountain spotted fever	x			
Rubella		x		
Smallpox and vaccinia		x		x
Tetanus	x		(x)	x
Tuberculosis		x		
Typhoid	x			
Typhus	x			
Varicella				(x)
Yellow fever		x		

(x) = Of limited improtance, value, application, or availability.
(From Dull, H. B. & Wehrle, P. F. Prevention of communicable diseases—general considerations. In P. F. Wehrle & F. H. Top, Sr. (Eds.), *Communicable and infectious diseases.* St. Louis: C. V. Mosby, 1981, p. 24.)

It is not necessary to achieve 100 percent immunity in the population to achieve control. A high degree of resistance by a group to invasion and spread of an infectious agent may be reached if a high proportion of individuals in the group are immune. This concept is termed herd immunity.

Secondary Prevention

Case-finding as a form of secondary prevention of an infectious disease also contributes to primary prevention. Case-finding can be done by following up on known contacts, as with sexual partners of those with venereal diseases or persons who may have eaten food prepared by someone with hepatitis. Once located, these contacts are tested for the disease and treated if disease is present. Case-finding can also occur through screening programs. Blood tests required for marriage licenses are one way of screening for venereal disease. Tuberculin testing in inner city schools is designed to detect cases of tuberculosis in a potentially high-risk population.

As a form of secondary prevention, case-finding detects the disease early so that treatment can be instituted and progression of the illness stopped. As a result of detecting and treating the disease early, spread to others in the community is limited.

Health education also plays a role in secondary prevention. Awareness of early signs and symptoms can enable an individual to seek care early. Knowledge of what behaviors contribute to spreading the disease may influence individuals with a disease to modify their behavior. Behavioral change may accomplish two things: (1) interrupt spread to other persons (primary prevention), for example, if an AIDS patient avoids sexual contact with well individuals, and (2) improve the prognosis for the sick person. Again, using AIDS as an example, the AIDS patient may prolong survival by avoiding situations, such as crowds, that are likely to expose him or her to infections.

Tertiary Prevention

As mentioned previously, residual disability is less common for diseases of infectious etiology than for those with noninfectious causal agents. Examples of infectious diseases resulting in disability can be found. Leprosy, stage-3 syphilis, impaired vision resulting from a severe conjunctivitis, hearing impairment caused by repeated or severe ear infections, and paralytic polio are illustrative of the variety of forms of disability possible. Tertiary prevention is aimed at minimizing the degree of disability and enabling the patient to live the fullest life possible within the limitations imposed by his or her illness. Medical technology, vocational rehabilitation, and physical rehabilitation are all aspects of tertiary prevention. Rehabilitation planning will be specific to the disease entity.

INVESTIGATION OF AN EPIDEMIC

The investigation of an epidemic, whether of an infectious communicable nature or not, follows basically the same process. The word *epidemic* refers to any marked upward fluctuation in disease incidence, whereas the term *endemic* implies the habitual presence of a disease or agent of disease within a given area. A third term, *pandemic* is used to describe epidemics that include large areas of the world, a worldwide epidemic.

Figure 5–3 illustrates the epidemic fluctuation of rates. The peak in January 1981 represents an epidemic as it is clearly in excess of normal rates, which fluctuate between the points marked by the upper horizontal line, representing the epidemic threshold, and the horizontal baseline of the table, representing the expected level.

The investigative process should proceed in an orderly fashion, encompassing the five basic steps discussed below, although the steps may not occur in this order depending on the particular circumstances of the outbreak. Sometimes, for example, it may be possible and desirable to institute measures to manage the epidemic and reduce the spread before results of hypothesis testing are obtained. These measures would be based on general principles of disease control and the best information available as to the probable source of infection.

Verification of the Diagnosis and Confirmation of an Epidemic. A standard definition of a case is needed. The criteria used to define a case can strongly affect rates. Further, inclusion of non-cases in a set of cases for study of an epidemic increases the difficulties in delineating a cause. Thus, while clinical

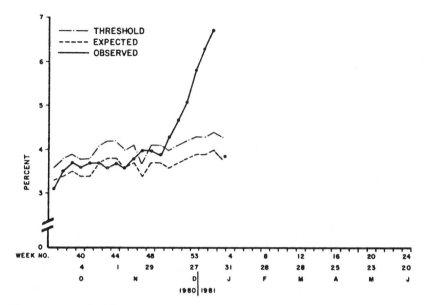

*Forecasts are made at 4-week intervals.

Figure 5–3. Observed and expected ratio of deaths attributed to pneumonia and influenza in 121 United States cities, 1980–1981. Forecasts are made at 4-week intervals. *(From Influenza.* Morbidity and Mortality Weekly Reports, 1981, 30(2), 22–24.)

knowledge and experience are necessary to make a diagnosis of an infectious disease, requiring laboratory evidence to confirm it is more precise. Rates based only on clinical diagnosis and those based on laboratory confirmation can be quite discrepant.

To establish the true epidemic nature of the disease, it is essential to have some estimates of previous incidence rates (preferably based on the same case criteria) in order to identify an apparent epidemic that is in fact due to better reporting of an endemic situation. The availability of a new treatment, for instance, may attract a large number of patients whose disease had not previously been reported.

An *epidemic or attack curve* is essentially an incidence curve on which the number of diseased persons in the population is plotted by time of onset of disease. The existence of an epidemic depends on the presence of a communicable agent and on the availability of susceptible individuals to be infected by the agent. Figure 5–4 illustrates the situation of a common source epidemic, also called a point source epidemic. This type of epidemic is characterized by the simultaneous exposure of a large number of susceptibles to a common infectious agent. Because nearly all the susceptibles have been infected at the same time, the epidemic terminates when the supply of susceptible persons is exhausted. The explosive increase in the number of cases of a disease over a short period of time, usually only hours, is characteristic of an epidemic of food poisoning originating from a single event, such as a church supper. Some epidemics related to a common source show a more scattered pattern of new cases. This occurs when the common source is a contaminated product that is widely distributed and consumed at different times by individuals or small groups. The 1985 epidemic of listeriosis caused by contaminated Mexican style cheese was of this type (MMWR, 1985).

Figure 5–5 illustrates a situation in which only a few susceptible individuals are initially infected. After an incubation period, however, these infected individuals are the source for secondary cases. A stepwise progression in the number of dis-

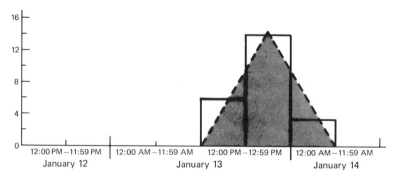

Figure 5–4. Example of an epidemic curve based on a point source epidemic. Graph based on approximate distribution of illness onset for an outbreak of illness due to Clostridium perfringens associated with a "Meals on Wheels" program for senior citizens in Victorville, California. Twenty-three persons who had meals delivered between 11 AM and 12:30 PM on January 13 became ill. The mean incubation period was 8.7 hours, with a range of 1–16 hours. The curve shows the abrupt rise in incidence with an equally abrupt dropoff, all within a matter of hours. *(From* Morbidity and Mortality Weekly Reports.)

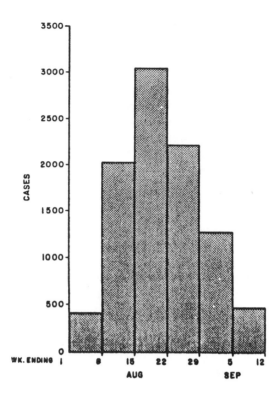

Figure 5–5. Example of an epidemic curve in a propagated epidemic. Persons with conjunctivitis reporting to government clinics, by week, in Belize, August 1–September 12, 1981, produce the typical stepped pattern seen in outbreaks where the disease is spread person to person. In this particular outbreak, the illness was thought to be introduced by a fisherman in a small fishing village in late July. The illness was spread primarily by hand–eye contact. The incidence of new cases in each district of the city peaked approximately 3 weeks after the first case was identified and new cases continued to be seen for one month. *(From Conjunctivitis in Central America.* Morbidity and Mortality Weekly Reports, 30*(39), 497–499.)*

eased persons is to be expected as persons exposed to each new group of infected individuals develop symptoms after an incubation period. The epidemic would continue as long as any susceptibles remained, especially if additional susceptible individuals were brought into the epidemic area. The dropoff in rates also is stepwise. This type of epidemic is called a *propagated epidemic.*

Identification of Affected Persons and Their Characteristics. Each case of the disease has to be identified in order to obtain a complete picture of the epidemic. In addition to the usual information about name, age, sex, occupation, place of residence, recent movements, symptoms of the disease, and time of onset, the epidemiological history-taking is concerned with the circumstances related to the illness and is guided by what is suspected as the cause (what has been eaten, in the case of suspected food poisoning). Also important is the individual's history of infectious diseases, immunization, recent travel, and associations with sick people and animals.

The search for additional cases of the disease helps complete the disease picture. Large scale serological surveys have been carried out on populations that have subsequently experienced epidemics of infectious diseases. A similar postepidemic serological survey would indicate the percentage of the population infected by the epidemic agent and who developed serum antibodies. If careful record of clinical illness was taken during the epidemic, results of such surveys provide useful data on the frequency of inapparent or asymptomatic disease. In addition to serological testing, which may be useful for the identification of asymptomatic cases, the epidemiologist attempts to identify environmental changes that set the stage for the epidemic.

Formulation and Testing of a Hypothesis. The descriptive characteristics of the population should make it possible to pinpoint a common experience shared only by the patients and also to obtain age and sex-specific incidence rates by knowing the total population at risk. Disease incidence is compared for persons exposed to the hypothesized cause and those not exposed. It might be instructive to study those individuals seemingly exposed but unaffected and compare their characteristics with those of the exposed and affected group. Statistical tests are helpful in evaluating the postulated source. All links in the infectious process should be included in the hypothesis: the agent, the reservoir, the mode of transmission to the human host, the mode of entry in the host, and host susceptibility to infection. In instances where the total population (or a representative sample) of exposed and unexposed individuals cannot be obtained, a case control approach must be used, comparing the ill population with well persons (controls) in regard to exposure to the hypothesized source.

Management of an Epidemic. In addition to the treatment of patients, control measures to reduce the spread of the epidemic (isolation measures) or to prevent its recurrence (improvement in the environment and vaccination of the population) are important. The success or failure of control measures may be helpful in confirming or refuting the hypothesis on which these measures were based. Health education leading to appropriate legislation is a long-range measure of great importance.

Continued surveillance and monitoring of infection, which can now be carried out, have been useful in defining thresholds, predicting outbreaks, and providing strategic information for health programs and economic deployment of resources. Surveillance requires data on:

Infective persons or sources
Susceptible persons at risk
Effective contact rate between susceptible persons and
    infective persons or sources
Time period of effective contact
Persons removed by isolation, immunity, or death
Removal rate

Surveillance systems have been useful in monitoring hospital infections as well as community-wide infections. Existing surveillance systems are discussed in Chapter 12.

Even when a disease has been virtually eradicated in one country, measures must be taken to prevent its entry from another region where it may be endemic. All links of the chain of transmission of a disease must be kept under scrutiny in order to maintain surveillance of a disease. WHO provides guidelines for surveillance of diseases that are likely to spread through international travel. Individual countries set up requirements for immunization and inspection of goods coming from endemic or epidemic areas of the world. In addition to the reporting of cases, which was discussed earlier, surveillance of diseases can utilize additional sources of information such as death certificates and data from public health laboratories, entomological and veterinary services, and estimates of the immune status of a young population based on the amount of DPT (diphtheria, pertussis, tetanus) vaccine used in relation to number of births. Infectious disease surveillance systems should also be designed for early identification of new problems. The emergence during the past ten years of Legionellosis, toxic shock syndrome, and AIDS serves as a reminder of the importance of surveillance systems.

REFERENCES

Barnes, A. M., & Poland, J. Plague in the United States, 1983. *Centers for Disease Control Surveillance Summaries, 1984*, 1985, *33*(155), 155–2155.

Benenson, A. (Ed.). *Control of communicable diseases in man.* Washington, D.C.: American Public Health Association, 1980.

Fox, J., Hall, C., & Elveback, L. *Epidemiology: Man and disease.* Toronto, Ontario: Collier-MacMillan Canada Ltd., 1970.

MMWR. Listeriosis Outbreak Associated with Mexican Style Cheese—California. *Morbidity and Mortality Weekly Reports, 34*(24), 357–359, 1985.

6

Epidemiology and Control of Diseases of Noninfectious Etiology

The major causes of death, serious illness, and disabilities in the United States today are chronic diseases of noninfectious etiology and violence. Chronic diseases of the heart, cancer, and stroke alone accounted for 68 percent of deaths in 1981. Accidents, suicide, and homicide accounted for another 7 percent. Table 6–1 shows rates for the ten major causes of death by age group. Although rates of these major killers are the highest among older age groups, these diseases represent a major proportion of deaths at younger ages as well. Calculation of "potential years of life lost" is one method of measuring the loss to society resulting from death at young or early ages. It has been estimated that three categories of deaths represent nearly 70 percent of potential years of life lost in the United States—diseases of the circulatory system, cancer, and accidents and violence. Figure 6–1 shows the percent contributions of various diseases to total years of life lost in 1982 to 1983. Diseases of the circulatory system and musculoskeletal system account for 38 percent of conditions causing limitation of activity (Somers, 1980).

These major health problems are not caused by infectious agents. Although the natural history differs for each, these dis-

TABLE 6-1. MORTALITY FOR TEN LEADING CAUSES OF DEATH BY AGE, UNITED STATES, 1981

	All Ages	1–14 Years	15–34 Years	35–54 Years	55–74 Years	75 + Years
All causes[a]	1,977,981	18,124	96,362	187,771	754,657	877,148
Heart diseases	753,884	1,424	4,336	51,467	292,566	403,945
Cancer	422,094	2,141	7,437	52,630	224,916	134,918
Cerebrovascular	163,504	258	1,383	7,831	46,598	107,406
Accidents	100,704	8,996	41,078	17,918	17,492	15,104
COPD	58,832	201	362	2,686	30,575	25,001
Influenza and pneumonia	53,731	1,210	898	2,541	12,382	36,686
Diabetes	34,642	46	703	33,083	15,461	15,341
Cirrhosis	29,308	54	1,291	9,619	15,368	3,214
Suicide	27,596	167	11,504	7,836	6,163	1,904
Homicide	23,646	1,023	12,508	6,514	2,222	791

[a]Where numbers do not add across, there are some deaths missing because age was unknown.
(Excerpted from NCHS. Advance report of final mortality statistics, 1981. Monthly Vital Statistics Report, 1984, 33,(3, Suppl.).)

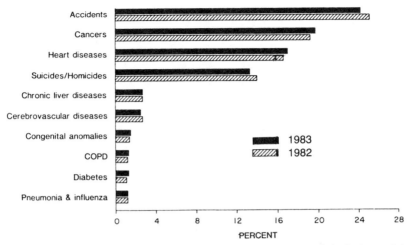

*These percentages of each year's total YPLL are calculated from age- and cause-specific death rates reported by the National Center for Health Statistics (*Monthly Vital Statistics Report*. vol. 32, no. 13, September 21, 1984, pp. 17–8) and population estimates from the Bureau of the Census.

Figure 6–1. Percent contribution to total years of potential life lost, by cause and year—United States, 1982 and 1983. *(From Changes in premature mortality—United States, 1982–1983.* Morbidity and Mortality Weekly Reports, *1985, 34 (2), 17.)*

eases as a group share certain commonalities of natural history not shared by diseases of infectious origin. Because we are using the natural history of disease as the basis for our discussion of disease control, we have chosen to classify all diseases as infectious or noninfectious. Although this approach is simplistic, we feel that it facilitates conceptualization of natural history and control issues, as well as approaches to research. It is necessary to recognize, however, that diseases classified here as noninfectious include acute and chronic conditions, physical and mental diseases, and conditions caused by numerous types of agents including physical, chemical, nutrient, and psychological, or a combination of these. In order to minimize the complexity of discussion, this chapter has been organized as follows: (1) major contrasts in the natural history of these diseases compared with those caused by infectious agents (2) methodological issues in the study of noninfectious etiology, (3) major categories of etiological agents, and (4) approaches to control of these diseases.

NATURAL HISTORY

As with infectious diseases, the natural history of chronic diseases involves interaction of host, agent, and environment. One can also view the progression of these diseases using the stages presented under our discussion of infectious disease: susceptibility, presymptomatic disease, and clinical disease. But although the framework for understanding the natural history applies to both infectious and noninfectious etiological agents, there are important differences. These are listed in Table 6–2 and discussed below.

One important difference is the absence of a single necessary agent. Infectious diseases cannot occur without exposure to the single infectious agent necessary to cause the disease. Although there may be additional agents or circumstances whose presence or absence increases or decreases the likelihood of acute infection, they are not necessary for the disease to occur. When diseases are caused by noninfectious agents, there is rarely, if ever, a single necessary agent. This is a function, in part, of the system used for disease classification. Although many infectious diseases are classified in terms of the causal agent, e.g., tuberculosis after the tubercule bacillus, most diseases caused by noninfectious agents are classified on the basis of manifestations rather than on the basis of etiology. Cardio-

TABLE 6–2. DIFFERENCES IN NATURAL HISTORY FOR INFECTIOUS AND NONINFECTIOUS DISEASES

Infectious Disease	Noninfectious Disease
Single necessary agent	No single necessary agent
Agent–disease specificity	Seldom agent–disease specificity
Causes are known	Causes unknown, intervention often based on risk factors
Short incubation period	Long latency period
Single exposure usually sufficient	May require multiple exposure to same or multiple agents
Usually produce acute disease	Most often produce chronic disease
Acquired immunity possible	Acquired immunity unlikely
Diagnosis based on tests specific to disease agent	Diagnosis often dependent on nonspecific symptoms or tests

vascular disease, renal disease, and neoplasm are all manifestation-based classifications. Numerous agents may lead to similar manifestations. Fire, chemicals, and the sun can all produce burns. Different chemical agents may produce cancer at the same site. Any of several combinations of life-style factors seem to produce the manifestations we call cardiovascular disease. But, in diseases of infectious etiology, even those classified by manifestation have a single necessary agent, e.g., rheumatic heart disease is caused by the staphylococcus.

A related difference between infectious and noninfectious diseases is that the known "causes" of noninfectious diseases are often really risk factors representing physiological states known to increase the individual's risk for developing the disease. As such, they represent physiological changes that have already begun. For example, obesity, elevated cholesterol levels, and hypertension are risk factors for coronary heart disease. These physiological states often involve cellular changes that are steps in the development of disease. Although some reversal of damage may occur with treatment, some residual is likely to remain

Another difference is the length of time required between initial exposure to causal agents and onset of detectible physiological signs and symptoms (latency period for noninfectious diseases; incubation period for infectious diseases). With most infectious agents, signs and symptoms of the related disease become evident in days or weeks, or at most a few months. In the case of most noninfectious agents, it will be years or decades before illness is apparent. The reason for the short time required by infectious agents is that, if the human host is not immune, then the agents are able to multiply rapidly until their number is sufficient to produce disease. Because the agents in conditions of noninfectious etiology are not living organisms, there is no multiplication. Therefore, multiple low-dose exposures may be required to cause illness; this is the case with certain chemicals. In other instances, such as asbestosis, only a single exposure is thought to be necessary, but the mechanism of physiological response seems to take as many as 40 years before damage to the lung is sufficient to produce signs and symptoms. In still other instances, such as cancers, it is suspected that the causal mechanism may require exposure to at least two agents that produce damage to the genetic material of cells. A final situation is exhibited by conditions such as cardiovascular or cerebrovascular diseases; these seem to evolve subsequent to chronic conditions or states of high risk such as obesity, smoking, diabetes, and high blood cholesterol.

Exceptions to the long latency periods of diseases of noninfectious etiology do occur, for example, in chemical agents that cause acute episodes of poisoning. Awareness of the probable latency period for a particular condition is important both in planning etiological investigations and in planning control measures, as we shall see later.

Another difference between diseases of infectious and noninfectious etiology is that more often than not, diseases of noninfectious or unknown etiology are chronic in nature. The term chronic disease is used in the sense defined by the 1957 Commission on Chronic Illness—all impairments or deviations from normal that have one or more of the following characteristics: is permanent, leaves residual disability, is caused by nonreversible pathological alterations, requires special training of the patient for rehabilitation, or may be expected to require long periods of supervision, observation, or care.

The high frequency with which chronicity is observed in those diseases of noninfectious etiology is probably a function of the long latency period characteristic of these conditions. When a disease process is proceeding slowly over time, the body is likely to make adaptive responses that will, in turn, contribute to the overall ability of the physiology to respond to stresses. These adaptive responses, although facilitating short-term function, may be detrimental over the long term. The residual disability of these diseases requires ongoing medical treatment and rehabilitation programs. For example, patients with cardiovascular disease are likely to require indefinite ongoing supervision of prescribed medications such as digitalis, control of diet, and modification of life-style.

In contrast, with diseases of infectious etiology the short incubation period required for multiplication and establishment of the infectious agent leaves little time for adaptive response, and an acute illness, often of rather abrupt onset ensues. Physiological response to the infection is agent specific; antibodies against the particular agent are produced and this immune response, when combined with drug treatment to aid in killing the organism, usually results in recovery. The patient may be ill for a period ranging from a few days to several months and recover without residual disability, or if the illness is severe or the patient is debilitated, he or she may die from the illness. Death is most frequently seen with debilitated or immune-compromised patients such as those found in hospital settings. Patients who recover rarely require long-term follow-up, except for diseases such as hepatitis that may have residual disability. As previously pointed out, there are infectious illnesses with chronic stages. These result either from residual damage, as with rheumatic heart disease, or from inactive stages of an organism that has survived the immune response of the host, as with the herpes simplex virus that produces shingles, and the syphilis organism that, if unrecognized and untreated with antibiotics, goes on to attack the neurological system.

Some noninfectious agents can produce both acute and chronic disease. Beryllium serves as an example. Beryllium may cause chronic disease characterised by granulomatosis lesions of the lung and enlarged lymph nodes in conjunction with the lesions. The chronic disease develops, in most cases, without being preceded by an acute phase. Beryllium can also produce acute episodes characterized by a pneumonia-like process that includes fever, chills, cough, sputum production, and shortness of breath with transient inflammation of the upper air passages and upper bronchi. The acute episodes can last up to 3 months and may cause death. It has been estimated that around 6 percent of acute cases will develop a chronic condition. The chronic condition is symptomatically characterized by a progressive shortness of breath, cough, slight sputum production, weight loss, occasional nausea, and low grade fever. Shortness of breath may be the sole symptom. Other cases are characterized by a rapidly progressive disease causing emaciation and death within moths. Some individuals with massive prolonged exposure show no clinical or radiographical evidence of any disease. The relationship between exposure and the natural history of beryllium lung disease is not well understood (Preuss, 1975; Waldbott, 1978).

Synergistic effects of two or more agents are frequently seen in causation models of noninfectious agents. In a recent example, workers in a grocery store in Ohio experienced an outbreak of phytophotodermatitis (MMWR, 1985). All cases occurred among cashiers, baggers, and produce clerks. None occurred among shelf-stockers, delicatessen clerks, meat clerks, or managers. Development of the rash was traced to contact with fresh vegetables and flowers, which contain psoralens. Risk of developing phytophotodermatitis, however, increased substantially among workers who used tanning salons. Risk of developing the rash was 4.2 times greater for exposure both to psoralen and ultraviolet light (tanning salons) than psoralen alone (Fig. 6–2).

In another example of synergism, non-smoking workers exposed to asbestos have been reported to have a risk of developing lung cancer eight times that of nonsmoking, nonexposed individuals. However, smokers who are exposed to asbestos have 90 times the risk of the nonsmoking, nonexposed individuals (Selikoff, Hammond, and Chung, 1968). This is of concern because control efforts often must settle for minimizing rather than eliminating the workplace exposures. The synergistic effect of other exposures could still incur substantial risk even with low level exposures.

The concepts of initiation and promotion are relevant. It is thought that one agent may initiate the process of cancer development and that numerous other agents, called promoters, can play the role of speeding up the process. It was hoped that if exposures to harmful environmental agents could be kept low, then the latency period before onset of symptoms would be so long that the average individual would not have problems until old age. This expectation was based on accumulating evidence that higher doses contribute both to increased disease risk and to length of the latency period (Seidman, Selikoff, and Hammond, 1979). The presence of synergism, however, may shorten latency periods and produce illness in the prime of life even with

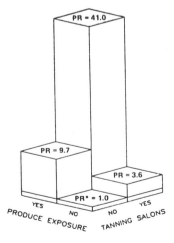

Figure 6–2. Risk of rash among grocery workers, by exposure to fresh produce and use of tanning salons: Ohio, April–August 1984. *(From Phytophotodermatitis in Ohio.* Morbidity and Mortality Weekly Reports, *1985, 34 (1), 13.)*

low level exposure. Additional research is needed to clarify these issues. In the meantime, lawmakers, planners of control programs, economists who consider the cost–benefit effects of control efforts, and many others concerned with the health of the public are forced to make decisions based on present levels of knowledge.

Methodological Issues in the Study of Diseases of Noninfectious Etiology

The natural history characteristics of diseases must be considered in the design of studies investigating etiology. The lack of a single necessary agent causing a disease makes it more difficult to isolate the effect of any individual factor. Synergistic effects of other agents and effects of known causes of a disease must be controlled. The long latency period between exposure and onset of disease increases the difficulties associated with obtaining information on exposure in retrospective study designs or in tracking exposed populations to assess disease incidence in prospective study designs. The chronic nature of many of these diseases, together with their relatively lower frequency of occurrence, means that often prevalence cases are studied rather than incidence cases. This produces a wide spectrum of stages in the natural history among the cases. Because factors may have independent effects and converse effects on the process of disease development, disease progression, and survival, interpretations of causality for prevalence may be difficult.

Also, identifying a case of disease of noninfectious etiology is more difficult than is defining a case of infectious disease. In the case of infectious diseases, definitive identification of a case is possible by obtaining a sample of the appropriate body fluid or secretion and growing the organism in a laboratory culture. If the criteria for case status demands a positive culture or a transformation to a positive antibody status, then separation of cases from noncases is possible with a high degree of validity. For most diseases of noninfectious etiology, definition of case status may depend on presence or absence of a cluster of symptoms with or without positive values on specified laboratory tests. Differentiation of specific diagnoses within a broad disease classification may be difficult, e.g., differentiating specific diagnosis, such as emphysema and asthma, within the broader category of chronic obstructive lung diseases. Particularly for research using medical records, the need to rely on stated diagnoses may be problematic because criteria for arriving at the recorded diagnosis may vary by institution or physician. Studies have demonstrated a lack of agreement among multiple psychiatrists making different psychiatric diagnoses based on the same information for patients with similar symptoms who differ by race, sex, or socioeconomic status. (Gross, et al., 1969; Haase, 1964). Similar, though probably less severe problems could be expected for different subcategories of cardiovascular and other noninfectious disease. Cutoffs for labeling blood pressure levels as hypertension or abnormal blood sugar values as diabetes vary from clinician to clinician and may vary over time as better data on the predictive valididty of various test levels indicating progression of clinical disease becomes available. These issues are discussed further in Chapters 11, 14, and 15. The importance of setting clear criteria for valid classification of cases versus noncases in studies of noninfectious diseases cannot be overemphasized.

The ability to accurately measure exposure is an important methodological consideration in the study of diseases of noninfectious etiology. Although investigations of infectious diseases require demonstration of exposure to a source of the infectious agent, quantity of the infectious agent is less of an issue than other agent qualities such as virulence or pathogenicity. In the case of noninfectious agents, whether life-style related agents like cigarette smoke or fat content of the diet, or occupational/ environmental agents like benzene, lead, or pesticides, the amount or level of exposure is important.

A single agent can produce acute illness with high dose exposures or can produce chronic illness with chronic low dose exposure. One does not lead to the other. The acute illness associated with lead intoxication is not an early stage of the disease associated with long-term low level chronic lead exposure.

Determination of dose of exposure is problematic. It must be decided whether dose is a function of the nature of the metabolite of the agent, enzymatic alteration, or level of the original xenobiotic agent. Should environmental levels be used as a measure of exposure or should levels in the body be used? If the latter, what is the appropriate place to measure the dose— plasma levels, brain concentration, kidney, some other organ? For agents with long tissue residence, biological measures reflecting cumulative burdens may be more appropriate.

An undifferentiated, broad range of exposures among an exposed population may make it more difficult to study effects because the exposed group may be diluted by the presence of substantial numbers of individuals with relatively low levels of exposure to the agent. Furthermore, precise identification of exposure levels enables the investigator to evaluate at what level of exposure hazard to health begins, an important piece of information in planning control measures. Demonstration of a dose–effect, i.e., increases in disease frequency associated with increasing levels of exposure, helps to establish a causal role for the agent.

Another important aspect of measuring exposure is the constancy of the exposure. Frequency or likelihood of effects may differ in constant exposure and intermittent exposure. For example, in our own work investigating health effects associated with the occupational exposure of nurses to antineoplastic drugs, this becomes a crucial factor. Although some antineoplastic drugs reach peak rates of excretion within 6 hours, others peak closer to 24 hours. A nurse who handles large amounts of these drugs only twice a week, on Monday and Thursday, has ample time between handling sessions to eliminate the drugs from his or her body. A nurse who handles a moderate amount of the drugs daily may never achieve total clearance of the drugs, thus experiencing a constant exposure. The constant exposure is more likely to be associated with effects than is the intermittent exposure even if the total dosage of exposure were the same.

It is not the intent of this text to discuss in depth such methodological issues related to epidemiological research. For those interested in designing epidemiological studies these issues are covered extensively in methodological texts (Kleinbaum, et al., 1982; Susser, 1973; Monson, 1980; Schlesselman, 1982). However, it has been the author's intent to raise issues that should be kept in mind when reading the epidemiological literature so that the reader can evaluate whether a study has addressed the important issues relevant to the particular study. The specific natural history characteristics discussed in this chapter for diseases of noninfectious etiology should be addressed.

Clinicians are often put on the spot by patients who have read a report of a medical study in the newspaper or in another lay publication. The questions usually relate to some agent that has been shown to "cause" a particular disease. The proliferation of such reports in the lay press puts considerable pressure on health professionals to keep up with their reading of the literature so that they can respond appropriately to requests for advice regarding the personal implications of such study reports. A dilemma arises, however, for many clinicians attempting to read the epidemiological literature because contradictory findings are often reported. It is probably useful to keep in mind, first of all, that there is a bias in favor of publication of studies with positive findings. Particularly if it is the first study to come along testing a particular hypothesis, editors are likely to find positive findings more interesting and are therefore more likely to publish such findings. Once positive findings have been published, negative findings on subsequent studies stand a greater chance of being published. As the literature develops with regard to a particular hypothesis, a variety of findings may therefore result. This is particularly true for studies of noninfectious causal agents. Some criteria for making inferences about causality are required.

For infectious agents, determining cause has been possible for many years, since Robert Koch (1843–1910) introduced his five postulates for demonstrating a causal relationship. These postualtes require that the organism be found in *all* cases of disease (possible because it is a single *necessary* agent); be isolated from patients and grown in pure culture; reproduce the disease when the pure culture is inoculated into a susceptible animal; be recoverable from the diseased animal; not be present as a nonpathogenic organism when the disease is not present. In general, these postulates have stood the test of time; carrier states are now known to exist, invalidating postulate number 5. Viruses cannot be grown on lifeless culture media, but require living cells. In addition, more recent technology had led to the identification of disease specific antibodies that can provide immunological proof of presence of an infection and case status.

Causality in disease of noninfectious etiology must rely more heavily on strictly epidemiological evidence. Epidemiological evidence requires well designed studies to demonstrate that the incidence of a disease is higher among those exposed than those not exposed (prospective studies) or that exposure to the putative causes should be present more commonly among those with the disease than among those without (case-control studies). Elimination or reduction of the putative cause should decrease the incidence of disease. The cumulative body of studies available must be reviewed as an entirety. After eliminating from consideration those studies in which the findings could be predicted a priori by the presence of biases in the design, the remaining study findings can be evaluated using the criteria discussed in Chapter 2—temporal correctness, consistency of findings, specificity of the relationship, strength of the relationships demonstrated (including dose–effect), and biological plausibility—to determine the level of evidence supporting an etiological role for the factor.

Major Categories of Etiological Agents

Noninfectious disease agents include physical, chemical, nutrient, genetic, and psychological agents. For purposes of the discussion to follow, these agents are considered as they relate to two specific areas of focus: (1) occupational health and (2) general environmental health. Discussion of life-style factors as disease agents is integrated in Chapters 7 through 10.

Occupational Health. Many human diseases can be traced to exposures associated with the work environment. A list of the leading work-related diseases and injuries is shown in Table 6–3. Control of work-related exposures that pose hazards to worker health is a major potential target for primary prevention. Epidemiological investigations play an important role in identifying chemicals, metals, or other substances associated with adverse health outcomes and in confirming as hazards to human health any substances initially implicated by animal studies. The cumulative body of evidence from laboratory and epidemiological studies provides a basis for control and regulatory decisions.

Chemicals are prime agents affecting the health of the working population. Each year thousands of new chemicals are developed. Many of these are potential mutagens, teratogens, or carcinogens. Chemicals can also cause respiratory inflammation, dermatitis, asthma, neurotoxicity, liver toxicity, and a variety of other adverse effects on human health. The World Health Organization's International Agency for Research on Cancer, which routinely evaluates evidence for carcinogenicity of chemicals, has identified 400 compounds as carcinogenic. A review of these results by Tomatis et al. (1978) identified 26

TABLE 6–3. THE 10 LEADING WORK-RELATED DISEASES AND INJURIES—UNITED STATES, 1982[a]

1. Occupational lung diseases: asbestosis, byssinosis, silicosis, coal workers' pneumoconiosis, lung cancer, occupational asthma
2. Musculoskeletal injuries: disorders of the back, trunk, upper extremity, neck, lower extremity; traumatically induced Raynaud's phenomenon
3. Occupational cancers (other than lung): leukemia; mesothelioma; cancers of the bladder, nose, and liver
4. Severe occupational traumatic injuries: amputations, fractures, eye loss, lacerations, and traumatic deaths
5. Cardiovascular diseases: hypertension, coronary artery disease, acute myocardial infarction
6. Disorders of reproduction: infertility, spontaneous abortion, teratogenesis
7. Neurotoxic disorders: peripheral neuropathy, toxic encephalitis, psychoses, extreme personality changes (exposure-related)
8. Noise-induced loss of hearing
9. Dermatologic conditions: dermatoses, burns (scaldings), chemical burns, contusions (abrasions)
10. Psychologic disorders: neuroses, personality disorders, alcoholism, drug dependency

[a]The conditions listed under each category are to be viewed as *selected examples*, not comprehensive definitions of the category.
(From Leading work-related diseases and injuries. *Morbidity and Mortality Weekly Reports, 34* (16), 219.)

chemicals having strong evidence of carcinogenicity in humans (Table 6–4).

Metals and naturally occurring minerals are a group of occupational agents. Mineral dusts and fibers, such as silica and asbestos, are physical agents that produce occupational disease. Silicosis and asbestosis are both respiratory conditions, each common to particular groups of exposed workers. Groups such as miners, quarry workers, tunnel drillers, excavators, and stonemasons experience a high incidence of silicosis. Asbestosis has been associated with workers in asbestos mines or processing plants, shipyard workers, construction workers, and auto repair workers. Lead, nickel, mercury, arsenic, beryllium, and tin are among the many metals associated with occupational diseases. Risk from these occupational exposures may extend beyond the work force at the particular exposure site. Asbestos dust carried home on the clothing of workers, for example, has been associated with asbestosis and mesothelioma among family members in the household of asbestos workers.

TABLE 6–4. CHEMICALS FOR WHICH EVIDENCE OF CARCINOGENICITY TO HUMANS EXISTS, TYPE OF EXPOSURE, AND TARGET ORGAN

| Chemical | Main Type of Exposure | | | Target Organs |
	Environmental	Occupational	Medical	
Aflatoxins	x	x		Liver
4-aminobi-phenyl		x		Bladder
Arsenic compounds	x	x	x	Skin, lung, liver
Asbestos		x		Lung, pleural cavity, GI track
Auramine (manu-facturing)		x		Bladder
Benzene		x		Hemopoietic system
Benzidine		x		Bladder
Bis (chloro-methyl) ether		x		Lung
Cadmium Oxide		x		Prostate, lung
Chloram-phenicol[a]			x	Hemopoietic
Chloro-methyl methyl ether		x		Lung
Chromium (Chromate-producing industries)		x		Lung, nasal cavities
Cyclophos-phamide			x	Bladder
Diethylstil-besterol			x	Uterus, vagina
Haematite (mining)		x		Lung
Isopropyl oil		x		Nasal cavity, larynx
Melphalan			x	Hemopoietic
Mustard gas		x		Lung, larynx
2-naphthyl-amine		x		Bladder
Nickel (nickel refining)		x		Nasal cavity, lung
N, N-bis(2-chloro-ethyl)-2-naphthyl-amine			x	Bladder

(continued)

TABLE 6–4. *(cont.)* CHEMICALS FOR WHICH EVIDENCE OF CARCINOGENICITY TO HUMANS EXISTS, TYPE OF EXPOSURE, AND TARGET ORGAN

| Chemical | Main Type of Exposure | | | Target Organs |
	Environmental	*Occupational*	*Medical*	
Oxymethal-one[a]			x	Liver
Phenacetin			x	Kidney
Phenytoin			x	Lymphoreticular tissues
Soot, tar, and oils (PAHs)	x	x		Lung, skin (scrotum)
Vinyl chloride		x		Liver, lung[a], brain[a]

[a]indicates strong suspicion
(Adapted from Tomatis, L. et al. Evaluation of the carcinogenicity of chemicals: a review of the monograph program of the International Agency for Research on Cancer (1971 to 1977). *Cancer Research*, 1978, *38* (4), 879–880.)

Four occupational exposures have potential impact on cardiovascular health: (1) metals, dusts, and trace elements, (2) occupational inhalants and other chemical exposures, (3) noise, and (4) psychosocial stress. Congestive heart failure resulting from restrictive lung disease (cor pulmonale) has been observed in occupational respiratory diseases such as silicosis and chronic beryllium disease. Other metals such as antimony, cobalt, and lead have also been implicated. Carbon monoxide may precipitate acute cardiovascular events, for example, changes in cardiac rhythm, in persons with preexisting coronary artery disease. Carbon disulfide, a common solvent, increases the risk of cardiovascular disorders, including coronary artery disease and hypertension. Other solvents, halogenated hydrocarbons, have precipitated sudden death, likely due to cardiac arrythmias, in workers exposed to high levels. Some of these solvents have been associated with arrhythmias at or below concentrations permitted by current occupational standards. Workers exposed to nitroglycerine and nitrates during manufacture of explosives experienced a "rebound vasospasm" effect with an increased risk of cardiac chest pain, myocardial infarction, and sudden death following withdrawal from exposure (MMWR, 1985).

Single exposures to noise leads to transient increases in blood pressure. Chronic occupational exposure to noise has been associated with sustained increases in blood pressure. Increases in serum cholesterol and changes in circulating hormones have also been observed in association with exposure of humans to noise. Evidence suggests that psychological stress in the work setting is related to cardiovascular disease, particularly hypertension. Work-overload, role conflicts, limited autonomy, non-supportive supervisors, and lack of job mobility have predicted cardiovascular disease risk in several studies (MMWR, 1985).

Agent factors to be considered in investigating occupational exposures include size and shape of particles (e.g., asbestos dust), route of exposure (e.g., lead by oral ingestion versus respiratory inhalation), and whether the substance is in free or compound form, organic or inorganic form, and liquid or vapor form.

Environmental factors pertinent to investigations of occupational disease include the conditions present in the work environment that influence the likelihood that workers will come in contact with an agent, for example, engineering containment measures, general cleanliness and ventilation of the work area, lighting of the work area, and temperature of the work area, which may affect volatility of certain chemicals and thus influence respiratory dose. Excessive temperature may, in itself be an agent. Male workers exposed to high temperatures on the job, for example, may experience infertility as a result of sperm mortality. The social and psychological aspects of the work environment may also play a role. Scheduled breaks, positioning of work stations for physical comfort of the worker, and the opportunity for conversation with co-workers may be related to morale and fatigue levels that are factors in ocupational accidents.

Host factors to be considered in occupational studies include life-style behaviors that may increase risk of disease from occupational exposure to an agent. Smoking is one such major factor that seems to have a synergistic effect on many exposures, leading, for example, to an enormous increase in risk for a variety of respiratory conditions when compounded by exposure to other agents that cause respiratory diseases. The increase in lung cancer for workers exposed both to asbestos and tobacco smoke was previously discussed. Smoking together with carbon monoxide exposure led to an incremental increase in the prevalence of angina pectoris among Finnish foundry workers (MMWR, 1985). Alcohol use, quality of personal relationships, sleeping patterns, eating patterns (e.g., eating on the job while handling hazardous chemicals), and diet can all affect risk for various occupational diseases or injuries. Genetic constitution may also affect susceptibility to a given occupational exposure.

Environmental Health. The field of environmental health encompasses exposures in the community or residential environment. Many of the same substances encountered in occupational settings may be present in the general community environment because of contamination of air, water, and soil by industrial activities or inadequate methods of waste disposal. Exposure to these substances is, in general, at a lower dose than is exposure to similar substances in occupational environments. Exceptions may occur near particular landfill or dump sites in which large quantities of waste substances have been disposed.

Other products produced by industry are distributed widely throughout the community as a function of their use. Pesticides, herbicides, and chemical fertilizers, for example, become airborne during spraying, drain off fields into streams, or soak into the ground after rain.

Some of those chemicals are subsequently ingested by fish, stored in fatty tissue, and later consumed by humans. They may also seep into underground aquifers or rivers used for drinking water by humans and many animals. Eventually the entire ecosystem can be exposed. Even the food we eat may be contaminated with these chemical products. Table 6–5 shows levels of

TABLE 6–5. ORGANOCHLORINE PESTICIDE IN THE DIET, U.S. MARKET BASKET SURVEYS

Pesticide	Daily Intake in Micrograms						
	1965	*1966*	*1967*	*1968*	*1969*	*1970*	*6 Years Average*
Aldrin	1	2	1	T	T	T	1
Dieldrin	5	7	1	4	5	5	5
DDT-T	62	87	56	45	32	29	53
Endrin	T	T	T	1	T	T	T
Heptachlor	T	—	T	T	T	T	T
Heptachlor epoxide	2	3	1	2	2	1	2

[a]T = trace

(From Krusé, C. Sanitary control of food. In J. Last (Ed.). *Maxcy-Rosenau public health and preventive medicine.* New York: Appleton Century Crofts, 1980, p. 883.)

organochlorine pesticide in the American diet for the years 1965 through 1970. These data are based on an FDA market basket survey of diets that simulate the daily intake for young males, 16 to 19 years of age, in five major cities. The DDT total (DDT-T), which shows high levels in food, consists of DDT, DDE, and DDD. These are fat soluble and therefore likely to be stored in body tissues and released slowly in the body over a period of time. Fortunately, use of DDT reached a peak in 1966 and began declining until 1973, when its use was banned for all but essential public health needs (Krusé, 1980).

Other potentially hazardous products are widely used in housing. Wood paneling and other products impregnated with formaldehyde, for example, are commonly used in residential dwellings. Such products have been associated with adverse health affects, particularly respiratory problems, in mobile homes or newer housing where better insulation decreases the exchange of indoor and outdoor air. As a result, the vapors of formaldehyde inside these dwellings can reach toxic levels during the winter months.

By-products of heating dwellings, factories, and other public buildings contribute to general environmental exposures. Burning coal, for example, produces emissions that pollute the air with particulates and SO_2. Automobile exhausts contribute to the air pollution problem. Such by-products also have contributed to acid rain and its widespread effects on tree growth and killing of fish and other life forms.

Radiation is another ubiquitous agent. In addition to the naturally occurring radioactive atoms within living plants and animals that come from natural radioactive substnaces found in rocks, soil, and cosmic rays, there are numerous forms of man-made radiation. Some of these are medical and dental x-rays, fallout from atomic explosions and weapons testing, and accidental radioactive leaks and wastes from nuclear power reactors. In the more developed countries, radiation from x-rays may reach 50 percent of the natural background radiation (Krusé, 1980). Although there has been a decrease in nuclear fallout from weapons testing since the 1963 Nuclear Test Ban Treaty, any such environmental radiation contaminates the food supply. Fallout on the land is absorbed and concentrated by plants that are eaten by humans and by animals subsequently consumed by humans. Similarly, fallout on the sea, lakes, and rivers is available to marine plants and animals that concentrate the substances. Radioactive concentration can cumulatively increase at every step of the food chain. The most important food contaminant is strontium 90, a long-life radioactive element that is deposited in bone (Krusé, 1980).

Many products used in the home for cleaning, redecorating or remodeling, or hobbies and crafts are potentially toxic agents if found by unsupervised children or if precautions during use, such as appropriate ventilation of the work area, are not followed. Some of these products may require use of protective garments, such as gloves, masks, or goggles, to prevent skin burns, eye irritation or damage, and other effects. Fumes from gas cooking stoves have been associated with respiratory diseases like asthma. Household dust can be a disease agent for susceptible individuals. Prescription and nonprescription drugs are other potential environmental agents in the home setting. Throw rugs, structural features like stairs, the temperature of the water, and a spectrum of other things in the home environment are potential agents for illness or injury.

The study of environmental agents uses methods similar to those discussed under occupational health. The major differences are in emphasis. Dose levels of many environmental exposures are considerably lower than those in occupational settings where workers are directly handling materials. Thus larger populations must be studied to detect the lower incidence of health effects likely to result. Also, routine availability of data on levels of contamination is less likely. Classification of persons as exposed or unexposed must often be done on the basis of residence in a contaminated or uncontaminated area. Mobility of individuals may complicate definition of an exposed population, particularly in ecological type studies; large numbers of individuals moving in or out of an area may lead to dilution of the population exposed and a major problem with misclassification of exposure. There may be more confounding variables to consider because individuals in a study may be scattered over a wide geographical area in which a variety of other exposures must be considered. Collection of data on health status and relevant behaviors may also be difficult and expensive.

Additional considerations in environmental studies include:

1. Wider ranges of ages exist among the exposed population than is true in occupational studies. Children and older people may be especially susceptible to a particular exposure.

2. Although workers are likely to be exposed for about 8 hours per day, residents of an area may be exposed 16 to 24 hours per day.
3. Meteorological conditions may play a much more important role in estimates of exposure. Air pollution levels may be much higher on the downwind side of a plant than on the upwind side.
4. Seasonal effects must be considered. A spring thaw may dilute pollutant levels in water, for example. People are more likely to be outdoors and in contact with soil, for example, in warmer weather.

Although this list is far from exhaustive, it does point out the kind of thinking that must go into the design of environmental studies. Environmental epidemiology has become an increasingly important field following the publicity focused in recent years on toxic waste sites such as Love Canal. The need to apply epidemiological methods to the identification of health effects in communities that may result from hazardous substances is becoming increasingly urgent.

CONTROL OF DISEASES OF NONINFECTIOUS ETIOLOGY

Primary Prevention

Because of the lack of a simple necessary agent, the lack of concrete evidence for causes other than risk factors indicative of existing physiological change, the ubiquitous distribution of many agents in the occupational and general environment, and the probable synergistic effects among agents, primary prevention of diseases of noninfectious origin is complex, difficult, and sometimes not possible. Basic approaches, similar to those for control of infectious agents, emphasize two methods:

1. Removal of agent(s) from the environment or minimizing the amount of the agent present and
2. Protection of the susceptible host from exposure.

These measures can be effective when a causal agent is known, although, because of the multiple cause problem, each and every agent must be eliminated to assure control of disease incidence. As mentioned before, however, often no specific agent(s) has been identified; the state of knowledge is such that only risk factors are known. In these instances, primary prevention may not be possible—for example, risk factors for breast cancer include early age at menarche, late age at first full-term pregnancy, and family history of breast cancer. It is difficult to intervene and change any of these risk factors, except perhaps, age at first full-term pregnancy. But if age at first full-term pregnancy is a risk factor because high-risk women have difficulty conceiving or carrying an infant to term, then intervention here is also difficult.

In other instances, such as with some of the risk factors for heart disease (e.g., obesity, elevated blood cholesterol, and high blood pressure), causal precedents might be diet, lack of exercise, and stress. Under these assumptions, efforts aimed at primary prevention of heart disease must focus on such things as maternal diet during pregnancy, the diet of the child during early life, regular exercise, and health education programs regarding the hazards of smoking, a known agent. Essentially, individuals must be persuaded to change their life-style. Success cannot be guaranteed.

Specific protection as an approach to primary prevention can be used when specific agents can be identified. In occupational settings, exposure to harmful substances may be eliminated or minimized by engineering equipment to enclose harmful substances or by designing safety equipment that can be worn by the worker. Right-to-know laws may influence worker awareness of potential hazards and motivate workers to seek means for self-protection. Injuries resulting from automobile accidents can be prevented by building and maintaining safe roads, engineeering safer cars, wearing seat belts, training drivers, and regulating speed. Much lung cancer can be prevented through health education programs aimed at convincing people not to begin smoking in the first place and, if they already smoke, to quit.

Secondary Prevention

As previously mentioned, because knowledge is limited regarding the etiology of many diseases caused by noninfectious agents, the best information regarding the natural history of these diseases often does not specify a particular agent, but rather physiological factors associated with higher risk of developing the disease. Because of this, secondary prevention assumes major importance. If tests or other means are available to identify persons at high risk, specific treatment can be instituted to halt the disease progression, and perhaps to reverse some damage. Thus, for breast cancer, where the current level of knowledge does not permit primary prevention, secondary prevention is crucial. Teaching self-breast examination to women, particularly those at high risk because of age, family history, prior benign breast disease, or other factors, may improve chances of detecting a lump before metastasis. Screening programs that may use mammography, tomography, or physician palpation also facilitate detection and diagnosis early enough that success of treatment is likely. The validity of the various screening procedures varies, both inherently and by personal characteristics such as age of the woman and build of the woman. Decisions need to be made with regard to the cost-effectiveness and ethical concerns relative to each procedure when planning a program. These issues are discussed in Chapters 13 and 15.

For diseases such as cardiovascular disease, early detection programs necessarily focus either on identification of early physiological risk factors, including the high density lipoprotein to low density lipoprotein ratio, obesity, high blood pressure, or diabetes, or on identification of behavioral risk factors like smoking, inactivity, or stressful life-styles. Changes in diet and activity, smoking cessation programs, stress reduction programs, and treatment of diabetes and high blood pressure are all interventions aimed at halting or slowing the rate of disease progression.

In the case of occupational or environmental exposures to known agents, secondary prevention is based on the screening or monitoring of exposed groups for early signs of disease. Worker notification programs may be required to alert former employees to their increased risk and to educate them regarding the appropriate action for them to take. Detection must be followed by prompt treatment.

Tertiary Prevention

Many of the diseases of noninfectious origin first present to the medical care system as advanced disease, e.g., the patient with atherosclerosis who first presents as an acute heart attack or the patient with chronic obstructive lung disease who seeks help only when he or she has an acute lung infection that overtaxes the limited function of the individual's severely damaged respiratory system. Because of this, tertiary prevention plays a crucial role in management of these diseases. Objectives of tertiary intervention are (1) to prevent further damage from ocurring, (2) to minimize the symptoms that interfere with daily life, and (3) to help the patient function maximally within the restrictions imposed by the disease.

Prevention of further damage is often accomplished through modifying harmful habits or states that contribute to a decline in function and to progression of the disease process, i.e., smoking cessation, weight reduction, regular physical activity, diet modification, and control of blood sugar levels in diabetics. These can all assist in preventing further damage for a patient with atherosclerotic heart disease. This same patient may require medications to minimize symptoms, such as angina, that interfere with normal daily activities. Vocational retraining may be required to enable the individual to secure a job that he or she is physically capable of performing.

Because of the chronic nature of many of the diseases caused by noninfectious agents, because the disease is often quite advanced before illness is diagnosed and treated, and because of the irreversible nature of many of these diseases, tertiary prevention must be the focus for a major portion of persons with these diseases. Improvements in medical technology during the past several decades have contributed greatly to the length and quality of life for many patients with these conditions.

REFERENCES

Commission on Chronic Diseases. *Chronic illness in the United States* (Vol. 1). Cambridge, Mass.: Harvard Univ. Press, 1957.

Gross, H., Herbst, M., Knatternd, G., & Donner, L. The effects on race and sex on the variation of diagnosis disposition in a psychiatric emergency room. *Journal of Nervous and Mental Disease,* 1969, *148,* 638.

Haase, W. The role of socioeconomic class and examiner class in examiner bias. In F. Riessman, I. Cohen, and A. Pearl (Eds.), *Mental health of the poor*. New York: Free Press, 1968.

Kleinbaum, D., Kupper, L. and Morgenstern, H. *Epidemiologic research, principles and quantitative methods.* Belmont, Calif.: Lifetime Learning Publications, Wadsworth, Inc., 1982.

Krusé, C. Sanitary control of food. In J. Last, (Ed.), *Maxcy-Rosenau public health and preventive medicine.* N.Y.: Appleton Century Crofts, 1980, pp. 875–919.

MMWR. Phytophotodermatitis in Ohio. *Morbidity and Mortality Weekly Reports* (CDC), 1985, *34*(1), 11–13.

Monson, R. *Occupational epidemiology.* Boca Raton, Fla.: CRC Press, 1980.

National Center for Health Statistics. Advance report of final mortality statistics, 1981. *Monthly Vital Statistics Report,* 1984, *33*(3, Suppl.). Washington, D.C.: PHS.

Preuss, O. Metals and mettaloids: Beryllium and its compounds. In C. Zenz (Ed.), *Occupational medicine: Principles and practical applications.* Chicago: Year Book Medical Publishers, 1975.

Schlesselman, J. J. *Case-control studies: Design conduct and analyses.* Oxford: Oxford University, 1982.

Seidman, H., Selikoff, I. J., & Hammond, E. C. Short-term asbestos work exposure and long-term observation. *Annals of the New York Academy of Sciences* 1979, *330,* 61–89.

Selikoff, I. J., Hammond, E. C., & Chung, J. Asbestos exposure, smoking and neoplasia. *JAMA* 1968, *204*(27), 106–112.

Somers, A. Life-style and health. In J. Last (Ed.), *Maxcy-Rosenau public health and preventive medicine.* N.Y.: Appleton Century Crofts, 1980, pp. 1046–1085.

Susser, M. *Causal thinking in the health sciences: Concepts and strategies in epidemiology.* Oxford: Oxford University, 1973.

Tomatis, L., Agthe, C., Bartsch, H., et al. Evaluation of the carcinogenicity of chemicals: A review of the monograph program of the International Agency for Research on Cancer (1971 to 1977). *Cancer Research* 1978, *38*(4), 877–885.

Waldbott, G. *Health effects of environmental pollutants* (2nd ed.). St. Louis: C. V. Mosby, 1978.

Section II

Epidemiology and the Life Cycle

Patterns of Morbidity and Mortality During Pregnancy and Infancy

The health of an infant cannot be separated from the health of the parents, particularly the mother. Health from infancy to adulthood is profoundly affected by conception, gestation, birth, and by the nurturing received early in life. This chapter describes the trends in reproductive health and childbearing in the United States and discusses the important health services that support healthy reproduction and healthy infants.

CHANGES IN REPRODUCTIVE BEHAVIOR AND FERTILITY

The most common and readily available measure of fertility is the crude birth rate (CBR), simply the number of births occurring in a given year divided by the total population at midyear and multiplied by 1000. Using this crude rate, a general picture of the course of fertility in the United States can be seen in Figure 7–1.

The crude birthrate in colonial America was 43 births per 1000 population, a rate as high as currently exists anywhere in

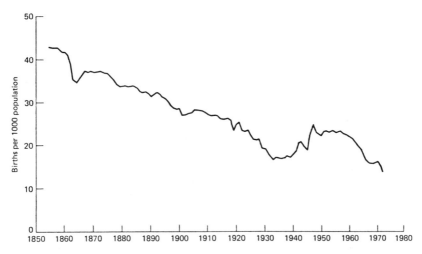

Figure 7–1. Estimated crude birth rate, United States, 1855–1970. *(From Romney, S. L., Gray, M. J., Little, A. B., et al.* Gynecology and obstetrics: The health care of women. *(2nd ed.). New York: McGraw Hill, 1981.)*

the developing world. The rate reflects the large families characteristic during that time in U.S. history. By the 1930s, the CBR had reached a low of 18 births per 1000 population and a high proportion of women of childbearing age remained childless. This low birth rate was interpreted as intrinsic to an industrial society and many sociologists predicted continued low fertility. Immediately after World War II there was an anticipated postwar "baby boom" as people compensated for delayed marriage and childbearing. What was unpredicted was the sustained period of increase in birth rate, peaking at a crude rate of 25 in 1957. This increase reflects an increase in the pace of childbearing. Women married earlier and had their first births earlier after marriage. It does not reflect a return to large families, but instead reflects the move to a two-child family from an earlier time when many women remained childless or bore only one child.

The fertility of American women decreased substantially between 1957 and 1976 (Fig. 7–2). In 1957 the fertility rate was 122 births per 1000 women aged 15 to 44 years. Since 1957, there has been an almost continuous decline in the rate at which women have been bearing children, resulting in a fertil-

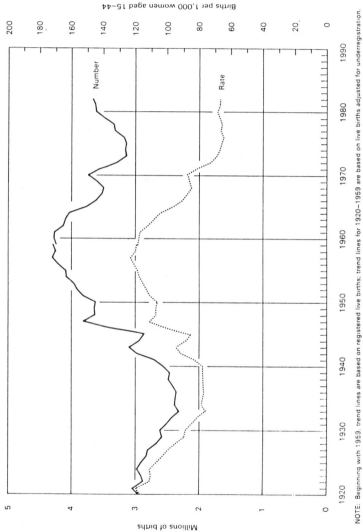

Figure 7-2. Live births and fertility rates; United States, 1920–1982. *(From NCHS. Advance report of final natality statistics, 1982.* Monthly Vital Statistics Report, *1984, 33(6, Suppl.).)*

NOTE: Beginning with 1959, trend lines are based on registered live births; trend lines for 1920–1959 are based on live births adjusted for underregistration.

ity rate of 65 per 1000 women age 15 to 44 in 1976. Between 1976 and 1982 the decline appeared to level off. The decline in fertility from 1957 to 1976 was due to women desiring fewer babies on the average and postponing conception of the first child. In 1967 the average American woman wanted to have three children, by 1976 most American women wanted and expected to have only two children (U.S. Bureau of the Census, 1978). The decline also reflects the increasing ability of women to prevent unwanted pregnancies and births by better accessibility to abortion services and effective contraceptive methods.

Age of Mother at Birth

Levels of childbearing among women aged 15 to 29 declined considerably in the early 1970s and have remained relatively stable since that time. (These changes are shown on Table 7–1.) Rates for women aged 30 to 39 also declined in the early 1970s, but since the mid 1970s have risen steadily. The birth rates for women aged 30 to 34 increased 23 percent from 1975 to 1982 and those for women aged 35 to 39 increased 8 percent during the same time period. The result of this trend has been an upward shift in the age of childbearing to later ages. This is most often attributed to more women entering the workforce and delaying pregnancies until their careers or financial stability has been established. As will be discussed later, this trend has important implications for health care providers because older women have more high-risk pregnancies.

Today's teenagers are less likely than teenagers 10 and 15 years ago to either marry or have a child while still in their teens. Adolescent fertility rates declined from 1972 until 1978, when they appear to have leveled off as shown in Table 7–1. The rate of decline has been greater among black than among white teenagers. Adolescent pregnancies are associated with higher rates of maternal and infant complications. Maternal morbidity and mortality is higher among adolescents, and their infants are more likely to be born prematurely or with a low birth weight. Adolescent motherhood is also associated with lower educational and occupational attainment. The younger the adolescent, the greater the risk for untoward complications.

Promoting the health of adolescents is a particularly difficult task because of the special physiological and psychological

TABLE 7-1. BIRTH RATES BY AGE OF MOTHER: UNITED STATES, 1970-1982

	Age of Mother						
Year	10–14 Years	15–19 Years	20–24 Years	25–29 Years	30–34 Years	35–39 Years	40–44 Years
1982	1.1	52.9	111.3	111.0	64.2	21.1	3.9
1981	1.1	52.7	111.8	112.0	61.4	20.0	3.8
1980	1.1	53.0	115.1	112.9	61.9	19.8	3.9
1979	1.2	52.3	112.8	111.4	60.3	19.5	3.9
1978	1.2	51.5	109.9	108.5	57.8	19.0	3.9
1977	1.2	52.8	112.9	111.0	56.4	19.2	4.2
1976	1.2	52.8	110.3	106.2	53.6	19.0	4.3
1975	1.3	55.6	113.0	108.2	52.3	19.5	4.6
1974	1.2	57.5	117.7	111.5	53.8	20.2	4.8
1973	1.2	59.3	119.7	112.2	55.6	22.1	5.4
1972	1.2	61.7	130.2	117.7	59.8	24.8	6.2
1971	1.1	64.5	150.1	134.1	67.3	28.7	7.1
1970	1.2	68.3	167.8	145.1	73.3	31.7	8.1

Birth rates are live births per 1000 women in a specified age group.
(Compiled from NCHS, Advance Report of Natality Statistics, 1982. *Monthly Vital Statistics Report,* 1984, *33*(6, Suppl.), p. 16.)

characteristics of this age group. In a 1979 study by the American Nurses Association on the health care of children in the United States, teenage pregnancy emerged repeatedly as an area of health needs unmet in our society; yet schools have traditionally been reluctant to allow health education programs on sex and contraception. This reluctance stems frequently from small but vocal parent groups who believe that sex education programs do not restrict themselves to the transmitting of information but also affect the development of personal values. Clearly parents should help plan health education programs in schools and should be aware of the content that is presented. Effective school programs providing information on sex and contraception, and content on risk taking and decision-making are needed to counteract the vast "pro-sex" influence of television, movies, recordings, and advertising.

Health services are needed to provide sexual counseling to adolescents. For that percentage of adolescents who choose to become sexually active, knowledge of and easy access to contraceptive methods is urgent. Family planning programs should be especially adapted to the needs of adolescents and to increase their utilization by this population.

Services for pregnant adolescents are crucial. Over 200,000 girls, 12 to 17 years of age, deliver infants each year (U.S. Select Panel for the Promotion of Child Health, 1981). An almost equal number have miscarriages or induced abortions. Early pregnancy detection is an important health service component because teenage pregnancies are at high risk of adverse outcomes for both the mother and the infant. Early diagnosis can lead to initiation of prenatal care at a time when it can be most effective. Once a pregnancy is diagnosed, the teenager needs assistance in making decisions as to continuing the pregnancy, keeping the infant, releasing the infant for adoption, or abortion. She should have counseling on the advantages or disadvantages of each of these alternatives. In the event that abortion is chosen, early diagnosis is more likely to permit abortion during the first trimester when a suction procedure or saline injection can be used. These procedures are safer for the mother than the alternative, dilatation and curettage (D & C).

Births to Unmarried Women

Marital status of the parent can affect the outcome of a pregnancy and the health of the infant. Almost 25 percent of women less than 25 years of age who married for the first time between 1972 and 1976 were pregnant or had an existing child at the time of marriage (U.S. Bureau of the Census, 1978b). The younger a woman is at the time of her first marriage, the more likely it is that she is already pregnant. Marriage subsequent to a pregnancy often predisposes couples to an economic disadvantage, because the traditional time in which a couple usually establishes an income and home prior to having children is lost. Economic disadvantage is associated with poor housing, malnutrition, and lack of health care, and may therefore be threatening to the health of the mother and the infant.

Historically, premarital conception has been much more prevalent among black than white women; however, in recent years the rate of childbearing by black unmarried women has declined whereas the rate in unmarried white women has increased. These converging trends have resulted in a sharp decline in the racial differential in birth rates among unmarried women. In 1975, the rate for black women was seven times the rate for white women. By 1982, this differential had declined to four (NCHS, 1984b).

In 1982, 20 percent of all births ocurred to unmarried women. The infants of unmarried women are associated with an increased rate of mortality, fetal death, and low birthweight. Unmarried pregnant women are younger and less likely to receive early prenatal care (NCHS, 1980b; Berkor & Sklar, 1976). Over one-half of all births to unmarried women are to teenagers. Unmarried women giving birth need social support, such as adequate housing and nutrition, and special medical care.

Timing and Spacing of Pregnancies

Other factors affecting pregnancy outcomes are the timing of pregnancy and spacing between children. Pregnancies at either end of the childbearing age range are at increased risk of complications. The spacing between pregnancies influences both the likelihood of complication and the ability of parents to meet the infant's needs. An interval between pregnancies of less than 24 months and longer than 48 months is associated with a higher incidence of low birth weight (Spiers & Wang, 1976).

When pregnancies occur at less than 24-month intervals, the mother has less time to restore her health, predisposing her to an increased rate of complications, and the family has less time to adjust to the stress introduced by new family members. On the other hand, when the interval between pregnancies is greater than 48 months the incidence of complications also increases. This increased incidence may be related to having unplanned pregnancies or perhaps to problems associated with infertility.

Black infants are more likely than white infants to be born at very short intervals and intervals between successive births tend to be shorter for young mothers than for older mothers (NCHS, 1984b). For example, 58 percent of second births to mothers 18 to 19 years of age followed the mothers' first birth by less than 24 months, compared with 12 percent to mothers aged 35 to 39 years. Overall there has been a gradual lengthening in the interval between births for both white and black women. Although the increase has been substantially greater for black women, 17 percent of newborn black babies in 1982 compared to 12 percent of white babies followed their mothers' previous live birth by less than 18 months (NCHS, 1984b).

Working Women

In recent years there has been a dramatic surge of women entering the workforce. Over 60 percent of women ages 25 to 34 and 60 percent of all wives are in the workforce (U.S. Bureau of the Census, 1979). In 1977, an estimated one million infants were born to women employed during pregnancy (Hunt, 1977). The risk entailed by pregnant working women and their working conditions merits careful examination. The developing fetus may be particularly susceptible to hazards present in the workplace environment. Some environmental hazards such as ionizing radiation, lead, and mercury have been clearly linked to poor pregnancy outcomes, but for other agents the risks are less clear. Hard physical labor may be detrimental to fetal development. Stress, whether in the workplace or caused by the joint responsibility of home and job could also affect fetal development. Research needs to be continued in assessing the health risks of pregnant women in specific work environments.

Maternal Mortality

In 1900, deaths of pregnant or newly delivered women were major contributors to overall population mortality figures. Large decreases in maternal mortality over the past 40 years have thus contributed to decreases in the overall mortality rate.

Maternal death is defined by the Committee on Maternal Mortality of the International Federation of Gynecologists and Obstetricians to be "death of any woman dying of any cause while pregnant or within 42 days of termination of pregnancy, irrespective of the duration or site of pregnancy" (Roehat, 1981). The completeness of reporting of maternal deaths in the United States has been reported to be a problem (Smith et al., 1984). Reasons for these reporting problems include:

1. Most state death certificates do not specifically ask for pregnancy status of the person who has died. The person certifying the cause of death may be unaware that a woman had a recent pregnancy.

2. If the information on the actual cause of a pregnancy-related death is not recorded accurately on the death certificate, misclassification of the cause of death will result when the death certificate is reviewed for entry into vital statistics registries.

3. The particular definition of maternal death can affect the reported incidence of maternal mortality. The definitions chosen by vital statistics registries, states, and other organizations are not always the same.

Despite the problems of reporting, the observed decreases in maternal mortality are so large that there can be no doubt that rates have dropped dramatically. The maternal mortality ratio has gradually decreased over the years as shown in Table 7–2. In 1940, maternal mortality was 320 per 100,000 live births to white and 782 to black women. By 1979 there were 9.6 maternal deaths for each 100,000 births in the United States. This decrease has resulted in large part from the greater use of hospitals for delivery, the recognition and special care of pregnant women at high risk, the availability of antibiotics, improvements in anesthesia, and intensive research on the preventable causes of maternal deaths.

Although substantial improvements have been made in the overall maternal mortality rates, improvements still need to be made in the rates for disadvantaged ethnic groups and mothers of low socioeconomic status. This is best reflected in the differences in maternal mortality ratios for whites and blacks, as shown on Table 7–2. Black women are more likely to be of a lower socioeconomic class and have less likelihood of receiving early and periodic prenatal care. They may also have poorer nutrition and more frequent exposure to infectious agents or

TABLE 7–2. MATERNAL MORTALITY RATIOS[a] BY RACE, UNITED STATES, 1940–1979

Race	1940	1950	1960	1970	1975	1976	1977	1978	1979
All	376.0	83.3	37.1	21.5	12.8	12.3	11.2	9.6	9.6
White	319.8	61.1	26.0	14.4	9.1	9.0	7.7	6.4	6.4
Black	781.7	223.0	105.6	59.8	31.3	29.5	29.2	25.0	25.1

[a]Deaths per 100,000 live births.
(From NCHS, *U.S. yearbook 1980*. Washington, D.C.: Department of Health and Human Services, 1984, Table 111.)

hazardous agents in their place of employment. Even though maternal mortality ratios in the United States have decreased dramatically during this century, the racial differentiation reflects significant inequality in the attainment of preventative health care services and socioeconomic status.

Maternal age may also affect the risk for maternal mortality. The lowest mortality is associated with the age group 20 to 29. Extremes of childbearing years, particularly those less than 15 years and those greater than 35 years, represent a higher risk for maternal mortality.

A total of 309 deaths in the United States were reported as pregnancy related during 1981. These deaths, shown in Table 7–3, were primarily of three categories.

1. Pregnancies with abortive outcome
2. Direct obstetrical causes
3. Indirect obstetrical causes

Direct maternal deaths result from obstetrical complications of the pregnancy, labor, or puerperium, and from interventions or any sequelae of the above. Indirect maternal deaths are not directly due to obstetrical causes, but result from previously existing diseases or a disease that developed during pregnancy, labor, or the puerperium, and that was aggravated by pregnancy.

During the 1970s the likelihood of deaths from illegally induced abortions was virtually eliminated. During this same time period, however, the rate of death from ectopic pregnancies increased. During the past 10 years there has been an epidemic in the number of ectopic pregnancies in the United States. The most commonly cited reason for this increase is the simultaneous increase in gonorrhea and the resultant pelvic inflammation and scarring. As shown in Table 7–3, in 1981 blacks were 4.6 times more likely than whites to die from all abortive outcomes and 6.2 times more likely to die from ectopic pregnancy. This difference is related both to a higher incidence of ectopic pregnancies in black women and to the reduced likelihood that diagnosis and treatment would be sought early on for the symptoms of an ectopic pregnancy.

The leading causes of maternal mortality in 1981 resulted directly from obstetrical complications of the pregnanacy, labor, or puerperium. Toxemia was the leading single cause of death.

TABLE 7–3. MATERNAL DEATHS AND MATERNAL MORTALITY RATES FOR SELECTED CAUSES BY RACE, UNITED STATES, 1981

Cause of Death	Number	All Races	White	Black
Pregnancy with abortive outcome	47	1.3	0.8	3.7
Ectopic pregnancy	34	0.9	0.5	3.1
Spontaneous abortion	4	0.1	0.1	1.2
Legal abortion	1	0.0	—	0.2
Other	8	0.2	0.2	0.3
Direct obstetrical causes	247	6.8	5.2	15.8
Hemorrhage	48	1.3	1.1	2.6
Toxemia	73	2.0	1.5	4.8
Puerperium complications	75	2.1	1.5	5.1
Other	51	1.4	1.1	3.4
Indirect obstetrical causes	15	0.4	0.3	0.9
All deaths	309	8.5	6.3	20.4

(Compiled from NCHS, Advance Report of Final Mortality Statistics, 1981. *Monthly Vital Statistics Report*, 1984, *33*(3) (Suppl. Washington, D.C.: PHS, 1984.)

This disease has often been associated with young maternal age, poor nutritional patterns, and lack of prenatal care. Clearly the maternal mortality rate could be further decreased by preventive health measures that would decrease the incidence of these known risk factors.

Prenatal Care

The importance of prenatal care in reducing maternal–infant morbidity and mortality has received increasing importance (NCHS, 1984b). In 1982, 76 percent of births were to women whose prenatal care commenced in the first trimester. Five percent of the mothers in the United States did not begin prenatal care until the third trimester or received no care at all. There is a substantial race differential in the use of prenatal care. In 1982, 79 percent of white mothers began care in the first trimester whereas 61 percent of black mothers began care this early.

Four percent of white mothers received delayed or no prenatal care, compared to 9 percent of black mothers. Married women began care much earlier than unmarried ones; only 40 percent of the latter had any care before the end of the first trimester even though they were predominantly very young, when the maternal and infant mortality risks are higher. Teenage girls are less likely than any other age group of women, except for mothers aged 45 years or more, to start prenatal care early in pregnancy. In 1975, only 53 percent of girls aged 15 to 19 began prenatal care in the first trimester and they were most likely to have no care at all (2.3 percent in 1975). Table 7–4 shows, by age of mother, the percent of live births in the United States, 1969 and 1975, for which the mother received late or no prenatal care (NCHS, 1978).

A major biological problem for pregnant teenagers is that the demands of the growing fetus are superimposed on the nutritional needs of the teenager. This competition for nutrients may result in a low birth-weight baby. In addition, toxemia is more common in young mothers. Depending on the age of the mother, the reproductive system may not be mature, predisposing her to fetopelvic disproportion. All of these factors make it even more desirable that pregnant teenagers receive appropriate counseling about sex education and contraception and be strongly urged to seek help at the earliest sign of pregnancy.

TABLE 7–4. PERCENT OF LIVE BIRTHS WHERE MOTHER RECEIVED LATE OR NO PRENATAL CARE, BY AGE OF MOTHER, 1969 AND 1975

Age of Mother	1969	1975
All ages	8.2	6.0
Under 15 years	26.9	21.1
15–19 years	13.9	10.8
20–24 years	7.7	5.8
25–29 years	5.5	3.6
30–34 years	6.7	4.2
35–39 years	8.7	6.7
40–44 years	10.4	10.5
45–49 years	12.8	13.4

(Adapted from NCHS. Prenatal care, United States, 1969–1975. *Vital and Health Statistics,* Series 21, *33.* DHEW Publication (PHS) 78-1911. Hyattsville, Md.: PHS, 1978.)

Infant Morbidity and Mortality

The chances of live birth and survival through the first year of life have steadily improved in the United States. As shown in Table 7–5, the 1979 U.S. infant mortality rate of 13.1 per 1000 live births was 4.4 percent lower than the previous year and 34.5 percent lower than in 1970. Despite these improvements, the United States ranks 16th in the world in infant mortality rates. This placement is due in part to better success in this country at bringing to term infants with defects and delivering alive infants of very low birth weight. In 1982, 248,104 infants were born weighing less than 5.5 pounds (NCHS, 1984b). In the same year in the United States, 43,305 infants died before the age of one (NCHS, 1984a). Clearly, despite progress, the fate of a child born in the United States today is by no means assured.

Black infant mortality rates in the United States remain almost twice as high as the rate of white infants. The gap between black and white infant mortality rates has been widening since 1973. It is useful to examine this gap more closely by comparing neonatal mortality rates (Table 7–6) and post-neonatal mortality rates (Table 7–7). Because neonatal mortality rates relate to deaths before the 28th day of life, they reflect deaths relating to problems at birth more so than do postneo-

TABLE 7–5. INFANT MORTALITY RATES BY RACE: UNITED STATES, 1940–1979 (DEATHS PER 1,000 LIVE BIRTHS EXCLUSIVE OF FETAL DEATHS)

Year	All Live Births	White	Black
1940	47.0	43.2	72.9
1950	29.2	26.8	43.9
1960	26.0	22.9	44.3
1970	20.0	17.8	32.6
1975	16.1	14.2	26.2
1976	15.2	13.3	25.5
1977	14.1	12.3	23.6
1978	13.8	12.0	23.1
1979	13.1	11.4	21.6

(From NCHS, *U.S. Yearbook 1980*. Washington, D.C.: Department of Health and Human Services, 1984, Table 111.)

TABLE 7–6. NEONATAL MORTALITY RATES ACCORDING TO RACE: UNITED STATES, 1970–1979 (INFANT DEATHS UNDER 28 DAYS OF AGE PER 1000 LIVE BIRTHS)

Year	All Races	White	Black	B/W Ratio
1970	15.1	13.8	22.8	1.65
1971	14.2	13.0	21.0	1.62
1972	13.6	12.4	20.7	1.67
1973	13.0	11.8	19.3	1.64
1974	12.3	11.1	18.7	1.69
1975	11.6	10.4	18.3	1.76
1976	10.9	9.7	17.9	1.84
1977	9.9	8.7	16.1	1.85
1978	9.5	8.4	15.5	1.84
1979	8.9	7.9	14.3	1.81

(From U.S. Select Panel for the Promotion of Child Health, *Better health for our children: A national strategy* (vol. 4). Department of Health and Human Services (PHS) Publication No. 79-55071, 1981.)

natal mortality rates; the latter rates include deaths occurring between 28 days and 1 year after birth and are therefore more likely to be related to factors in the infant's environment.

The ratio of black to white neonatal deaths appears to be increasing whereas the ratio of postneonatal deaths appears to have a slight decrease. This ratio of neonatal deaths in the United States went from 1.65 in 1970 to 1.81 in 1979. The corresponding rate for postneonatal deaths went from 2.45 in 1970

TABLE 7–7. POSTNATAL MORTALITY RATES BY RACE: UNITED STATES, 1970–1977 (INFANT DEATHS 28 DAYS TO 365 DAYS OF AGE PER 1000 LIVE BIRTHS)

Year	All Races	White	Black	B/W Ratio
1970	4.9	4.0	9.9	2.45
1971	4.9	4.1	9.3	2.27
1972	4.9	4.0	8.9	2.23
1973	4.7	4.0	8.8	2.20
1974	4.4	3.7	8.1	2.19
1975	4.5	3.8	7.9	2.08
1976	4.3	3.6	7.6	2.11
1977	4.2	3.6	7.6	2.11

(From U.S. Select Panel for the Promotion of Child Health, *Better health care for our children: A national strategy* (vol. 4). Department of Health and Human Services (PHS) Publication No. 79-55071, 1981.)

to 2.11 in 1977. If one assumes that neonatal deaths reflect prenatal and perinatal circumstances and that postneonatal deaths result from environmental factors, different preventive health strategies are needed to decrease the number of deaths in each of these categories.

It is important to note that much, if not all, of the racially-related differences in mortality are socioeconomically associated. Infant mortality declines as socioeconomic class rises. The racial difference observed in infant mortality rates could be considerably offset by improving the quality of health care available to impoverished families.

Low Birth-Weight Infants

The low birth weight of an infant has been associated with an elevated risk of infant mortality, congenital malformations, and other physical and neurological impairments. Though only an approximate 7 percent of all newborns are of low birth weight, this group of infants accounts for more than half of all infant deaths and nearly three-fourths of all neonatal deaths (NCHS, 1972). Either low birth weight or gestational age can be used to estimate the physical maturity of a newborn infant. Weight at birth is more commonly used in epidemiology because it is accurately and completely recorded. Although accurate physical assessment of gestational age may be done in some birth settings, often the accuracy of gestational age depends on the mothers correct recollection of the date of her last menstrual period. Infants weighing 2500 grams (5.5 pounds) or less at birth are considered to be of low birth weight. Low birth-weight infants may be preterm, that is born before 37 weeks gestation, or full term but small for their gestational age.

Trends in the incidence of low birth weight are shown by Figure 7–3. Between 1950 and the mid-1960s there was a gradual increase in the United States from 7.5 to 8.3 percent, followed by a decrease in the next decade. The risk of low birth weight in 1976 was twice as great for infants of other races (1.2 percent) as for white infants (6.1 percent). Most nonwhite infants in the United States are black.

The socioeconomic status of the family as measured by the mother's highest year of educational attainment is strongly associated with birth weight. The proportion of infants of low

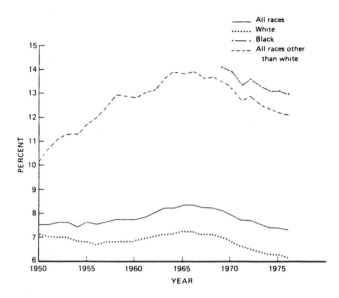

Figure 7–3. Percent of infants of low birth weight by race:
United States, 1950–1976. *(From NCHS. Factors Associated
with Low Birth Weight, U.S., 1976.* Vital and Health Statistics,
*Series 21, No. 37. DHEW Publication No. (PHS) 80-1915.
Hyattsville, Md.: PHS, 1980, p. 3.)*

birth weight born to mothers with 16 years or more of education
(4.9 percent) was half that of infants born to mothers with less
than nine years of education (9.9 percent) (NCHS, 1980a).

Differences between the birth weight of infants in the two
major racial groups in the United States have been well recognized. In 1976, black babies were more than twice as likely as
white babies to be of low birth weight (13.0 percent compared to
6.1 percent (NCHS, 1980a). Other characteristics such as previous stillbirths and miscarriages, short intervals between pregnancies, late or no prenatal care, and mothers under 18 years of
age or over 35 years of age are associatd with low birth weight.
Clearly the problem of low birth weight is one that merits particular emphasis in health-promotion programs in the United
States.

Even though the incidence of low birth weight decreased in
the decade of the 1970s, infant mortality rates declined much
more sharply. This disproportionate decline in rates can be

explained by the fact that low birth weight contributes greatly to the infant mortality rates and that any small changes in the incidence of low birth weight will result in a large improvement in infant survival. Also, advances in perinatal and neonatal medicine have increased the survival of many low birth-weight infants.

Changes in the incidence of low birth weight among newborns have been attributed to programs since the 1960s that have improved the health status and nutrition of pregnant women. In addition, there has been improvement in the outcome of infants of all given birth weights, but particularly of those infants weighting 1000 to 2500 grams. These improvements have been largely due to better intrapartum and neonatal care. Decline in the incidence of low birth weight and neonatal mortality coincided with the introduction of a series of federally-funded programs introduced in the late 1960s and early 1970s that targeted for intervention those socioeconomic factors associated with low birth weight. These included prenatal care and nutrition programs, such as the Maternal and Infant Care (MIC) projects, community health centers, Medicaid, food stamps, and Women, Infant, and Children supplemental feeding (WIC). Increased availability of effective contraceptive methods, as well as increased access to family planning and abortion services, also occurred during this time period, resulting in a decrease in the proportion of births to high-risk women.

Survival of low birth-weight infants has been greatly improved as a result of advances in intrapartal care including fetal monitoring techniques and neonatal care. The late 1960s brought about efforts to regionalize prenatal and neonatal services to ensure that all pregnant women and their newborn infants would have rapid access to an appropriate level of care. These efforts appear to have decreased both mortality and morbidity rates.

Leading Causes of Death During Infancy

The recent decline in the infant mortality rate has been phenomenal. The neonatal period, the first 7 days after birth is the time when the risk of infant death is greatest; 58 percent of all infants who died in 1978 died during the first 7 days (Hunt, 1977). The decline in deaths in the postneonatal period has not been as great, only 14 percent from 1970 to 1978. The leading causes of death in children less than 1 year and the related mortality rates are shown on Table 7–8. Clearly, complications of pregnancy and birth, such as respiratory distress syndrome, low birth weight, and hypoxia, are major factors contributing to infant mortality. Congenital anomalies are the largest single cause of death in infants (NCHS, 1980c). The leading congenital defects causing death are listed in Table 7–9.

Advances have been made in the prenatal diagnosis of congenital defects. Diagnostic ultrasound may be used to detect fetal anomalies such as hydrocephaly, microcephaly, anencephaly, ascitis, myelomeningocele, and polycystic kidneys. Amniotic fluid analysis can provide information on chromosomal aberrations and the detection of neural tube defects through α-fetoprotein analyses. Prenatal diagnosis enables one to prevent the birth of an affected infant. Use of birth control can prevent conception of future affected infants if desired. Screening of fetuses of high-risk pregnant women could result in a savings of the cost of the lifetime care of severely retarded

TABLE 7–8. LEADING CAUSES OF DEATH, 1981, UNDER 1 YEAR OF AGE

Cause of Death	No. of Deaths	Death Rate[a]
All causes	43,305	1,193.2
1. Congenital anomalies	8,914	245.6
2. Sudden infant death syndrome	5,295	145.9
3. Respiratory distress syndrome	4,319	119.0
4. Disorder relating to short gestation and unspecified low birth weight	3,658	100.8
5. Newborn affected by maternal pregnancy complications	1,458	40.2
6. Hypoxia/birth asphyxia	1,405	38.7
7. Accidents/adverse effects	981	27.0
8. Newborn affected by complications of cord placenta and membranes	977	26.9
9. Birth trauma	918	25.3
10. Neonatal hemorrhage	909	25.0
11. All other causes	14,471	298.7

[a]per 100,000 live births.
(From NCHS. Advanced Report of Final Mortality Statistics, 1981. *Monthly Vital Statistics Report, 33*(3, Suppl.) Washington, D.C.: PHS, 1984.)

TABLE 7–9. FIVE LEADING CAUSES OF DEATH FROM CONGENITAL DEFECTS; UNITED STATES, 1981

1. Congenital anomalies of heart/circulatory system
2. Anencephalus and similar anomalies
3. Congenital anomalies of respiratory system
4. Down's syndrome and other chromosomal anomalies
5. Musculoskeletal system anomalies

or handicapped individuals. What cannot be accurately estimated in dollars is the emotional and psychological savings to the family when such diseases are prevented.

Rapid advances are being made in fetal medicine. Surgical techniques have been performed on fetuses with congenital defects that surely would have led to death in utero or at birth if intervention had not taken place. Clearly, the area of fetal medicine and prenatal diagnosis opens new prospects for primary and secondary prevention in the coming years.

Significant improvements have occurred in the diagnosis and treatment of other congenital defects, and many deaths can now be prevented. Significant advances in palliative care and open heart surgery have decreased the mortality of those with congenital heart defects. In recent years, organ transplants for defects such as biliary atresia have increased the survival of infants who otherwise would not survive past the first year of life.

As shown in Table 7–8, the second leading single cause of death in infants is the sudden infant death syndrome (SIDS). In the United States it is the number one cause of death in infants after the first week of life. It occurs five times more frequently in the low birth-weight infant. The cause of the disease is still unknown though its occurrence was recorded as early as the New Testament. Preventive efforts toward SIDS have recently begun; such efforts became possible with the identification of high-risk groups, premature infants and siblings of children who have died from SIDS. Apnea monitors have been installed in homes to permit closer surveillance of high-risk infants and possibly to prevent some of the deaths from SIDS.

Health problems developing after the neonatal period are most often related to environmental factors. Parent–child bonding has been shown to be a crucial attachment process during the early days and weeks of life, and can affect the subsequent physical and emotional growth of the infant (Klaus & Kennel, 1976). Significant changes have occurred in our health care system during the last decade to decrease the time that parents and infants are separated after birth. Infants with inadequate attachment appear to have more growth problems or to be more prone to develop failure to thrive. An infant who fails to thrive is one in whom no clear organic etiology can be demonstrated for the growth failure. Instead the problem seems to arise from situations of environmental, sensory, or parental deprivation. Placement of a child in a nurturing environment often brings improvement, but prevention of the problem by thorough prenatal and postpartum assessment and anticipatory guidance is clearly more desirable.

Lastly, respiratory diseases and other conditions, such as diarrhea, result in many visits to the physician by infants. In the past, these diseases were major causes of death during infancy. There is today less mortality from these causes, but a tremendous amount of time is spent by the health industry in controlling these acute illnesses.

MAJOR FOCI OF PREVENTIVE EFFORTS

Prepregnancy Health Services

The health of our infants is largely dependent on the health of mothers and fathers. Health services are needed throughout the stages or periods of gestation, birth, early life, and parenting. The optimal type of health service begins in anticipation of pregnancy. Nurses should develop and implement health education programs in schools and in health care settings. Mass media sources should be used to promote health practices beginning at the preschool level and continuing throughout life. Areas to be emphasized in such programs of primary prevention include needs of the body for maintaining health, activities that promote health and prevent disease, family planning and sex education, knowledge of the menstrual cycle and pregnancy, harmful factors during pregnancy such as smoking, infections, drugs, and radiation, and the need for early prenatal care.

Food supplementation programs to ensure the health of the women and children in our society should be maintained.

Nurses must become aware of the political process and be active in or support lobbying efforts to maintain these programs. Medical services to detect and treat diseases such as sexually transmitted diseases and communicable diseases, and chronic problems such as hypertension should be accessible to the entire population regardless of socioeconomic class. Mental health services should also be accessible to those with predictable or nonpredictable life stresses. The relationship between increased accessibility to family planning services and decreased infant and maternal mortality is clear. These sources, including an outreach component, should be available to all persons contemplating or engaging in sexual activity. Nurses have historically been in the forefront of family planning efforts and should continue to be there. Pregnancy testing services should be readily available with referral for counseling, genetic screening, family planning, and infertility services as requested or needed.

Prenatal Services and the Recognition of High-Risk Pregnancies

Much research has accumulated in the past two decades as to the identification of those pregnancies with the greatest risks for maternal or infant problems. Figure 7–4 illustrates that services to identify and treat any conditions existing before pregnancy should begin with comprehensive health services for all adolescents and young women. Hopefully, women or adolescents

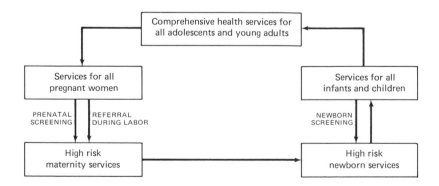

Figure 7–4. Health services network to improve maternal-infant health status.

TABLE 7–10. FACTORS INFLUENCING NEONATAL OUTCOME

Socioeconomic

  Age <16 and >35
  Emotional stress or history of emotional instability
  Smoking
  Drug and alcohol use
  Low socioeconomic status
  Marital status—single
  No or late prenatal care

Pregnancy History

  Parity ≥5
  Previous abortion, stillbirth, neonatal death or anomaly
  Previous C-section

Maternal Health

  Endocrine disturbances (e.g., diabetes, thyroid dysfunction)
  Hypertension
  Repeated UTI
  Chronic renal disease
  Cardiac disease
  Pneumonia, asthma
  Malnourished nutritional state
  Underweight or obese
  Infection

Anatomical

  Incompetent cervix
  Abnormal uterus
  Small pelvis

Pregnancy Complications

  Toxemia
  Placental abnormality
  Multiple pregnancy
  Rh isommunization
  Failure to gain adequate weight
  Excessively large fetus
  Premature rupture of membranes

Labor and Delivery

  1st stage over 12 hours, under 3 in primigravida
    over 8 hours in multigravida

  2nd stage over 2 hours in primigravida
    over 30 minutes in multigravida

  Midforceps
  Compressed or prolapsed cord
  C-section
  Breech, face, shoulder, or transverse presentation
  Meconium before delivery
  General anesthesia
  CNS depressants < 30 minutes before delivery
  $MgSo_4$

(Adapted from Oehler, J. M. *Family-centered neonatal nursing care*, Philadelphia: Lippincott, 1981.)

carrying the greatest risk for abnormal pregnancy and outcome could be identified at this point, whereupon appropriate counseling and family services would be provided so that this population can make responsible decisions regarding the timing of childbearing. Table 7–10 outlines those factors associated with a higher likelihood of a high-risk pregnancy. These are danger signals of potential threats to the mother and newborn. Optimally, primary prevention should begin prior to conception. Nurses functioning in school and community settings with adolescents can be particularly helpful in recognizing individuals with potential or actual risk factors and in providing or referring these individuals to appropriate resources and services.

Failing that approach, initial screening would occur at the time of pregnancy diagnosis. The woman and fetus should have continual assessment to detect potential threatening conditions such as hypertension, diabetes, or abnormal fetal development. Screening, diagnosis, and counseling for fetal genetic disorders should be available along with second trimester abortion services if desired by the parents. Nurses should make available education on behaviors promoting healthy pregnancies and also information on the labor and delivery process. Childbirth education classes should remain available to all couples. Education on breastfeeding and parent–child bonding should be available prenatally. Parents can also be taught early infant development, stimulation techniques to promote development, and accident prevention measures with infants. Special prenatal programs could be developed for adolescents, particularly those programs geared to permit the teenager to continue her educational or vocational training. Social and legal services are needed to assist women and families with proper housing and food. Adoption services and counseling should also be available.

Appropriate referrals need to be made for all women diagnosed as high risk during this prenatal period. Approximately two-thirds of high-risk newborns can be anticipated through careful prenatal evaluation. In addition to the services needed by all pregnant women, the high-risk mother needs constant, careful surveillance of herself and infant. Such monitoring can include periodic amniotic fluid analyses to detect stress in the fetus, sonography or fundal height measures to assess fetal maturity, and careful management of medical problems or problems arising from the pregnancy. In addition to those who develop problems during pregnancy, women who develop problems in late pregnancy or during labor should have access to the high-risk maternity services. This high-risk population should be followed in a prenatal care center that also has services for the infants of these women. Clearly, some infants will enter the perinatal system without first appearing in the high-risk prenatal group.

Services During the Intrapartal Period

The birth setting, the qualifications of the birth attendants, and the management of the birth and postpartum period are all important determinants of the health of the mother and the infant. The woman in labor needs continuing observation by a trained attendant. Fetal monitoring may be used to augment but not replace the observation of the nurse or physician. Back-up services should be available, including transportation to a perinatal center if indicated. The mother and family unit should be provided with optimal privacy and physical and emotional support during this time. Services to assess the newborn's status and to make referrals to a perinatal center, if necessary, are crucial to the health of the newborn. Opportunities to bond with and care for the infant in a "rooming-in" situation should be available to the family, provided the newborn's physical condition does not necessitate transport to a perinatal center. In that instance, supportive care should be given to the family, and visitation with the infant promoted as soon as possible. All families should receive postpartum instruction on recovery and care of the mother and newborn, including breastfeeding and recognition of illness in the newborn. Home visitation services should be made available not only to high-risk families, but also to any family requesting such services. Counseling and legal services for adoption, foster care, or financial support may be indicated. Information on family planning and self-care should be provided prior to the 6-week postpartum visit.

Newborn Services

The newborn period, particularly the first 7 days of life, is critical in determining the outlook for the infant. A newborn needs immediate evaluation postdelivery, with appropriate treatment to prevent complications from heat loss or respiratory difficulty.

Equipment for resuscitation should always be available, even in uncomplicated labors and deliveries. Safe, rapid transportation to a perinatal center should be provided if needed. The normal newborn also needs screening for certain genetic diseases during the neonatal period. Screening for relatively rare diseases, like PKU, during the neonatal period benefits the infant, the family, and society. The costs of detection and prevention have been estimated to be only one-tenth of the cost of lifetime institutional care. Breastfeeding should be encouraged whenever possible to provide the mother's immunities to the infant during the first months of life. Adequate nutritional services, such as WIC, and education on the infant's nutritional needs should be available to needy families. Early and periodic check-ups for the newborn should be accessible and encouraged. The importance of infant immunizations should be recognized and provided free of charge to needy families. Nurses should educate parents on the benefits of breastfeeding, the nutritional needs of infants, and the importance of immunizations. In addition, nurses can provide information on the normal development of infants and changes in family systems that result from the addition of a new family member. Comprehensive anticipatory guidance by nurses can reduce the incidence of infant mortality and morbidity.

SUMMARY

A preventive program as described above would lead to a decrease in maternal mortality, particularly in the disadvantaged socioeconomic groups, and also a decrease in the incidence of infant morbidity and mortality. Improvements of the health of mothers and infants can only be achieved by focus on each of the following areas:

1. Improving the knowledge of men and women of childbearing age on reproduction and fertility. This would increase the likelihood of more planned and wanted pregnancies in our society.
2. Insuring that every pregnant woman receives early prenatal care. These services should be available to all of our population, and especially to teenage mothers and economically disadvantaged women.

3. Continuing research on causes of death in women and children, particularly toxemia of pregnancy, ectopic pregnancies, congenital malformations, and sudden infant death syndrome.

4. Continuing advancement of knowledge in the areas of prenatal screening, fetal medicine, fetal surgery, and neonatology.

5. Advocating social programs to enhance the quality of life of all people in the United States, but with particular emphasis on women and infants who, although they are the future of any society, are traditionally the weakest members and those most in need of assistance from others.

REFERENCES

American Nurses Association. *A report on the hearings on the unmet health needs of children and youth,* Kansas City, Missouri, 1979.

Berkov, B., & Sklar, J. Does illegitimacy make a difference? A study of the life chances of illegitimate children in California. *Population & Development Review,* 1976, 2(2); 201–217.

Hunt, V. *The health of women at work.* Evanston, Ill.: Northwestern University Program on Women, 1977.

Klaus, M. H., & Kennel, J. H. *Maternal-infant bonding.* St. Louis: Mosby, 1976.

National Center for Health Statistics. A study of infant mortality from linked records by birth weight, period of gestation, and other variables, United States. *Vital and Health Statistics,* Series 20, No. 12. DHEW Publication No. (HSM) 72-1055. Health Services and Mental Health Administration. Washington, U.S.: Government Printing Office, 1972.

National Center for Health Statistics. Prenatal care, United States, 1969–1975. *Vital and Health Statistics,* Series 21, No. 33. DHEW Publication No. (PHS) 78-1911. Hyattsville, Md.: PHS, 1978.

National Center for Health Statistics. Factors associated with low birth weight, United States, 1976. *Vital and Health Statistics.* Series 21, No. 37. DHEW Publication No. (PHS) 80-1915. Hyattsville, Md.: PHS, 1980a.

National Center for Health Statistics. Trends and differentials in births to unmarried women: U.S. 1970–76 by S. J. Ventura. *Vital and Health Statistics,* Series 21, No. 36. DHHS Publication No. (PHS)

80-1914. Washington, D.C.: U.S. Government Printing Office, 1980b.

National Center for Health Statistics. Final mortality statistics, 1978. *Mortality Vital Statistics Report. 29* (Suppl 2.) DHHS Publication No. (PHS) 80-1120. Hyattsville, Md.: PHS, 1980c.

National Center for Health Statistics. Advance Report of final mortality statistics, 1981. *Monthly Vital Statistics Report, 33,* (3, Suppl.), Washington, D.C.: PHS, 1984a.

National Center for Health Statistics. Advanced report of final natality statistics, 1982. *Monthly Vital Statistics Report, 33,* (6 Suppl.) Washington, D.C.: Public Health Service, U.S. Department Health and Human Services, 1984b.

Roehat, R. W. Maternal mortality in the United States of America. *World Health Statistics Quarterly,* 1981, *34;* 2–13.

Smith, J. C. Hughes, J. M., Pekow, P. S., & Roehat, R. W. An assessment of the incidence of maternal mortality in the United States. *American Journal of Public Health,* 1984, *74;* 780–783.

Spiers, P. S., & Wang, L. Short pregnancy interval, low birth weight and the SIDS. *American Journal of Epidemiology,* 1976, *104;* 15–21.

U.S. Bureau of the Census. *Current Population Reports,* Series P-20, No. 315, Trends in child-spacing, June 1975. Washington, D.C.: U.S. Government Printing Office, 1978a.

U.S. Bureau of the Census. Fertility of American women; June 1977. *Current Population Reports,* Series P-20, No. 325. Washington, D.C.: U.S. Government Printing Office, 1978b.

U.S. Bureau of the Census. Population profile of the U.S.: 1978. *Current Population Reports,* Series P-20. No. 336. Washington, D.C.: U.S. Government Printing Office, 1979.

U.S. Select Panel for the Promotion of Child Health. *Better health for our children: A national strategy* (Vol. IV). DHHS (PHS) Publication No. 79–55071, 1981.

8

Patterns of Morbidity and Mortality in Childhood and Adolescence

The health of young people is of crucial importance to any society because children represent the future of a society. As a result of high childhood mortality rates, parents in much of the world have had to bear many children so that a few survive to adulthood. In these countries, children under 15 still constitute the majority of the population. For the world as a whole, children under 15 comprised 35 percent of the total population in 1980 (NCHS, 1984b). Because of declining birth rates and declining mortality at older ages, it is projected that by the year 2000, children under 15 will comprise only 30.7 of the total world population.

In the United States, children under 15 years of age comprised 26.8 percent of the total population in 1980. Projections for the year 2000 are that this proportion will drop to 25.1 percent. Maintaining the health of these children, who represent the next generation of workers and parents, must be a national priority. Health status throughout the remainder of the life span depends on the health status and life-style established during the childhood years.

Table 8–1 summarizes the leading age-specific health prob-

TABLE 8–1. LEADING AGE-SPECIFIC HEALTH PROBLEMS OF
CHILDREN 1–19 YEARS, GEORGIA, 1975–1977

Early Childhood (1–4 Years)	Childhood (5–12 Years)	Adolescence (13–19 Years)
Accidents	Accidents	Adolescent pregnancy
Infectious diseases	Cancers, including	Alcohol
Child abuse	leukemia	Drug abuse
Lead poisoning	Influenza and pneumonia	Accidents
Development lag	Homicide	Suicide
	Infections of ear, nose, throat, other	Homicide
	Malnutrition	Venereal disease
	Dental disease	Dental disease
		Mental/emotional problems
		Sports injuries

(Adapted from Dever, A. *Epidemiology of Health Services Managment.* Rockville, Md.: Aspen Systems Corp., 1984.)

lems of children 1 to 19 years of age. Although the table is based on data from the state of Georgia for the time period 1975 to 1977, it is a reasonable representation of health problems for children of these ages in the United States as a whole. Some of the health problems listed, for example, accidents, are a problem at all childhood ages, whereas others are particular to a single age subgroup, for example, lead poisoning, which is a problem primarily among low income children under 4 years of age; lead poisoning is often attributable to the eating of peeling lead-based paint found in many slum apartments.

Some of the health problems shown in Table 8–1 are primarily causes of mortality (e.g., homicide, suicide), others are primarily associated with morbidity (e.g., sports injuries, developmental lag, respiratory infections). Still other health problems contribute substantially both as a cause of morbidity and mortality; accidents are the most striking of these.

This chapter presents major causes of morbidity and mortality among children and adolescents. The first section of the chapter deals with causes of mortality by age, sex, and race. This is followed by presentation of acute and chronic diseases common in children. The final section of the chapter is devoted to interventions that are important to maintenance of health from 1 year of age through adolescence.

MORTALITY IN CHILDHOOD
AND ADOLESCENCE

Variation in Mortality by Age

As might be expected death rates among children are low in comparison to death rates for older age groups. Within ages 1 to 14, rates are higher from 1 to 4 years than they are from 5 to 14 years (NCHS, 1984a). To some extent, this higher mortality continues to represent exposures in utero (e.g., deaths from congenital malformations, neoplasms and heart disease); a high accident rate is the major cause of the remaining deaths. Preliminary data for 1981 indicate mortality rates of 67.3 per 100,000 for boys between 1 and 4 years of age and 52.8 per 100,000 for girls of that age. In the 5- to 14-year age group, rates are 35.7 for boys and 22.9 for girls. After this age, death rates begin to rise in the 15- to 29-year group (157.7 men; 54.6 women) and continue to increase with each decade of age throughout the remainder of the life span (NCHS, 1984a).

There are proportionately more boys relative to girls at ages under 15 years than at any subsequent age of the life cycle. The male to female ratio under 15 years was 104.6 in the United States in 1980. For the 15- to 24-year age group it was 101.7. Above that age it dropped below 100 and continued to decline with increasing age. By 65 years of age, it was 67.6. This is due to the higher mortality rates for men compared to women that begin in childhood and continue throughout the life cycle.

The major causes of death for three age subgroups, 1 to 4, 5 to 14, and 15 to 24 years, are shown in Table 8–2. Because most mortality statistics include ages 15 to 24 as one subgroup spanning late childhood and young adulthood and because causes of death in this age group resemble those of ages 5 to 14 more than those of the age group 25 to 34, this age subgroup is included in this chapter. Accidents are the leading cause of death in all three of the age subcategories, accounting for 49.97 percent of all deaths between ages 1 and 24. Congenital anomalies at 7.6 per 100,000 are the second leading cause of death in the youngest age category. Rates of 1.6 and 1.4, respectively, drop this cause to third in the 5- to 14-year age group, and seventh in the 15- to 24-year group. Malignant neoplasms, about half of which

TABLE 8–2. RATES PER 100,000 FOR FIVE MAJOR CAUSES OF MORTALITY UNDER AGE 29 BY SUBCATEGORIES OF AGE, UNITED STATES, 1981

Rank Order of Cause	Age					
	1–4		5–14		15–24	
	Cause	Rate	Cause	Rate	Cause	Rate
1.	Accidents	23.6	Accidents	14.2	Accidents	56.0
2.	Congenital anomalies	7.6	Malignant neoplasms	4.1	Homicide	14.7
3.	Malignant neoplasms	4.9	Congenital anomalies	1.6	Suicide	12.3
4.	Homicide	2.6	Homicide	1.3	Malignant neoplasms	5.7
5.	Heart disease	2.5	Heart disease	0.9	Heart disease	2.6
6.	Pneumonia and influenza	1.8	Suicide	0.5	Symptoms, signs, and ill-defined conditions	2.2
7.	Meningococcal infection	0.8	Pneumonia and influenza	0.5	Congenital anomalies	1.4
8.	Septicemia	0.7	Symptoms, signs, and ill-defined conditions	0.5	Cerebrovascular disease	0.9
9.	Benign neoplasms, carcinoma in situ and neoplasms of uncertain and unspecified nature	0.4	Chronic obstructive pulmonary disease	0.3	Pneumonia and influenza	0.8
10.	Cerebrovascular disease, chronic obstructive pulmonary diseases and allied conditions	0.3	Cerebrovascular disease	0.3	Chronic obstructive pulmonary disease	0.4

(Compiled from NCHS Advance report of the final mortality statistics, 1981. *Monthly Vital Statistics Report*, 1984, 33 (3, suppl.), pp. 15–17.)

are leukemias, are among the top five causes of death in all three age categories, as are homicide and heart diseases. Suicide moves into the top five causes for those in the 15- to 24-year category and ranks among the top 10 for the 5- to 14-year group.

Although the numbers of deaths are relatively small for most individual causes of death (for example, 505 for cerebrovascular diseases and 360 for malignant neoplasms between ages 1 and 24), many deaths in this age group are theoretically preventable. Since the late 1960s, mortality from natural causes has been lower than mortality from accidents and violence (U.S. Public Health Service, 1982); the latter causes could be prevented. Motor vehicle accidents accounted for 45.1 percent of accidents (3611 deaths) between ages 1 and 14 and for 73.6 percent of the accidents (17,363 deaths) between 15 and 24. The other major accidental causes of death vary among the three age subcategories. Between 1 and 4 years of age, fires or burns, drowning, and ingestion of food or objects are the major accidental causes of death after motor vehicle accidents. Between 5 and 14 years, the other major accidents are drowning, fires or burns, and firearms, in that order. Among those 15 to 24 years, the other major accidents are drowning, firearms, and poison (National Safety Council, 1984).

Use of child restraint seats is a proven lifesaver. By 1983, child restraints were required by law in 21 states and legislation was pending in 25. Tennessee, the first state to pass such a law has had a decrease in childhood motor vehicle deaths. Prior to the 1978 child restraint law, motor vehicle deaths in Tennessee among the 0 to 4 age group averaged 20 to 25 per year. In 1980 there were 14 deaths. In 1981, injuries were down 30 percent and deaths were down 55 percent (Fisher, 1983). Other accidents are preventable if the environment is structured to deny children access to hazardous substances. Some accidents could be prevented if an adult were present to supervise play activities such as swimming or water play. Primary prevention is essential to accident prevention. Accident prevention for this age group is discussed more fully in the final section of this chapter.

Of the other nine of the ten major causes of death under age 14, four are clearly candidates for primary prevention: homicide, suicide, pneumonia and influenza, and meningococcal infections. Cancer and congenital anomalies may also be prevented in some instances by eliminating maternal exposure to hazardous sub-

stances during pregnancy. Because the cause of these conditions
is often unknown, early detection and prompt treatment can
reduce the case–fatality rates. Heart disease and cerebrovascular disease in this young age group may be inherited or related
to maternal diet during pregnancy and compounded by a high
fat, high sodium diet during childhood.

The improvement in childhood mortality in the United
States has been dramatic during this century. Elimination of
the major childhood infections as causes of death was accomplished during the early part of the century. Even during the
last decade (1970 to 1981), mortality rates in this age group
have dropped substantially, by 28.6 percent for ages 1 to 4, by
26.5 percent for ages 5 to 14, and by 16.7 percent for ages 15 to
24 (calculations based on data from U.S. Public Health Service,
1982). These reductions are due to improved survival of children
with congenital anomalies, with cancer, particularly leukemia,
and with influenza and pneumonia, which showed an 89 percent
decline since 1950. This decline, relative to rates for accidents,
is shown for the age group 5 to 14 years in Figure 8–1. Clearly,
it is possible to further reduce mortality in this age category.

Variation in Mortality by Sex and Race

Available 1981 data comparing mortality in the United States
by race show higher rates for blacks than for whites of both
sexes at all childhood ages. These rates are listed in Table 8–3
(NCHS, 1984a). Differences in black and white sex ratios reflect
the disproportionate mortality among very young black males.
The sex ratio under age 15 for blacks in 1980 was 101.6, for
whites it was 105.3 (NCHS, 1984b).

Variation in mortality rates by sex reflects, to some extent,
traditional sex differences in life-style, although death rates for
boys tend to be higher among all causes including those not
related to life-style. Greater differences between the sexes are
observed, for example, in accidents, homicides, and suicide;
these are causes that should be preventable and that are related
to life-style and societal conditions. Sex differences in rates are
greater for non-motor vehicle accidents than they are for motor
vehicle accidents—a mortality sex ratio of 2.7 versus 1.8 in 1979
(U.S. Public Health Service, 1982). These excess non-motor
vehicle accidents among boys may reflect the more active and

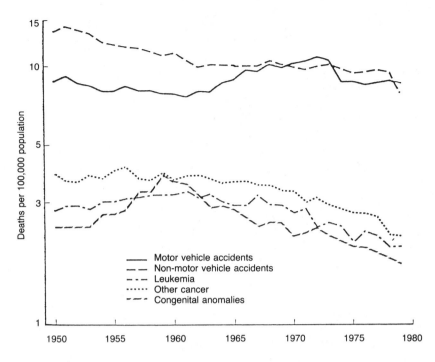

Figure 8–1. Death rates for children 5 to 14 years of age, according to selected causes of death: United States, 1950–1979. *(From U.S. Public Health Service.* Health, U.S., 1980–81, *Rockville, Md., 1982.)*

TABLE 8–3. DEATH RATES PER 100,000 BY AGE, SEX, AND RACE, UNITED STATES, 1982

	Race and Sex					
	All Races		**White**		**Black**	
Age Category	*Male*	*Female*	*Male*	*Female*	*Male*	*Female*
1–4	67.3	52.8	60.5	47.7	105.3	81.6
5–9	34.4	23.6	32.4	22.4	34.8	30.7
10–14	36.9	22.1	35.7	20.9	43.8	29.4
15–19	129.7	50.2	130.9	51.1	125.3	45.9
20–24	185.6	59.0	176.6	55.1	253.0	82.1

(Compiled from NCHS. Advance report of the final mortality statistics, 1981. *Mortality Vital Statistics Report,* 1984, *33* (3, Suppl.), p. 8.)

daring play of male children. Reasons for higher rates of homicide and suicide deaths among male children are unclear. Use of alcohol likely plays a role. There have been reports of higher rates of child abuse among male children than among female children. The social and psychological factors contributing to aggression toward male children and self-destructive tendencies among male children need further investigation.

Large racial differences in mortality are observed for non-motor vehicle accidents, particularly fire and drowning, with black children more than 1.9 times as likely as whites to die from such accidents (U.S. Public Health Service, 1982). For motor vehicle accidents, death rates for black children are 17 percent higher than for white children. Whether the higher mortality rates are due to higher accident rates, higher case–fatality rates, or both is not entirely clear. Since 1950, however, the racial differences have been narrowing.

Declines in mortality from natural causes occurred in both racial groups—fairly equally for congenital anomalies and cancer and slightly faster among white children than among black children for influenza and pneumonia. This latter difference could be related, in part, to blacks seeking care at a later stage in the natural history of the illness. In 1979, mortality from influenza and pneumonia among white children was about half of that for black children (U.S. Public Health Service, 1982).

Mortality rates for those under age 25 have been declining much faster for black females than for black males. As a result, among those under 25 years of age, gaps in mortality between the races have closed much faster for females than for males. The excess mortality among black males is seen primarily in the rates of deaths from accidents, homicide, and suicide. These are potentially preventable.

MORBIDITY IN CHILDHOOD AND ADOLESCENCE

In general, childhood is a time of good health in the United States. Children have much less illness than do older persons. Data from the National Health Survey indicate that only 3 percent of white children under 17 rated their health as fair or poor; 6 percent of Hispanics and 8 percent of nonwhites rated their health fair or poor (Fig. 8–2). All other children of this age group rated their health as good or excellent.

The majority of illnesses among children are acute in nature. Chronic conditions are relatively rare. In the following sections of this chapter, data relating to major causes of acute and chronic illness are presented.

Acute Conditions

Acute conditions, as presented in data from the National Center for Health Statistics, generally refer to illness or injury of short duration, typically less than 3 months, that has involved either medical attention or 1 day or more of restricted activity. Acute conditions usually include respiratory conditions, infective and parasitic diseases, injuries, digestive system disorders, and miscellaneous conditions, including diseases of the ear, headaches, skin diseases, genitourinary and musculoskeletal diseases, and disorders of pregnancy or delivery. A classification system for acute disorders is shown in Table 8–4. Acute conditions are

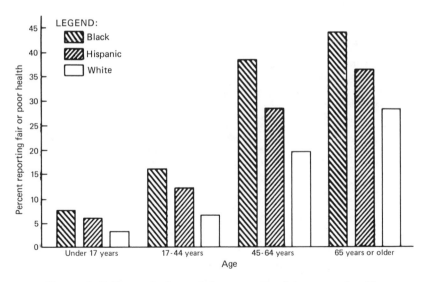

Figure 8–2. Percent of population reporting fair or poor health, by ethnic group and age: 1976–77. *(From U.S. Public Health Service. Health, U.S., 1980–81, Rockville, Md., 1982.)*

TABLE 8–4. CLASSIFICATION OF ACUTE CONDITIONS

I. Respiratory conditions
   A. Upper Respiratory
      Common cold
      Other upper respiratory
   B. Influenza
      With digestive manifestations
      Other
   C. Other respiratory
      Pneumonia
      Bronchitis
      Other

II. Infective and parasitic
   A. Common childhood diseases
   B. Virus
   C. Other

III. Injuries
   A. Fractures and dislocations
   B. Sprains and strains
   C. Open wounds and lacerations
   D. Contusions and superficial injuries
   E. Other

IV. Digestive system disorders
   A. Dental conditions
   B. Functional and symptomatic upper gastrointestinal conditions
   C. Other

V. Other
   A. Diseases of ear
   B. Headaches
   C. Genitourinary
   D. Deliveries/disorders of pregnancy
   E. Skin diseases
   F. Musculoskeletal diseases

(From Bloom, B. Current estimates from the National Health Interview Survey: United States, 1981. *Vital and Health Statistics,* Series 10, No. 141. DHHS Publication No. (PHS) 83-1569. Washington, D. C.: U.S. Government Printing Office, 1982.)

reported in terms of the annual number of acute conditions per 100 persons, for example, 241 per 100 persons. One could think of this figure as an annual average of 2.41 conditions or episodes per person.

Acute conditions are most common in the group under 6 years of age, declining continuously as age increases to a low of

111.0 conditions per 100 persons per year by 65 years of age. The incidence of acute conditions for 1977 to 1978 is shown in Table 8–5 for ages less than 6 years and those 6 to 16 years of age. In 1977 to 1978 those under age 6 had an annual incidence of 381.6 acute conditions per 100 persons, compared with 278.7 for the 6- to 16-year group. Most in both age groups were respiratory conditions. Although the number of acute conditions decreases with age, the duration of restricted activity caused by acute conditions increases with age (Ries, 1983); in other words, each episode lasts longer in older persons than in children.

Acute conditions accounted for 169,126 days of school lost among children aged 6 to 16 in 1981. This represents a rate of 436.2 days per 100 children, an average of 4.36 days per child per year. Fully 62 percent of these days lost were due to respiratory conditions (NCHS, 1982b).

Consistent with the incidence rates for acute conditions is the proportional distribution of conditions seen during visits to physicians' offices. Visits to the school nurse could be expected to be for similar conditions. Fully 29 percent of office visits among children under 15 years of age and 14.3 percent among 15- to 24-year olds were for respiratory conditions. Accidents,

TABLE 8–5. INCIDENCE OF ACUTE CONDITIONS PER 100 PERSONS PER YEAR BY AGE, CHILDREN UNDER 15, UNITED STATES, JULY 1977–JUNE 1978, AND PERCENTAGE OF PHYSICIAN'S OFFICE VISITS ATTRIBUTED TO THESE CONDITIONS

Condition	< 6 Years	6–16 Years	Percentage of All Office Visits Under 16 Years
Respiratory conditions	203.6	158.9	29.0
Upper respiratory	130.3	90.2	
Influenza	56.1	61.3	
Other respiratory	16.6	7.5	
Infective and parasitic	61.4	34.9	7.3
Injuries	38.0	40.9	8.2
Digestive system disorders	14.1	12.1	1.5
Other acute conditions	65.1	31.9	5.4

(Adapted from Ries, P. *Acute conditions: Incidence and associated disability.* DHEW Publication No. (PHS) 79-1560, Series 10, No. 132. Hyattsville, Md.: Public Health Service, 1979, p. 14.)

poisons, and violence were the second most frequent diagnoses, accounting for 8.2 percent of visits among those under 15 years of age and 10.6 percent between 14 and 24 years. Infective and parasitic disease was the principal diagnosis for 7.3 percent of visits among those under 15 years, 5.3 percent of those 15 to 24 years. Digestive diseases accounted for only 1.5 and 2.4 percent, respectively, of visits among these age groups (Table 8–5, Ries, 1983).

In general, the annual incidence of all respiratory conditions in children has been decreasing for sometime, dropping from 183.8 in 1961 to 1962 to 104.0 in 1981. The most dramatic change was in the subcategory of upper respiratory conditions, which dropped by almost half from 119.7 in 1961 to 1962 to 59.9 in 1981 (Ries, 1983). Infective and parasitic diseases have also been declining over time, also by almost 50 percent from 54.2 per 100 persons in 1961 to 1962 to 28.4 per 100 persons in 1981. Of the defined categories of acute conditions, injury is the one showing the least decline between 1961 and 1981, decreasing by only 10.7 per 100 persons. Digestive system disorders have declined nearly 50 percent.

For certain of the infective conditions reporting to public health authorities is mandatory (discussed in Chapter 12 on Disease Control and Surveillance). The 1979 incidence of the top ten of these mandatory-notice (notifiable) diseases in the age group 0 to 24 is shown in Table 8–6. Gonorrhea is by far the major infection in this age group; this condition potentially could be controlled through early detection, prompt treatment, and follow-up of sexual contacts. In the 1950s and 1960s large amounts of money were channeled into venereal disease control programs. The effectiveness of such programs was reflected in decreasing rates of gonorrhea and syphilis during that time. Later, as funds were diverted to other programs, rates began increasing again. This was probably due to a number of factors, including the introduction of the birth control pill, which led to greater sexual freedom, to evolvement of penicillin resistant strains of venereal organisms, to the return of Vietnam veterans, many of whom were infected, and to poorer case identification and follow-up of contacts as a result of cuts in funding to control programs.

Other mandatory-notice conditions are preventable through appropriate schedules of immunization. Cases of measles and mumps are few in number because most schools require immu-

TABLE 8–6. TOP TEN NOTIFIABLE DISEASES IN 1979 FOR 0–24 YEAR OLDS, UNITED STATES

1. Gonorrhea	642,325	6.16
2. Salmonellosis	17,913	0.17
3. Hepatitis A	14,128	0.14
4. Shigellosis	12,074	0.12
5. Measles	11003	0.11
6. Syphilis	10,517	0.10
7. Rubella (German measles)	6,859	0.07
8. Hepatitis B	6,199	0.06
9. Hepatitis, unspecified	5,424	0.05
10. Mumps	4,906	0.05

(From Annual summary 1979: Reported morbidity and mortality in the United States. *Morbidity and Mortality Weekly Reports,* 1980, *28* (54).)

nization for school entry. Some diseases covered by school immunization requirements have become so rare that they no longer fall among the top ten, for example diphtheria, pertussis, tetanus, and polio. In 1978, among children entering kindergarten in the United States, 93 percent were immunized against measles, 92 percent against polio, diphtheria, pertussis, and tetanus, 91 percent against rubella and 83 percent against mumps (U.S. Public Health Service, 1981). In the early part of the century before immunizations were available, childhood infections were major killers of children as well as major causes of morbidity. Current recommendations for preventive immunization of children are discussed in the last section of this chapter.

Table 8–7 shows incidence of acute conditions and related activity limitations by sex for those under 6 years and 6 to 16 years of age using various measures of acute illness that are commonly found in the National Health Survey. Although boys under age 6 have a lower incidence of acute conditions than do girls under 6 years of age, they have more restricted activity associated with acute conditions than do girls. From 6 to 16 years, girls have more activity restriction.

The largest percentage of office visits by those under 15 years of age were, not surprisingly, to pediatricians (48.6 percent). Another 3.24 percent were to practitioners of general and

TABLE 8-7. INCIDENCE OF ACUTE CONDITIONS AND RESTRICTED ACTIVITY FOR ACUTE CONDITIONS BY SEX, UNITED STATES, 1980

| | Age | | | | | |
| | Under 6 Years | | | 6–16 Years | | |
	Male	Female	% Difference	Male	Female	% Difference
Acute conditions per 100 persons per year	394	406	Female 3% higher	284	292	Female 3% higher
Restricted activity days / 100 persons per year	1266	1122	Male 13% higher	945	1015	Female 7% higher
Bed disability days per 100 persons per year	603	559	Male 8% higher	416	512	Female 23% higher
Restricted activity days per condition	3.2	2.8	Male 14% higher	3.3	3.4	Female 3% higher
Bed disability days per condition	1.5	1.4	Male 7% higher	1.5	1.7	Female 13% higher
School lost days per 100 persons/year	—	—	—	432	544	Female 26% higher

(Adapted from Verbrugge, L. Sex differentials. *Public Health Reports*, 1982, 97(5), 418.)

family practice. The third highest percent of visits was to otolaryngologists, presumably related in large part to swallowing foreign objects or substances (3.3 percent). This is followed closely by orthopedic surgery (2.8 percent), general surgery (2.7 percent), and ophthalmology (2.7 percent) (Ezzoti & McLemore). Clearly, because more than half of the office visits made by children are to sites other than pediatricians' offices, nurses in other treatment settings need to have some knowledge in the care of children.

Hospitalization

Only 5.3 percent of children under 17 years of age were hospitalized in 1978, a typical year (Haupt, 1982). Acute illness, as reflected in hospital discharge data, is shown in Table 8–8 for the age group under 15 years of age. Consistent with previously presented data on incidence of acute diseases and reasons for physicians' office visits, respiratory diseases top the list. Among the respiratory diseases, pneumonia and those affecting the tonsils and adenoids are the two most frequent; asthma and acute bronchitis and bronchiolitis are third and fourth. Diseases of the digestive system, seventh among diagnoses in physicians' office visits, was second most frequent among hospitalization diagnoses; particularly frequent in this complex of illnesses were enteritis and colitis, inguinal hernia, and appendicitis. These acute conditions can be life threatening and therefore usually require hospitalization rather than office treatment.

Injury and poisoning was the third most frequent set of diagnoses among hospital discharges. Fractures were the most frequent type of injury. Ear-related problems were the most common of the conditions included under the fourth most frequent diagnostic category, diseases of the nervous system and sense organs.

The fifth through seventh most frequent diagnostic categories, infectious and parasitic diseases, congenital anomalies, and diseases of the genitourinary system, respectively, have similar rates, ranging from 34.4 to 37.1 per 10,000 population.

Length of hospital stay is generally short in this age group. The longest length of stay is for diseases of the central nervous system, at 7.6 days. Congenital anomalies at 5.7 days are second. Injury and poisoning is in third place, at 4.8 days.

TABLE 8–8. RATE OF DISCHARGE (PER 10,000 POPULATION) FROM SHORT-STAY HOSPITALS FOR THE FIRST LISTED DIAGNOSIS AND AVERAGE LENGTH OF STAY FOR PATIENTS UNDER 15 YEARS OF AGE, UNITED STATES, 1980

Diagnostic Category by Rank of First Listed Diagnosis	First Listed Diagnosis	Average Length of Stay
1. Diseases of the Respiratory system	201.9	3.5
Acute upper respiratory infections except influenza	(32.8)	(3.3)
Chronic disease of tonsils and adenoids	(58.8)	(1.7)
Pneumonia	(44.4)	(4.9)
Asthma	(24.3)	(3.9)
Acute bronchitis and bronchiolitis	(19.7)	(4.2)
2. Diseases of the digestive system	100.9	3.9
Noninfectious enteritis and colitis	(38.8)	(4.3)
Inguinal hernia	(18.0)	(2.3)
Appendicitis	(14.8)	(5.2)
3. Injury and poisoning	94.2	4.8
Fractures	(30.4)	(3.7)
Intracranial injuries	(14.8)	(3.6)
Lacerations and open wounds	(8.6)	(3.3)
4. Diseases of the nervous system and sense organs	70.8	3.4
Diseases of the ear and mastoid	(43.1)	(2.4)
Diseases of the central nervous system	(12.9)	(7.6)
5. Infectious and parasitic diseases	37.1	4.3
6. Congenital anomalies	36.4	5.7
7. Diseases of the genitourinary system	34.4	3.6
8. Symptoms, signs and ill-defined conditions	23.3	3.4
9. Disease of the skin and subcutaneous tissue	14.9	4.4
10. Diseases of the blood and blood forming organs	13.8	4.0

(Compiled from Haupt, B. *Utilization of short-stay hospitals: Annual summary for the U.S., 1980.* DHHS Publication No (PHS) 82-1721, Series 13, No. 64. Hyattsville, Md.: Public Health Service, 1982.)

Chronic Conditions

Chronic conditions are not common among children. This is because chronic conditions usually develop over long periods of time after exposure to environmental hazards or an unhealthy life-style. The bodies of children have not had a lifetime of exposure to such hazards and to the general stresses and strains of living. Nor has sufficient time passed between any harmful exposure and onset of these conditions because latency periods are quite long. Incidence of chronic conditions thus increases with age. Because most children do not have chronic conditions, the vast majority of children (96.1 percent) have no activity limitation related to such conditions. Of the 3.9 percent with activity limitation, about half are limited in major activity. Major activity refers to ability to work, keep house, or engage in school or preschool activities. Girls are more often limited in activity than boys, although differences are not striking, 4.2 percent versus 3.6 percent, respectively (Feller, 1981). Data from the 1950s and 1960s showed that the major causes of activity limitations in children under 17 seen by physicians were for asthma or hay fever (affecting 20.0 percent of children), impairments of lower extremities and hips (8.3 percent), paralysis (7.4 percent), chronic bronchitis and sinusitis (5.5 percent), mental and nervous conditions (3.8 percent), and heart conditions (3.7 percent). The ability to treat asthma, bronchitis, and heart conditions has improved; thus, they are now less frequently associated with limitation of activity than in the past. New technology has also improved functional ability in those with orthopedic impairments.

Major handicapping conditions in the under-17 age group include vision, hearing, and speech deficits, crippling emotional disturbance, mental retardation, and learning disability. Table 8–9 shows rates for selected orthopedic conditions and speech, visual, and hearing impairments in 1977 for children under 17 years of age by sex and race. Clearly, orthopedic impairments of the lower extremity or hip and the speech, hearing, and visual impairments are the most common of these handicapping conditions. Vision deficits, some hearing deficits, and crippling usually can limit physical function. Equally as important for children as physical function is the ability to function well in school and social settings. Emotional disturbances, mental retardation, learning disability or developmental lag, and speech deficits, as

TABLE 8–9. RATES OF SELECTED ORTHOPEDIC CONDITIONS AND OTHER IMPAIRMENTS BY SEX AND RACE, UNITED STATES, 1977

Impairment	Rate per 1000			
	Male	*Female*	*White*	*Nonwhite*
Orthopedic impairment				
of lower extremity or hip (except paralysis or absence)	20.8	16.7	19.5	15.2
of back or spine (except paralysis or absence)	3.0	7.4	5.7	2.8
of upper extremities or shoulder (except paralysis or absence)	2.3	1.2	1.9	1.0
paralysis, complete or partial	2.2	1.9	2.0	2.2
Speech impairments	19.8	10.5	14.3	19.9
Hearing impairments (including tinnitus)	16.0	12.5	14.9	11.2
Visual impairments	14.3	8.2	11.8	8.8

(From: Feller, B. *Prevalence of selected impairments, U.S., 1977.* DHHS Publication No. (PHS) 81-1562, Rockville, Md.: NCHS, 1981; excerpted from Tables 11 (p. 23), 9 (p. 30), 10 (p. 31), 6 (p. 27), 5 (p. 26), 4 (p. 25), 1 (p. 22).)

well as vision and hearing deficits, affect function in school and social settings.

MAJOR FOCI FOR PREVENTIVE EFFORTS

Prevention of Accidents

Because accidents affect more children than any other cause of morbidity and mortality, they are addressed first. Although changing human behavior has been considered, at times, as a potential method to reduce accidental injuries, this approach is probably less effective than some other strategies; this is so because modification of human behavior is expensive, time-consuming, and marginally effective, perhaps because the element of human error still remains. Passive measures requiring no action on the part of the individual are preferred. Airbags and passive seatbelts protect the individual without any action on his or her part. Sprinkler systems that turn on automatically in response to elevated air temperature are another example. A comprehensive approach employing countermeasures aimed at the three phases of the injury control sequence offers the most hope. The three phases are (1) preventing potentially injurious events, (2) minimizing the chance that injury will result in the event an accident occurs, and (3) reducing unnecessary consequences of injury (Haddon & Baker, 1981). Table 8–10 gives examples of these three types of interventions for various types of injuries that commonly affect children.

The measures for primary prevention bypass dependence on the human element of the moment and focus on structuring the

TABLE 8–10. STRATEGIES FOR REDUCING INJURIES DUE TO ACCIDENTS AMONG CHILDREN AND ADOLESCENTS

Event Type	Prevent Phase	Event Phase	Postevent Phase
Electrocution	Covered electric outlets Insulation on electrical tools	Circuit breakers Fuses	Portable defibrillators
Drowning	Fences around pools Stable watercraft Grading slopes of man-made lakes Swimming training	Lifelines, poles, rings, and jackets	Training public in resuscitation
Burns	Elimination of floor heaters Matches that burn with less heat and self-extinguish when dropped	Smoke detectors Flame retardant clothing and furnishings Alternate escape routes	Burn centers Skin grafting Occupational and psychological rehabilitation
Motor vehicle	Road design and maintenance Driver training Drunk driving laws Vehicle design and regular maintenance	Passive seat belts Air bags Paramedic teams	Emergency centers Rehabilitation centers
Poisoning	Childproof caps Locked storage	Poison control center emergency information lines Administration of antidotes	Emergency centers

environment through safer product design or designing safety features into the environment. For example, fences around swimming pools make unsupervised access difficult. Swimming instruction for children, while not a design feature, does reduce the likelihood of drowning because the child is better prepared to cope with water. These measures do not eliminate the need for adult supervision of children; they do, however, reduce the likelihood of accident when the attention of a supervisory adult is diverted.

The event-phase interventions focus on immediate response when an accident occurs; circuit breakers or fuses, for example, can cut off current. Throwing a rope, lifeline, or other aid to a swimmer in trouble can save a life. Smoke detectors alert occupants of a burning building to danger.

Once an accident has occurred, e.g., a child has been burnt or electrocuted, intervention strategies aim at restoring function. Defibrillators can restore the heartbeat of an electrocuted child, emergency transport services can maintain life on the way to the hospital treatment center, skin grafting and special care procedures at burn centers can save lives and minimize resulting morbidity and disability.

Health education is important to all three phases. If the general public is unaware of safer products they will not be used. Similarly, the public needs to be aware of behavioral means for reducing the likelihood of accidents; educating parents about growth and development of children gives them a basis for structuring the environment and the child's play activities appropriate to the child's ability. Parents need also to know basic facts that can correct misimpressions, for example, that it is possible for a child to drown in even a few inches of water. Instructions on first aid measures and where to call in the event of an emergency are also important.

Prevention of Infection

Prevention of the infectious causes of childhood morbidity and mortality begins with childhood immunizations during infancy and maintenance of booster immunizations during early childhood. Table 8–11 presents the schedule of recommended childhood immunizations, the effects of each disease, and the common reactions to the immunizations. Such artificial, active

TABLE 8–11. RECOMMENDED SCHEDULE OF CHILDHOOD IMMUNIZATIONS, EFFECTS OF DISEASE, AND REACTIONS TO IMMUNIZATIONS

Disease	Vaccine and Recommended Times of Administration	Disease Symptoms and Effects	Case-Fatality Rate	Reactions to Immunization
Diphtheria	Diphtheria, persussis, and tetanus toxoid (DPT), 2 months, 4 months, 6 months, 1½ years, and 4–6 years	Difficulty breathing Damage to heart, kidneys, and nerves	10%	Sore arm or lump at injection site Occasional fever 12–24 hours after vaccination
Tetanus (lockjaw)	Tetanus and diphtheria toxoid, 14–16 years Tetanus toxoid whenever contaminated puncture injury occurs—if no booster in 5 years	Painful muscular contractions Ear infections, pneumonia	50%	
Pertussis		Convulsions Brain disorder (rare)		
Polio	Trivalent oral polio-virus vaccine (TOPV)	Paralysis of arms or legs and respiratory muscles	10%	No common reactions
Measles	Measles vaccine, 15 months	High fever and rash (103°–105°) Pneumonia and ear infection Deafness, blindness, convulsions Brain disorders (1/1000 cases)	10%	Mild fever and rash within 10 days (10–20% of those vaccinated)
Rubella	Rubella vaccine, 15 months	Mild fever, rash and swollen glands Joint pains (especially in teens) Pregnant women—miscarriage, stillbirth, multiple birth defects		Occasional rash Low incidence of arm, leg, joint pains
Mumps	Mumps vaccine[a], 15 months	Fever and swelling of salivary glands Permanent deafness Inflammation of testicles in adolescent and adult males Temporary brain disorders		Fever and swelling of salivary glands (rare)

[a]May be given at 15 months as measles–rubella or measles–mumps–rubella combined vaccines.
(Adapted from data in Barrett-Connor, E. Immunization. In L. Schneiderman (Ed.), *The practice of preventive health care*. Menlo Park, Calif.: Addison-Wesley, 1981, pp. 64–65; and Rafers, K. Prevention in the medical care of children. In D. Clark & B. MacMahon (Eds.), *Preventive medicine and the community*. Boston: Little, Brown, 1981, p. 525.)

187

immunization against communicable disease confers protection directly on the recipient and indirectly on his or her associates by interfering with the chain of disease transmission, thus controlling infection in the community as well as in the individual (herd immunity). In the United States and Canada, routine active immunization of children against pertussis, poliomyelitis, measles, rubella, mumps, tetanus, and diphtheria is recommended. Active immunization against rabies is advocated after exposure. Although fewer than 5 cases per year are reported in the United States, the rate of case-fatality from this encephalitic disease approaches 100 percent. The frequency of the disease is increasing in wild animals, decreasing in domestic animals. More than 30,000 people nationally receive the rabies vaccine each year after possible exposure. Immunization against influenza is recommended in major epidemics and routinely for children who have special health problems likely to make the impact of the disease more severe, for example, children with cystic fibrosis or muscular dystrophy. BCG immunization is sometimes recommended for children with high exposure to tuberculosis, particularly repeated household exposures to patients with ineffectively treated sputum-positive tuberculosis.

General hygiene measures, including food and water handling practices, maintaining a clean house, teaching children basic hygiene practices like handwashing, and avoiding contact of infected individuals with children, particularly with a very young child or with ill children, can be helpful in primary prevention of many childhood gastrointestinal and respiratory infections. Plenty of rest and a well-balanced nutritionally adequate diet can also contribute to primary prevention of childhood infections. Health and sex education programs aimed at young teens can play an important role in preventing venereal diseases as well as teenage pregnancies.

Secondary prevention of childhood infections includes screening in high-risk groups for those infections with high prevalence, e.g., tuberculosis among inner city children. Because the incidence of even the commonest infections is low in the under 17-year age group, early case-finding is often more useful and cost-effective than is population screening. A complete history (including sexual history) and physical examination may be an effective method of detecting conditions such as gonorrhea; diagnosis can be confirmed by testing and treatment promptly instituted.

Prevention of Stress-Related Morbidity and Mortality

Included as stress-related conditions in childhood are child abuse, homicide, suicide, alcohol and drug abuse, and mental–emotional problems. Although accidents may, in some instances, be stress-related, they are discussed separately because they often have causes that are clearly not stress-related and because they account for such a large proportion of childhood morbidity and mortality.

Abuse of children is most often inflicted by a parent. Many homicides are also commited by family members. Suicides, alcohol and drug abuse, and other mental or emotional problems often arise out of difficult, unsupportive home environments. Add the pressures of peer relationships, and problems result. Primary prevention should begin before a child is born, perhaps as early as before a couple marries. Marriage requires maturity, a sense of self, and the ability to deal with the daily pressures of life. It is possible that high school family-living courses can help prepare young persons to approach marriage and family with more realistic expectations. More realistic expectations, by leading to a more supportive family environment for future children, could in turn contribute to decreasing the frequency of child abuse and other problems associated with a stressful family environment.

Similarly, pregnant women and their partners should be taught about child growth and development so they are prepared to deal with the demands of a growing child and the pressures on their own relationship that a child can produce. Approaches to maintaining the relationship of the parents can be discussed with the couple at this time. Such preparation can reduce family tension and create a more supportive atmosphere for both parents and children.

Health education programs in schools, on television, and for parents regarding drug, alcohol, and cigarette use and abuse may be of some help to youngsters who are tempted to try these substances. Enforcement of laws forbidding sale to and public consumption of these substances by underage children can prevent exposure of their bodies during childhood and thus at least postpone by a few years the onset, in adulthood, of acute and chronic health conditions caused by use and abuse of these substances. If a life-style free of use of these substances can be established prior to 18 years of age, perhaps young adults will be less prone to initiate use. An active community program of extracurricular activities offers children an opportunity for involvement in interesting activities that can build self-esteem and keep children sufficiently busy and involved that drugs, alcohol, and cigarettes offer little competition.

Secondary prevention of stress-related illness can involve both the parents and a spectrum of health-related professionals. Parents can be taught to watch for early signs of emotional problems and learn what resources are available to treat these problems. When effective communication between parent and child has been established early, the child may come to the parent for help before serious problems develop. Teachers, nurses, and the child's physician are all in a position to detect problems early and to provide the family with a referral for counseling. Counseling and rehabilitation centers, as well as medical facilities for treatment of physical effects of stress-related illness, are important in tertiary prevention of stress-related conditions.

Prevention of Sports Injuries

Participation in sports involves movements of the body that are exaggerations of those ordinarily performed and those not ordinarily performed, or movements performed in such a way that they place an unusual stress on the affected body parts. They may also call on performance qualities such as strength, speed, flexibility, coordination, agility, balance, or endurance. Although qualities may be essential to the sport, they may be poorly developed in an individual. Thus, physical preparation for any sport must be based on the particular demands and hazards of the sport and sufficient time must be permitted to develop adequately the necessary qualities. Types of potential injuries must be analyzed and equipment and environment structured to minimize injury. Thus, primary prevention involves five strategies: (1) preparticipation evaluation of prospective participants for suitability and documentation of status, (2) preparation of participants through careful training and conditioning, (3) provision of appropriate protective equipment, (4) development of correct participation techniques; and (5) control of the environment in which the sport will be practiced, particularly elimination of physical hazards, careful monitoring of climatic conditions, and control of spectators (Ryan, 1981).

Secondary prevention involves education of coaches and athletes to recognize signs of injury and the importance of reporting injury immediately. Prompt treatment may entail a brief period of disability from the sport, but allowing an injury to go untreated likely will lead to a longer period of disability at a later time. Athletes who have previously suffered an injury are at higher risk for subsequent injury. Treatment for sports injuries must continue over an adequate period of time to heal, and rehabilitative measures to restore strength, agility, and endurance, must be completed before returning to sports activity to prevent future injury.

Prevention of Dental Diseases

A complete set of healthy teeth is rare in adults. The measure of dental disease most frequently used, the sum of decayed, missing, and filled teeth (DMF), rises steadily with age due to the cumulative nature of the index. However, it is during the years following tooth eruption that susceptibility to dental caries is the greatest; subsequently it declines. Whites experience more dental caries than nonwhites, women slightly more than men.

Modifiable factors that affect the incidence of dental caries include the gross constituents of the diet, use of cigarettes, and fluoride. Table 8–12 lists the types of dental problems among children and strategies for prevention. Primary and secondary prevention strategies during childhood lead to improved dental health at older ages.

Nutrition has been mentioned in the previous discussions on prevention of infection and prevention of dental diseases. A good diet is essential to provide the necessary nutrients for general growth and development during childhood. Poor diet is also associated with specific conditions later in life, including obesity, high blood pressure, coronary heart disease, certain types of cancer, and diabetes. Since the seeds for development of these conditions may originate during childhood, a diet high in saturated fats, salt, sugar, and excess calories is to be avoided. The advent of more highly processed foods in supermarkets, and the increasing use of convenience foods or meals in fast-food restaurants, concurrent with the increased number of working women who have children, reduce the likelihood that children will get

TABLE 8–12. STRATEGIES FOR PREVENTION OF DENTAL DISEASE

Disease	Strategies for Primary Prevention
Dental caries	Appropriate diet
	Rough, fiberous components for mechanical cleansing of tooth surface
	Avoidance of sticky sweets
	Reduction or elimination of refined sugars
	Reducing bacterial population in mouth
	Oral hygiene
	Eliminate smoking
	Minimizing solubility of tooth enamel
	Fluoride
	Good prenatal nutrition
Malposition	Guide teeth into proper position as they erupt
	Prevent spaces from extraction of deciduous teeth
Trauma	Protective mouth guards for sports

proper preventive nutrition. Between 1958 and 1978 sales in fast food restaurants increased by 305 percent (DHHS, 1981). Information on nutrient content of foods and public education regarding healthy diets are imperative.

SUMMARY AND RECOMMENDATIONS

Many diseases of adulthood have their roots in the health status and ways of living developed during childhood. Arteriosclerotic heart disease and hypertension, for example, are thought to begin with plaque deposition in childhood that continues throughout adult life. Lung cancer and chronic respiratory disease due to smoking are to some extent time dependent; the earlier smoking begins, the sooner the disease onset. The minimum latency period is passed at an earlier age because tissues in youngsters are thought to be more susceptible than those of adults and because the number of packs of cigarettes smoked tend to increase over time. Thus, good diet, regular exercise, and obesity control in childhood may contribute to lower adult rates of arteriosclerotic heart disease. Not smoking reduces the risk for lung cancer, heart disease, and chronic respiratory diseases.

Similarly, disability resulting from childhood injury will carry over and affect the quality of adult health and life.

For these reasons, efforts toward developing positive health-related behaviors in children are crucial. Health education efforts cannot be limited to the children. Other sources of influence on their health-related behaviors include the family, school, peers, television, and the socio-economic and political community in which they live. Efforts must be made to encourage positive health behaviors in the family and in the wider community. Because of the enormous number of hours of exposure to television experienced by most children, efforts must be directed toward changing the negative images portrayed on television. The average preschooler spends more than 30 hours per week watching television, more than 6,000 hours before starting first grade. By the time of high school graduation, the average child has viewed 15,000 hours of television, about 4,000 hours more than was spent on formal education. Thus, the child is continually exposed to advertisements for foods that often offer empty calories or high fat content. Other negatives of television include emphasis on aggressive behavior, sex-stereotyping, over-the-counter drug use, and drinking (DHHS, 1981). Television potentially is a medium for promoting positive health messages. Until television provides more positive health emphases, all other avenues for promoting good health behavior in children must be pursued.

We have earlier outlined preventive approaches to some specific childhood health problems. In closing, we should like to advocate a regular program of preventive care. Pediatricians, school nurses, nurses in well-child clinics, school psychologists, teachers, and others who have regular contact with children should be aware of the recommended components of preventive and health maintenance procedures for children. Recommendations consistent with the Committee on Standards of Child Health Care of the American Society of Pediatrics (American Academy of Pediatrics, 1974) and the School Health Guide of the Committee on School Health of the American Academy of Pediatrics (American Academy of Pediatrics, 1977) are shown in Table 8–13. These recommendations are data based in that they are built on epidemiological evidence of normal growth and development, risk factors, and incidence and prevalence of childhood illness. The author would like to note, however, that she

TABLE 8–13. PREVENTIVE AND HEALTH MAINTENANCE PROCEDURES FOR CHILDREN BY AGE CATEGORY

12–23 Months

1. Up-to-date medical history recorded in permanent record, each visit
2. Physical examination recorded in permanent record, each visit
3. Record of length and weight recorded on standard growth chart, each visit
4. Age appropriate immunizations (measles, rubella, mumps, DTP, and TOPV)
5. Parental counseling and education on each visit concerning accidents, behavior, feeding, and social and emotional development
6. Developmental screening test, each visit

2 Years–School Entry

1. Up-to-date medical history recorded in permanent record, each visit
2. Physical examination recorded in permanent record, each visit
3. Height and weight recorded on standard growth chart, each visit
4. Vision screening test, each visit
5. Hearing screening test, each visit
6. Developmental screening test, each visit
7. Urine culture, females only
8. Age-appropriate immunizations (DTP, TOPV)
9. Dental screening examination, each visit (and dental supervision starting at age 3 years)
10. Parental education and counseling, each visit, concerning accidents, behavior, and social and emotional adjustment. Toward the end of this period, the child's school readiness should be discussed

For High-Risk Patients Only: 12 Months–School Entry

1. Blood–lead determination (screening test)
2. Tuberculin test
3. Serum lipid determination

School Entry–11 Years

1. Up-to-date medical history recorded in permanent record, each visit
2. Physical examination recorded in permanent record, each visit
3. Height and weight recorded on standard growth chart, each visit
4. Vision screening test (distant vision, eye–muscle balance), each visit
5. Hearing screening test (sweep–check audiometry), each visit
6. Immunizations, if not already acquired
7. Patient and parent counseling and education concerning water safety and swimming courses, bicycle safety instruction, and use of automobile safety devices; inquiry about adjustment problems (e.g., school phobia) and learning problems
8. Tuberculin test, for high-risk populations, each visit

TABLE 8–13. *(cont.)* **PREVENTIVE AND HEALTH MAINTENANCE PROCEDURES FOR CHILDREN BY AGE CATEGORY**

12–20 Years

1. Up-to-date history recorded in permanent record
2. Physical examination recorded in permanent record
3. Hemoglobin or hematocrit determination, optional, females
4. Tetanus and diphtheria booster immunization
5. Screening test for visual acuity
6. Patient education and counseling concerning safety (driver training, water safety), drug use, cigarette smoking, and sexual development and activity
7. Tuberculin test (high-risk population)

(Adapted from Rogers, K. Prevention of medical care of children. In D. Clark & B. MacMahon (Eds.), *Preventive medicine and the community.* Boston: Little, Brown, 1981, pp. 545–546.)

feels that certain recommended procedures, for example, counseling as to drug use, smoking, and sexual development and sexual activity need to begin between the ages of school entry and 11 years rather than beginning at 12 to 15 years as in the original recommendations. Physicians and nurses in clinical practice who follow this basic schedule of primary and secondary prevention can do much to contribute to healthy children and healthy adults. It is particularly important that such programs be readily accessible to disadvantaged groups in our society, those whose children are at higher risk for childhood morbidity and mortality. These same groups, also at higher risk of illness and death at older ages, would derive considerable long-term health benefit from such programs. In conjunction with public health efforts to control environmental hazards and to educate the public about healthful living and social programs in maternal–child health and nutrition, these efforts could do much toward assuring the optimal health of children.

REFERENCES

American Academy of Pediatrics. Committee on Standards of Child Health Care. *Recommendations for Preventive Health Care.* Evanston, Ill.: American Academy of Pediatrics, 1974.

American Academy of Pediatrics. Committee on School Health. *School Health Guide*. Evanston, Ill.: American Academy of Pediatrics, 1977.

Barrett-Conner, E. Immunization. In Schneiderman, L. (Ed.), *The practice of preventive health care*. Menlo Park, Calif.: Addison-Wesley, 1981.

Bloom, B. Current estimates from the National Health Interview Survey: United States, 1981. *Vital and Health Statistics,* series 10, No. 141. DHHS Publication No. (PHS) 83-1569. Washington, D.C.: U.S. Government Printing Office, 1982b.

Dever, A. *Epidemiology of Health Services Management*. Baltimore, Md.: Aspen Systems, 1984.

Ezzati, T., & McLemore, T. *The national ambulatory medical care survey, 1977 summary U.S., Jan.–Dec. 1977*. DHHS Publication No. (PHS) 80-1799, Series 13, No. 44. Hyattsville, Md.: National Center for Health Statistics, April 1980.

Feller, B. *Prevalence of selected impairments, U.S. 1977*. DHHS Publication No. (PHS) 81-1562. Hyattsville, Md.: National Center for Health Statistics, Feb. 1981.

Fisher, L. A. Fact Sheet #1 on the Child Passenger Protection Bill (HB-605)—Fisher (D-16), handout to Ohio Senate. Columbus, Ohio, 1983.

Haddon, Jr. W., & Baker, S. Injury control. In Clark, D. & McMahon, B. (Eds.), *Prevention and community medicine*. Boston: Little, Brown, 1981, pp. 109–140.

Haupt, B. *Utilization of short-stay hospitals: Annual summary for the U.S. 1980*. DHHS Publication No. (PHS) 82-1721, Series 13, No. 64. Hyattsville, Md.: National Center for Health Statistics, March 1982.

National Center for Health Statistics. Advance Report of Final Mortality Statistics, 1981, *Monthly Vital Statistics Report, 33*(3, suppl.) Washington, D.C.: PHS, 1984a.

National Center for Health Statistics. *U.S. Yearbook 1980*, Rockville, Md.: PHS, 1984b.

National Safety Council. *Accident Facts, 1982,* New York, 1984.

Ries, P. *Americans assess their health: U.S. 1978*. Publication No. (PHS) 83-1570, Series 10, No. 142. Hyattsville, Md.: National Center for Health Statistics, March 1983.

Rogers, K. Prevention in Medical Care of Children. In D. Clark, & B. McMahon (Eds.). *Preventive medicine and the community*. Boston: Little, Brown, 1981, pp. 523–550.

Ryan, A. Prevention of Sports Injuries. In L. Schneiderman (ed.), *The practice of preventive health care*. Menlo Park, Calif.: Addison-Wesley, 1981, pp. 96–123.

U.S. Department of Health and Human Services.. *Better health for our children: A national strategy*, The Report of the Select Panel for the

Promotion of Child Health (vol. III). DHHS (PHS) Publication No. 79-55071, 1981.

U.S. Public Health Service. *Health, U.S., 1980–81.* Rockville, Md., 1982.

Verbrugge, L. Sex differentials in health. *Public Health Reports,* 1982, *97* (5), 415–421.

Patterns of Morbidity and Mortality in Young and Middle Adulthood

The health of young and middle-aged adults is of critical importance, both because of the desire for assuring high quality of life during the adult years, and also because of society's need to maintain an active and healthy labor force. Because persons 25 to 64 years of age constitute most of the labor force, they provide the economic security base for themselves as well as for dependent children, adolescents, disabled persons, and older adults.

As of 1982, there were approximately 110 million Americans who were 25 to 65 years of age. These working-age adults accounted for about 48 percent of the total U.S. population (U.S. News and World Report, 1984), 3 percent less than the total proportion of working-age adults in 1940, but 4 percent more than the proportion of working-age adults in 1970 (NCHS 1978). The number of adults in the 24 to 44 age group in 1982 was approximately 66 million, whereas the number of adults in the 45 to 64 age group was approximately 44 million.

According to national health surveys conducted in 1978 and 1981, young and middle-aged adults, overall, perceive themselves to be relatively healthy. Ninety-two percent of the young adults report "good or excellent" health for these years, whereas only 3 percent of this age group report "fair or poor" health. Seventy-eight percent of the 45- to 64-year olds rated their health status as "good or excellent", whereas 22 percent rated their health status as "fair or poor" (NCHS, 1983b; Reis, 1983).

There are no major differences in the self-reported health ratings for men and women in middle adulthood, despite the fact that men have much higher rates of mortality from debilitating conditions such as heart disease, cerebrovascular disease, and malignancies. Black Americans in young and middle adulthood report "fair or poor" health almost twice as frequently as do white Americans during these years, and their higher mortality and morbidity rates correspond to these ratings (NCHS, 1981). Life tables also suggest that white persons, overall, are healthier than black persons. At age 45, the average white person in the United States has 31.8 remaining years of life, whereas the average black person has 29 remaining years of life (NCHS, 1978).

MAJOR CAUSES OF MORTALITY

Overall, mortality during the young and middle adult years has markedly declined over the decades, from rates of 1200 per 100,000 persons in 1900 to a rate of 566 per 100,000 persons in 1981 (DHEW, 1979; NCHS, 1984). Since 1950, mortality among young adults of 25 to 44 years of age has decreased by one-third, primarily because of decreasing numbers of deaths due to cancer and heart disease. Mortality rates have declined by one-fourth during this 30-year period for adults in the 45- to 64-year age group, and the decreased rates have mostly been for heart disease and strokes (NCHS, 1982a).

Current mortality rates for persons in young and middle adulthood are higher than the rates for children and adolescents, though they are much lower than the rates for persons 65 years of age and older. Compiled vital statistics data for 1981 (NCHS, 1981) show mortality rates for persons 25 to 44 years of age to be 178.8 per 100,000 population and rates for persons 45 to 64 years of age to be 954.0 per 100,000 population. As might be expected, mortality rates consistently increase for each age decade, with 132.2 deaths per 100,000 for the 25- to 34-year olds, 225.4 deaths per 100,000 for the 35- to 44-year olds, 570.3

deaths per 100,000 for the 45- to 55-year olds, and 1337.7 deaths per 100,000 for the 56- to 65-year old group. These rates are shown in Table 9–1.

Variations in Mortality by Sex and Race

A comparison of the 1981 mortality rates for young and middle-aged adults across gender and race (Table 9–1) show an unequal distribution of mortality for men and women as well as for blacks and whites. Men have higher death rates than do women for each decade of adulthood, with an overall rate of 758.8 deaths per 100,000 persons versus a rate of 392.4 per 100,000 persons for women. The higher mortality among young adult males is primarily due to excessive deaths from accidents, homicides, and suicides, whereas the higher mortality rates among men in the middle adult years are primarily due to deaths from heart disease and malignancies, especially cancer of the lung (Table 9–2).

During the middle adult years, men are three times as likely as women to die of heart disease (NCHS, 1982a, 1983a). This gender difference is partly due to the higher levels of smoking, hypertension, and cholesterol among men. Preventive health programs during the 1970s have begun to be successful in lowering such risk factors as well as in reducing mortality from cardiovascular disease (DHEW, 1979).

TABLE 9–1. MORTALITY RATES PER 100,000 FOR 5-YEAR PERIODS WITHIN YOUNG AND MIDDLE ADULTHOOD, WITH COMPARISONS ACROSS GENDER AND RACE, 1981

Age	All	Men	Women	Blacks	Whites
25–29	128.7	190.5	67.4	231.1	115.1
30–34	137.7	190.8	81.6	284.8	117.3
35–39	180.1	240.6	121.5	293.7	155.7
40–44	270.6	353.4	191.0	560.0	236.5
45–49	441.8	575.6	315.4	842.6	397.1
50–54	698.8	920.9	493.1	1247.4	644.8
55–59	1066.4	1427.8	744.4	1783.9	1002.1
60–64	1608.9	2171.1	1124.8	2469.0	1537.9
(25–64)	566.4	758.8	392.4	976.6	525.9

(From Advanced report of final mortality statistics, 1981. *Monthly Vital Statistics Report,* 33(3, Suppl.) Washington, D.C.: National Center for Health Statistics, 1984, Table I.)

TABLE 9–2. MORTALITY RATES PER 100,000 BY SELECTED CAUSES FOR YOUNG AND MIDDLE-AGED ADULTS, ACROSS RACE, GENDER, AND AGE, 1980

	Age 25–34					Age 35–44				
Cause	All	White Male	White Female	Black Male	Black Female	All	White Male	White Female	Black Male	Black Female
Diseases of the heart	8.3	9.1	3.9	30.3	15.7	44.6	61.8	16.4	136.6	61.7
Malignancies	13.7	13.7	13.5	14.1	18.3	48.6	41.8	50.9	73.8	73.5
Cerebrovascular diseases	2.6	2.0	2.0	7.7	7.0	8.5	6.5	6.7	29.2	21.6
Motor vehicle accidents	29.1	46.6	12.2	44.9	10.6	20.9	30.7	10.6	41.2	8.3
Homicides and legal interventions	19.6	18.9	4.3	145.1	25.8	15.1	15.5	4.1	110.3	17.7
Suicides	16.0	25.6	7.5	21.8	4.1	15.4	23.5	9.1	15.6	4.6

	Age 45–54					Age 55–64				
Cause	All	White Male	White Female	Black Male	Black Female	All	White Male	White Female	Black Male	Black Female
Diseases of the Heart	180.2	269.8	71.2	433.4	202.4	494.1	730.6	248.1	987.2	530.1
Malignancies	180.0	175.4	166.4	333.0	230.2	436.1	497.4	355.5	812.5	430.4
Cerebrovascular diseases	25.2	21.7	18.7	82.1	61.9	65.2	64.2	48.7	189.8	138.7
Motor vehicle accidents	18.6	26.3	10.2	39.1	9.1	17.4	23.9	10.5	40.3	9.3
Homicides and legal interventions	11.1	11.9	3.0	83.8	12.5	7.0	7.8	2.1	55.6	8.9
Suicides	15.9	24.2	10.2	12.0	2.5	15.9	25.8	9.1	11.7	2.3

(From National Center for Health Statistics. Health, United States, 1983. DHHS Publication No. (PHS) 83–1232, Washington, D.C.: U.S. Government Printing Office, December 1983, Tables 16–22.)

The different mortality patterns of blacks versus whites in young and middle adulthood are as striking as the differences between men and women. For each decade of the adult years, black persons have a higher percentage of deaths, with an overall mortality rate of 976.6 per 100,000 persons versus a rate of 525.9 per 100,000 persons for whites (Table 9–1). Among young adults in the 25 to 34 age group, violent deaths from homicides and legal interventions account for much of the higher mortality of blacks. Black males in this age group are eight times as likely as white males to die from violence, whereas black females are six times as likely as white females to die from violence (NCHS, 1982a). Among 25- to 34-year-old adults, blacks also have much higher death rates from heart disease, and in the 35 to 44 age group blacks more frequently die of malignancies and heart disease.

In comparison with white persons, black persons in the middle adult years traditionally have had higher death rates from certain malignancies, e.g., stomach and esophogeal, as well as from heart disease, strokes, and cirrhosis of the liver (Rudov and Santangelo, 1979). Fortunately, the death rates for many of these diseases have declined in the 1970s, and although the rates for blacks are still much higher than for whites, preventive programs have begun to demonstrate some success in reducing excessive risk factors for chronic disease (such as high blood pressure and cigarette smoking) among the black population (NCHS, 1983a).

Variations in Mortality by Age

Reviewing the ten major causes of death for each decade of young and middle adulthood (Table 9–3), one sees that many of the diseases or conditions that cause high mortality are represented in each of the different age groups. The ranking of the conditions by mortality rates within each age group does differ, however.

Accidents, suicides, and homicides and legal interventions are the three leading causes of death among the 25- to 34-year-olds. Overall, the death rates for these causes have increased since the 1950s, though they have declined during the 1970s (NCHS, 1982a). Currently, the three causes account for 80 deaths per 100,000 adults in the 25 to 34 age group, whereas the

TABLE 9-3. DEATH RATES PER 100,000 FOR THE TEN LEADING CAUSES OF MORTALITY IN EACH DECADE OF YOUNG AND MIDDLE ADULTHOOD, 1981

Age 25–34		Age 34–44		Age 45–54		Age 55–64	
Cause	Rate	Cause	Rate	Cause	Rate	Cause	Rate
Accidents and adverse effects	45.1	Malignancies	47.2	Malignancies	128.1	Heart disease	481.5
Homicides and legal interventions	18.5	Heart disease	43.2	Heart disease	177.7	Malignancies	434.8
Suicide	16.3	Accidents and adverse effects	35.7	Accidents and adverse effects	37.7	Cerebrovascular diseases	62.9
Malignancies	14.0	Suicide	15.9	Liver disease	28.3	Chronic obstructive pulmonary disease	43.3
Heart diseases	8.4	Homicides and legal interventions	14.4	Cerebrovascular diseases	24.9	Accidents	40.4
Liver disease	3.1	Liver disease	12.2	Suicide	16.6	Liver disease	39.3
Cerebrovascular diseases	2.6	Cerebrovascular diseases	8.4	Homicides and legal interventions	11.3	Diabetes	25.6
Pneumonia and influenza	1.5	Diabetes mellitus	3.5	Chronic obstructive pulmonary disease	10.0	Pneumonia and influenza	18.4
Diabetes mellitus	1.4	Pneumonia and influenza	3.3	Diabetes mellitus	9.6	Suicide	16.4
Congenital anomalies	1.3	Chronic obstructive pulmonary disease	1.7	Pneumonia and influenza	7.4	Kidney diseases	8.8

(From Advanced report of final mortality statistics, 1981. *Monthly Vital Statistics Report*, 33(3, Suppl.). Washington D.C.: National Center for Health Statistics, June 22, 1984, Table 4.)

other seven causes of death account for 32.3 deaths per 100,000. Malignancies are still the fourth leading cause of death among the 25- to 34-year-olds, though mortality from most malignancies has been steadily declining for young adults since the middle 1960s (NCHS, 1982a).

Malignancies and diseases of the heart are the two current leading causes of death for persons 35 to 54 years of age. Women are more likely to die from breast cancer, whereas men have high death rates from lung cancer and from heart disease (NCHS, 1982a). Fatal accidents are the third leading cause of death for 35- to 54-year old adults, with a mortality rate of 35.7 per 100,000 for persons 35 to 44 years of age and a rate of 37.7 per 100,000 for persons 45 to 54 years of age (Table 9–3).

In the last decade of middle adulthood (55 to 64 years), heart disease is the leading cause of death and malignancies are the second most frequent cause of death. Other chronic diseases, such as strokes, chronic lung disease (COPD), and diabetes mellitus, also kill many persons in the 55- to 64-year age group. Although accidents rank as the fifth cause of death in late middle adulthood, the actual rates of accidents are quite constant throughout the young and middle adult years, decreasing only 5 percent from young adulthood to late middle age (Table 9–3).

Overall, the ten leading causes of death for young and middle-aged adults reflect a combination of acute and chronic illness conditions, with a pattern of increasing chronicity emerging over the 40-year period. From a public health perspective, many of the deaths, including those due to accidents, homicides, and suicides, as well as those caused by chronic illness, are largely preventable. About 50 percent of the deaths from accidents, for instance, are motor vehicle casualties (NCHS, 1981). To the extent that these accidents are alcohol-related, stricter enforcement of drinking laws should result in fewer deaths. Fatal automobile accidents related to other causes, as well as accidents in the home and in recreational areas, may also be curtailed by more effective health education programs in the schools, other institutions, and public media. Interventions to prevent fatal work-related accidents may necessitate more effective education efforts as well as more strict monitoring of the Occupational Safety Health Administration (OSHA) requirements.

The cardiovascular diseases are still the leading causes of death for young and middle-aged Americans, though mortality from these disease conditions steadily has decreased since the mid-1960s (NCHS, 1983a). Advances in medical research, diagnoses and treatment, and prevention programs, which have focused on the identification and alleviation of chronic disease risk factors, have all contributed to this decrease (DHEW, 1979). Because the prevalence and mortality rates due to the cardiovascular diseases, as well as many other diseases, are highest among black Americans and persons of low income groups, these high-risk groups should be given priority in prevention efforts (DHEW, 1979; Rudov and Santangelo, 1979).

Fatalities from suicide and homicide during the adult years present a very challenging problem. Better understanding of the direct causes of violence, as well as the possible predisposing factors such as social stressors, mental illness, and childhood abuse is probably necessary in order to plan effective prevention programs. Stronger economic support for mental health and social service programs as well as legislation to control handguns and other means of violence may help to lower the death rates from homicide and suicide.

MAJOR CAUSES OF MORBIDITY

Acute Conditions

As noted in the previous chapter, acute conditions refer to illnesses of short duration that are serious enough to require medical attention or that result in brief periods of restricted activity. The estimated incidence rates for specific types of acute illness episodes are available from the National Health Interview Survey data published by the Center for Health Statistics (Givens, 1979), the National Ambulatory Medical Care Survey (Cypress, 1981), and listings of reportable infectious diseases (CDC, 1981). Diagnostic listings for short-stay hospitalizations are also available (Haupt, 1982).

The classifications of acute illnesses in the National Health Interviews include (1) respiratory conditions, (2) infectious and parasitic diseases, (3) injuries and poisonings, (4) digestive system disorders, and (5) other miscellaneous conditions. The number of acute conditions reported by young and middle-aged adults for 1978 is shown in Table 9–4, and the number of work

TABLE 9–4. NUMBER OF ACUTE ILLNESS EPISODES REPORTED BY YOUNG AND MIDDLE-AGED ADULTS, 1977–1978 (RATES PER 100 PERSONS)

Type of Illness Episode	Age					
	17–44			45 and over		
	All	*Men*	*Women*	*All*	*Men*	*Women*
Respiratory conditions	116.6	107.7	125.0	66.7	58.3	73.7
Upper respiratory	55.9	51.0	60.5	29.8	26.6	32.5
Influenza	55.5	52.3	58.4	31.9	27.5	35.6
Other	5.3	4.4	6.1	5.0	4.2	5.6
Infective and parasitic diseases	22.3	17.2	27.1	9.4	7.7	10.7
Injuries	36.4	44.0	29.2	24.5	24.1	24.9
Digestive system disorders	11.2	10.6	11.9	7.4	6.5	8.2
Other acute conditions	37.9	23.2	51.7	21.1	17.7	23.4
All acute conditions listed	224.5	202.7	244.9	129.1	114.4	141.4

(From Givens, J. *Current estimates from the health interview survey: United States, 1978.* DHEW Publication No. (PHS) 80–1551, Series 10, No. 130. Hyattsville, Md.: National Center for Health Statistics, November 1979, Table 2.)

days lost because of these conditions is shown in Table 9–5. Overall, the young adults, aged 17 to 44, report many more acute illness episodes than do adults who are 45 years of age and older, with 224.5 episodes per 100 persons versus 129.1 episodes per 100 older persons. Women report more acute conditions than do men, with an average of 193.7 acute illnesses per 100 versus the male average of 158.6 acute illnesses per 100 persons.

Among the young adult group, the respiratory conditions are the most frequently reported type of acute illness for both men and women. Upper respiratory tract infections and influenza account for about equal numbers of these illness episodes. Although the respiratory illnesses rarely have fatal consequences in young adulthood, they do cause much discomfort as well as loss of work days. In 1978, young adult males lost 149.2 days of work per 100 employed persons because of respiratory illnesses, and young females lost 183 days of work per 100 employed persons, an average of 1.5 and 1.8 days per person, respectively.

TABLE 9–5. DAYS LOST FROM WORK FOR ACUTE ILLNESS EPISODES, REPORTED BY YOUNG AND MIDDLE-AGED ADULTS, 1977–1978 (DAYS PER 100 EMPLOYED PERSONS)

Type of Illness Episode	Age					
	17–44			45 and over		
	All	Men	Women	All	Men	Women
Respiratory conditions	163.4	149.2	183.0	151.8	140.4	169.5
Infective and parasitic diseases	29.7	28.9	30.8	15.0	13.9	16.8
Injuries	111.3	121.4	97.4	109.9	99.5	126.1
Digestive system disturbances	24.4	22.6	27.0	19.3	21.3	16.3
Other acute conditions	59.7	31.7	98.0	56.0	41.7	78.3

(From Givens, J. *Current estimates from the health interview survey: United States, 1978.* DHEW Publication No. (PHS) 80–1551; Series 10, No. 130. Hyattsville, Md.: National Center for Health Statistics, November 1979, Table 8.)

Injuries are the second most frequently reported of the acute conditions among young adult males (44 injuries per 100 persons), and they are the third most frequently reported acute condition among young females (29.2 injuries per person). The work days lost because of injuries almost equals those lost because of the respiratory conditions, 121.4 days per 100 working males and 97.4 days per 100 working females.

Infectious and parasitic diseases and digestive system disorders account for only moderate numbers of the acute illness episodes in early adulthood. Young females report a greater number of infections than do men (27.1 per 100 women versus 17.2 per 100 men), though their loss of work days because of the infections are only slightly higher than those for men. Women also report greater numbers of miscellaneous acute conditions, and they lose three times as many work days because of these conditions as do their male counterparts. Overall, acute illness episodes among young adults during 1978 resulted in a loss of 388.6 work days per 100 working persons, or approximately 4 work days per person.

The pattern of acute illness reported in 1978 by persons who were 45 years of age and older is similar to that reported by the younger adults, though persons in the older age group had fewer episodes of acute illness and fewer loss of work days. As in the young adult group, the respiratory conditions were the most frequently reported type of acute illness. These illnesses may pose greater risks for older adults than for younger adults because complications are more likely to occur. The work days lost because of older adults' respiratory illness episodes were almost equal to the number of work days lost in the younger population, despite the fact that fewer illness episodes were reported by older persons. For men 45 years of age and older 140.4 work days per 100 persons were lost, whereas for men under 45 years of age 142.2 work days per 100 persons were lost.

Physicians' reports of patients' ambulatory office visits provide additional information concerning acute illness episodes that usually are not serious enough to require hospitalization. The five most frequent symptom-related reasons for office visits during 1977 and 1978, for each decade of young and middle adulthood, are shown in Table 9–6. The listing is a shortened version of the National Center for Health Statistics publication of the principal reasons for office visits (Cypress, 1981), excluding the visits for general medical examinations, for routine gynecological and prenatal examinations, and for postoperative examinations.

Table 9–6 demonstrates the pattern of increasing chronicity with advancing age in young and middle adulthood. Many of the office visits of young adults, aged 25 to 34 years, are for acute illness symptoms such as sore throats, headaches, colds, skin problems, and abdominal pain, whereas the visits of persons 55 to 64 years of age are more frequently for blood pressure testing and control of diagnosed hypertension. Young and middle-aged adults made about equal numbers of symptom-related office visits during 1978, though when visits for examination and prenatal and postpartum care are included, young adults much more frequently visited physicians.

There are definite differences in the physician visit patterns for men versus women in the young and middle adult years (Table 9–7). Women in this age group more frequently visit physicians than do men, and many of their symptom visits are for headaches and weight gain problems. Men have fewer visits, but the visits are for more ominous symptoms such as chest pain and high blood pressure (Table 9–6). Back symptoms appear to pose a persistent problem for both men and women in the middle adult years, and they are the number one reason for physi-

TABLE 9–6. FIVE MOST FREQUENT SYMPTOM-RELATED REASONS FOR PHYSICIAN OFFICE VISITS, FOR YOUNG AND MIDDLE-AGED ADULTS, 1977–1978

Reason for Visit	No. of Visits in Thousands	Reason for Visit	No. of Visits in Thousands
Men, Age 25–34		*Women, Age 25–34*	
Back symptoms	2270	Throat symptoms	2959
Throat symptoms	2051	Weight gain	2813
Headache	1237	Abdominal pain	2730
Chest pain	1138	Skin problems	2002
Colds	1132	Headache	2001
Men, Age 35–44		*Women, Age 35–44*	
Back symptoms	1725	Weight gain	2571
Chest pain	1220	Headache	1857
Blood pressure test	1097	Throat symptoms	1836
Throat symptoms	1024	Back symptoms	1818
Headache	902	Anxiety or nerves	1639
Men, Age 45–54		*Women, Age 45–54*	
Blood pressure test	2176	Blood pressure test	2341
Back symptoms	1955	Back symptoms	2109
Hypertension	1554	Headache	2039
Chest pain	1207	Weight gain	2037
Low back pain	1035	Hypertension	1762
Men, Age 55–64		*Women, Age 55–64*	
Blood pressure test	2671	Blood pressure test	3812
Chest pain	2261	Hypertension	2623
Hypertension	2119	Back symptoms	2025
Back symptoms	1955	Headache	1660
Diabetes mellitus	1184	Abdominal pain	1611

Listings exclude visits for routine physicals, prenatal and postopertive examinations.
(Adapted from Cypress, B. *Patients' reasons for visiting physicians: National ambulatory medical care survey, United States 1977–78.* DHEW Publication No. (PHS) 82–1717, December 1981, Tables 3–4.)

cian office visits for young men, 25 to 34 years of age (Cypress, 1981). More effective education messages regarding prevention of back injuries are obviously needed.

The number of physician-reported notifiable diseases for young and middle-aged adults during 1980 is shown in Table 9–8. The table shows a higher rate of acute infections among

TABLE 9–7. TOTAL PHYSICAL OFFICE VISITS AND PERCENT OF EXAMINATION VISITS FOR MEN AND WOMEN IN YOUNG AND MIDDLE ADULTHOOD, 1977–1978 (NUMBER OF VISITS IN THOUSANDS)

Age	All Visits	Male Visits	% Exam Visits	Female Visits	% Exam Visits
25–34	177,100	54,675	4.8	122,425	26.9
35–44	123,884	47,124	3.7	76,760	6.1
45–54	138,327	54,608	4.7	83,719	4.5
55–64	145,344	60,826	5.1	84,518	5.0
Total	584,655	217,233		367,422	

(Adapted from Cypress, B. *Patients' reasons for visiting physicians: National ambulatory medical care survey.* United States 1977–78. DHEW Publication No. (PHS) 82–1717, December, 1981, Tables 3 and 4.)

younger adults. As in the adolescent population, the incidence of gonorrhea cases is far greater than that for any of the other reportable diseases. There were 329,097 cases among the 25- to 39-year-old adults and 26,994 cases among the 40- to 59-year-old adults. Hepatitis A, salmonellosis, and shigella infections had the second, third, and fourth highest incidence rates in the middle adult years, though the rates for these infections were significantly lower than those among the adolescent population (CDC, 1981).

TABLE 9–8. MOST PREVALENT NOTIFIABLE DISEASES AMONG YOUNG AND MIDDLE-AGED ADULTS, 1980

Disease Condition	Number of Reported Cases	
	Ages 25–39	*Ages 40–59*
Gonorrhea	329,097	26,994
Salmonellosis	3,480	2,415
Hepatitis A	9,270	3,159
Shigellosis	2,351	910
Measles	300	35
Mumps	154	67
Typhoid fever	106	54

(From Annual summary, 1980: Reported morbidity and mortality in the United States. *Morbidity and Mortality Weekly Reports,* 1981, 29(54).)

Chronic Conditions

Listings of the ten most prevalent chronic health problems for young and middle-aged adults in 1981, as identified in the National Health Interview Survey, are shown in Table 9–9. Among the 17- to 44-year-old adults, chronic sinusitis, hay fever, and orthopedic impairments were the three most prevalent chronic conditions, whereas hypertension, arthritis and rheumatism, and hearing impairments were the fourth to sixth most prevalent problems.

Of the five most prevalent chronic health problems reported by young adults in 1981, the prevalence rate had increased only for sinusitis and hay fever since 1979. The prevalence rate had decreased for orthopedic impairments, hypertension, and arthritis and rheumatism. Heart conditions were the ninth most prevalent type of chronic health problem for young adults in 1979, but they had dropped to the eleventh most prevalent type of problem by 1981 (NCHS, 1981, 1981a).

The 1981 prevalence rates for chronic conditions were generally higher for the 45- to 64-year-old adults than for the young adults, with the middle-aged persons having more disabling conditions such as arthritis and rheumatism, hypertension, hearing impairments, heart disease, and diabetes. The most prevalent chronic conditions among the middle-aged adults were the arthritic and rheumatoid diseases. The combined prevalence rate for these two conditions was 246.5 cases per 1000 persons (Table 9–9).

From 1979 to 1981, there was a slight decrease in the prevalence rates for chronic sinusitis, heart disease, arthritis and rheumatism, and diabetes among adults 45 to 64 years of age. The prevalence rates for hypertension and hearing impairments in this age group increased during this period (Table 9–9). Much of this increase is believed to be due to improved diagnosis and public awareness, however. Intensive national educational efforts have led to the diagnosis and treatment of many cases of hypertension that normally would not have been detected (DHEW, 1979), and screening for hearing impairments also has improved.

In assessing functional disabilities related to chronic health problems during the years of 1978 and 1979, 8.5 percent of adults in the 17 to 44 age group and 23.6 percent of the adults in the 45 to 64 age group reported activity limitations (Givens, 1979). About 5.1 per 1000 of the young adults and 20.6 per 1000

TABLE 9–9. LISTINGS OF THE TEN MOST PREVALENT CHRONIC HEALTH PROBLEMS FOR YOUNG AND MIDDLE-AGED ADULTS IN 1981, WITH COMPARISONS OF PREVALENCE RATES FOR 1979

Young Adults: 17–44			Middle-Aged Adults: 54–64		
Rank by Prevalence in 1981	Prevalence Rates		Rank by Prevalence in 1981	Prevalence Rates	
	1979	1981		1979	1981
Chronic sinusitis	148.4	158.4	Arthritis and rheumatism	252.7	246.5
Hay fever (without asthma)	92.3	100.2	Hypertension	214.4	243.7
Orthopedic impairments	95.2	90.5	Chronic sinusitis	189.2	177.5
Hypertension	58.8	54.2	Hearing impairments	119.2	142.9
Arthritis and rheumatism	47.8	47.7	Heart conditions	128.5	122.7
Hearing impairments	44.9	43.8	Orthopedic impairments	117.9	117.5
Hemorrhoids	48.5	43.7	Hay fever (without asthma)	69.3	77.5
Eczema, dermatitis	37.2	39.8	Hemorrhoids	64.7	66.6
Migraine headaches	—	38.7	Diabetes	57.9	56.9
Acne	46.7	38.5	Visual impairments	58.2	55.2

(From *Vital and Health Statistics*, Series 10, No. 136 Hyattsville Md.: National Center for Health Statistics, 1979; and unpublished data from the National Center for Health Statistics, 1981.)

of the middle-aged adults needed help with at least one basic physical activity such as walking, bathing, dressing, using the toilet, going outside, or eating. Walking was the primary physical activity affected by chronic illness during middle adulthood. About 1.5 percent of men 45 to 64 years of age and 1.2 percent of women in this age group reported that they needed assistance with walking. Home management activities, especially those activities requiring ambulation, were also difficult for many middle-aged adults. About 24.9 per 1000 adults in the 45 to 64 age group reported need for help with shopping, household chores, preparing meals, or taking care of finances (Feller, 1983).

Hospitalization Episodes for Acute and Chronic Illness

Eleven percent of young adults and 15 percent of middle-aged adults polled in health interviews of 1978 reported hospitalizations for the previous year (Givens, 1979). The rates of "first listed diagnoses" for adults discharged from short-stay hospitals during 1980 are shown in Table 9–10. These diagnoses may represent single, acute illness episodes or recurrent exacerbations of more chronic serious illnesses.

According to the data in Table 9–10, adults in the 15 to 44 age group were primarily hospitalized for acute conditions, with genitourinary tract problems, injuries and poisonings, and digestive system disturbances accounting for most hospitalizations. Other problems requiring short-stay hospitalizations in this age group included mental disorders (with 284,000 admissions for psychotic episodes and 233,000 admissions for alcoholism treatment), complications of pregnancy, and diseases of the musculoskeletal system.

Adults in the 45 to 64 age group were hospitalized with a variety of acute and chronic illness conditions during 1980 (Table 9–10). The cardiovascular diseases (circulatory system diseases) required the largest numbers of short-stay hospitalizations among this age group, with 1,711,000 persons hospitalized for treatment. Other frequent reasons for hospitalization included digestive problems, genitourinary tract diseases, neoplasms, diseases of the musculoskeletal system, and injuries and poisonings. Of the 897,000 admissions for neoplastic disorders,

TABLE 9–10. NUMBERS OF FIRST-LISTED DIAGNOSES FOR
YOUNG AND MIDDLE-AGED ADULTS DISCHARGED FROM
SHORT-STAY HOSPITALS, 1980

| First-Listed Diagnosis (Primary reason for hospitalization) | Numbers of Patients Discharged (in thousands) | |
	Young Adults: 15–44	Middle-Aged Adults: 45–64
Infections and parasitic diseases	250	88
Neoplasms	471	897
Malignant neoplasms	181	691
Endocrine, nutritional and metabolic	299	368
Diabetes mellitus	137	245
Diseases of the blood	93	56
Mental disorders	954	450
Psychoses	284	127
Alcoholism	233	169
Diseases of the nervous system	384	410
Diseases of the circulatory system	535	1711
Diseases of the respiratory system	755	669
Diseases of the genitourinary system	1812	919
Complications of pregnancy	999	3
Diseases of the skin	238	150
Diseases of the musculoskeletal system	917	727
Congenital diseases	98	39
Conditions originating in the perinatal period	85	4
Symptoms, signs, undefined illnesses	276	145
Injuries and Poisonings	1780	628

(From Haupt, B. *Utilization of short-stay hospitals: Annual summary for the United States, 1980.*
DHHS Publication No. (PHS) 82–1721, Series 13, No. 64; Hyattsville, Md.: National Center for
Health Statistics, March 1982, Table 13.)

691,000 (or about 77 percent) of the diagnosed tumors were
malignant (Table 9–10).

Comparisons of the hospitalization rates for young and middle-aged adults (Table 9–10) demonstrate the increasing prevalence of the serious chronic conditions with advancing age.
Adults in the 45- to 64-year-old age group accounted for many
more of the hospitalizations necessitated by neoplasms, diabetes, and cardiovascular (circulatory) diseases. The difference in
the rates of hospitalizations for malignancies was particularly
striking. In 1980 there were approximately 105,720,000 adults

in the 14 to 44 age group (Madden et al., 1982), and these persons accounted for 252,000 of the diagnosed malignancies (Haupt, 1982). In contrast, there were only 43,909,000 adults 45 to 64 years of age (Madden et al., 1982), but this age group had over a million diagnosed malignant conditions (Table 9–10).

The average length of short-stay hospitalizations for young and middle-aged adults provides additional information for assessing the seriousness of illness in adulthood. Conditions requiring the longest hospital stays were mental disorders, with acute psychotic episodes requiring an average of 13.2 days and alcoholism requiring an average of 10.2 days (Table 9–11). Neoplasms required the second longest hospitalization periods—an average of 7 days for the 15- to 44-year-old adults and an aver-

TABLE 9–11. AVERAGE LENGTH OF HOSPITALIZATIONS FOR YOUNG AND MIDDLE-AGED ADULTS, BY CATEGORIES OF FIRST LISTED DIAGNOSES, 1980

First-Listed Diagnoses (Primary reason for hospitalization)	Average Length of stay (Hospital days)	
	Young Adults: 15–44	Middle-Aged Adults: 45–64
Infections and parasitic diseases	6.2	8.7
Neoplasms	7.0	10.3
Endocrine, nutritional and metabolic	7.3	9.3
Diseases of the blood	5.7	8.6
Mental disorders	11.1	11.3
Psychoses	11.9	14.5
Alcoholism	9.8	10.5
Diseases of the nervous system	5.8	5.8
Diseases of the circulatory system	7.2	9.0
Diseases of the respiratory system	4.4	7.5
Diseases of the genitourinary system	4.5	5.7
Complications of pregnancy	2.5	2,7
Diseases of the skin	5.7	9.4
Diseases of the musculoskeletal system	6.6	8.3
Congenital diseases	6.7	8.5
Conditions originating in the perinatal period	2.0	9.0
Symptoms, signs, undefined illnesses	3.9	4.7
Injuries and poisonings	6.1	8.2

(Adapted from Haupt, B. *Utilization of short-stay hospitals: Annual summary for the United States, 1980.* DHHS Publication No. (PHS) 82–1721, Series 13, No. 64. Hyattsville, Md.: National Center for Health Statistics, March 1982, Table 13.)

age of 10.3 days for the 45- to 65-year-old adults. Other illnesses that required more than a week of hospitalization for adults in middle age included endocrine disorders (diabetes and others), diseases of the circulatory system and musculoskeletal system, and injuries and poisonings (Haupt, 1982).

PREVENTIVE EFFORTS

Young and middle adulthood covers a span of approximately forty years, and it is apparent from the previous discussion that many different types of health problems occur during these years. In young adulthood, acute illnesses, accidents, and violence present the greatest threats to health. By the third and fourth decades, malignancies and other chronic disease conditions begin to take their toll, and by the fifth and sixth decades, these conditions have caused many deaths and have left large numbers of Americans permanently disabled.

Interventions for maximizing positive health, as well as for curtailing morbidity and mortality in the adult years, must be broad in scope yet appropriately targeted toward specific health risks. In the Surgeon General's report on health promotion and disease prevention, the Secretary of DHEW summarized the major risks to health and longevity by stating:

> We are killing ourselves by our careless habits; we are killing ourselves by carelessly polluting the environment, and we are killing ourselves by permitting harmful social conditions to persist . . . (DHEW, 1979)

These statements are particularly relevant for health problems of the adult years. Although the etiology of most adult health problems is not perfectly understood, many risk factors and preventive interventions are well known.

Cardiovascular Diseases

The cardiovascular diseases account for the greatest morbidity and mortality among young and middle-aged Americans. Heart disease is the leading cause of death for men over 40 years of age and the second cause of death for women over 40 years of age. It also causes the greatest work disability and activity limitations for men in the middle adult years (DHEW, 1979).

The major identified risk factors for the cardiovascular diseases include smoking, hypertension, elevated blood cholesterol, and diabetes. Physical inactivity, overweight, personality factors related to stress, and use of estrogen medications may also increase the risk of heart disease (DHEW, 1979). For young adults in the 25 to 44 age group, prevention should focus on the complete elimination or at least the control of these risk factors. Because many adults in the 45- to 65-year-old age group may already have symptoms of cardiovascular disease, secondary and tertiary interventions, which focus on early dignosis, treatment, and provisions of supports for physical and social role functioning, are parmount.

Primary prevention efforts over the past decade have been fairly successful in reducing cardiovascular risks, especially among young adults. From 1960 to 1980, one-third of the young adult smokers quit smoking. Smoking cessation rates were greater for men than for women, with the percentage of male smokers decreasing from 71 to 43 percent and the percentage of female smokers decreasing from 57 to 33 percent. Unfortunately, young persons with heavier smoking habits (over 15 cigarettes per day) were less likely to quit smoking, as were persons with less education. As of 1980, 52 percent of young adults with less than a high school education still smoked, compared with 31 percent of the young adults with a college education (NCHS, 1982a). This suggests that in the present decade, prevention programs need to be directed more toward meeting the needs of heavy smokers and less educated persons.

The increased emphasis on blood pressure control in the 1970s has resulted in a decline in the prevalence of hypertension, especially among black persons who are at a higher risk for cardiovascular disease. Cholesterol levels have generally declined for men but not for women. The percentage decline in cardiovascular disease mortality, which is attributable to the decrease in smoking, hypertension, and cholesterol levels among adults, has been estimated to be 41 percent for white males, 44 percent for white females, 81 percent for black males, and 67 percent for black females (NCHS, 1983a). Continued focus on these risk factors should further lower the number of early cardiovascular deaths.

The contribution of health promotion programs, both in work settings and in the community, in decreasing the risk of cardiovascular disease should not be underestimated. Such programs can be very helpful by supporting healthy life-styles as well as by providing opportunities for early detection and control of risk factors. Such programs should also maximize the effectiveness of clinical health services because they encourage early diagnosis and better regimen adherence.

Strokes

Strokes or "cerebrovascular accidents" continue to be major hazards of the middle adult years. Although about 85 percent of the deaths from strokes occur after the age of 65, these conditions nevertheless are the third leading cause of death for adults in the 55 to 64 age group and they are the fifth leading cause of death for persons in the 45 to 54 age group. Disability from strokes also imposes tremendous physical, emotional, and economic burdens on families and society. As of the late 1970s, about 10 percent of the nursing home admissions for persons under 65 years of age were due to these conditions (DHEW, 1979).

Because atherosclerosis is the underlying disease process for both heart disease and cerebrovascular accidents, the major risk factors for strokes are those previously discussed. Control of hypertension is the most crucial preventive activity. Well-designed and well-implemented prevention programs can be very effective in controlling hypertension and its potential harmful effects. In Milwaukee, for instance, a major public health program was initiated in the schools, industry, and other community organizations, and within 4 years, there was a 34 percent reduction in the death rates from strokes (DHEW, 1979).

Early detection and treatment of diabetes may help to prevent strokes because diabetics in each age group have about twice as many strokes as do nondiabetics. This may be partially due to the fact that diabetics are more likely to be hypertensive and overweight (DHEW, 1979). Elimination of smoking is also very important for these individuals, both for controlling their primary disease process and for decreasing the risk of strokes and heart attacks.

The higher morbidity and mortality from strokes among black Americans is believed primarily to be due to untreated hypertension (Rudov & Santangelo, 1982). As in heart disease prevention programs, special efforts should be made to screen for high blood pressure in this group. Supportive services to assist individuals with high blood pressure to cope with environmental stressors, in addition to needed medical treatment, may help to prevent complications such as strokes.

Malignancies

Malignancies are the leading cause of death for both young and middle-aged women, and among men 35 to 64 years of age they are only surpassed by heart disease as the major cause of death. Although death rates for the malignancies generally decreased during the 1970s for adults under 50 years of age, a third of all cancer deaths still occurred in the 35 to 64 age group. The most prevalent malignancies among adult females are cancers of the breasts and genital organs, whereas lung cancer is the most common type of cancer among men (DHEW, 1979). For each decade of adulthood, black persons have higher mortality from malignancies, with the rate differential increasing for each decade (see Table 10–2).

The malignancies are a group of many different diseases, each with its own unique etiology and developmental history. Risk factors that have been identified as potential contributors to cancer development include cigarette smoking and excessive alcohol intake, occupational exposures to carcinogenic agents, water and air pollution, over-exposures to radiation and sunlight, heredity factors, and other predisposing medical conditions. At the present time, the most effective prevention efforts against these malignancies include the maintenance of individuals' positive health and resistance, limitation of exposures to known carcinogenic substances, and early diagnosis and treatment (DHEW, 1979).

Of all the risk factors, cigarette smoking is responsible for more malignancies and cancer deaths than any other known carcinogenic agent. Smokers are about 10 times as likely as nonsmokers to develop lung cancer, and it has been estimated that 80 percent of the cases of lung cancer and 50 percent of the cases of bladder cancer could be prevented by smoking cessation alone. The risk of dying from cancer quickly multiplies when an individual smokes and is exposed to other carcinogens in the living environment or work setting. The combination of cigarette smoking and exposure to asbestos, for example, increases the lung cancer risk 90 times (DHEW, 1979).

Efforts to decrease the prevalence of cigarette smoking include educational programs to motivate and assist individuals and groups to quit smoking as well as legislative sanctions against smoking. Broad-based educational programs during the 1960s and 1970s, which focused on instructing the public about the hazards of smoking, provided the impetus for current anti-smoking programs. During the 1980s, increased emphasis should be placed on providing individuals with actual behavioral skills for long-term smoking cessation. Health promotion programs in industry, schools, and other community settings will play an increasingly important role in assisting persons to gain these behavioral skills as well as to develop more healthy lifestyles. Physicians, nurses, and other health practitioners also have a major responsibility for encouraging smoking cessation, especially because persons may have stronger motivation for smoking cessation when they are first diagnosed with a life-threatening illness. If feasible, behaviorally oriented smoking cessation guidance should be offered in the clinical setting itself, and if not, appropriate referrals to community-based educational programs should be made.

Legislative efforts to influence smoking behaviors, although quite controversial, should also continue to be pursued. An important consideration for determining the reasonableness of smoking restrictions in public areas is the effects of smoking on nonsmokers. Given the overwhelming evidence concerning the health hazards of smoking, higher taxes on tobacco products also seem warranted. Finances from increased taxation could be channeled into research to further establish the health effects of smoking or into health education programs.

Establishing and enforcing appropriate environmental controls on water and air pollution as well as on direct occupational exposures is also critical for preventing malignancies. According to the Surgeon General's report (1979), 80 percent of Americans live in urban areas where toxic gases or particulate matter pollute the air. The National Institute of Occupational Safety and Health also estimates that nine of ten American industrial workers are inadequately protected from exposures to at least one common hazardous industrial chemical (DHEW, 1979). Although a strong preventive focus on individual health behaviors, such as smoking, is very positive, there is danger of under-emphasizing the risks of such environmental hazards.

Responsibility for improving the quality of the environment must be shared by individuals, health professionals, and community groups as well as by industry and governmental agencies. On the individual level, cooperative attitudes toward legislated standards such as those for automobile emissions and waste disposal is critical. Educational messages that focus on both the personal and social consequences of sabotaging environmental control efforts are needed, as are stronger penalties for infringements. Industrial regulations can be expected to continually be challenged, especially when such regulations increase an industry's immediate financial burden. Increased public demand for industrial controls as well as improved public awareness of legislative and lobbying skills are necessry to counteract organized efforts of special interest groups who attempt to thwart regulatory controls.

Specific risk factors for some types of malignancies are unknown, and in such cases secondary preventions that focus on early diagnosis and treatment are the most effective intervention strategies. Breast cancer, for example, is the most common malignancy among American females, affecting nearly 1 in 13 women. Most breast cancers are found by women themselves rather than in physician examinations, and monthly breast self-examination can greatly enhance early detection. Periodic physical examinations and mammography can also help to assure early diagnosis and treatment.

Other screening procedures that are very effective include the Pap smear for detection of cervical cancer, rectal examinations for detection of prostatic cancer, and x-rays for detection of lung and abdominal tumors. Useful guidelines for establishing a clinically based health monitoring program for individuals, based on age-specific health problems and needs, have been published by Breslow and Somers (1977). Preventive screening and treatment, as well as counseling concerning risk factors for the specific age group, are recommended. A listing of Breslow and Somers' goals and recommended health services for adults in the 25 to 39 and 40 to 59 age groups is shown in Table 9–12.

Accidents and Acts of Violence

Motor vehicle casualties and other accidents such as falls, burns, and poisonings account for most of the deaths among

TABLE 9–12. LIFETIME HEALTH MONITORING

Young Middle Age (25–39 years)

Health goals	To prolong the period of maximum physical energy and to develop full mental, physical, and social potential
	To anticipte and guard against the onset of chronic diseases through good health habits and early detection and treatment where effective
Professional services	Two professional visits with the healthy person—at about 30 and 35—including tests for hypertension, anemia, cholesterol, cervical and breast cancer, and instruction in self-examination of breasts, skin, testes, neck and mouth
	Professional counseling regarding nutrition, exercise, smoking, alcohol, marital, parental and other aspects of health-related behavior and life-style
	Dental examination and prophylaxis every two years

Older Middle Age (40–59 years)

Health goals	To prolong the period of maximum physical energy and optimum mental and social activity, including menopausal adjustment
	To detect as early as possible any of the major chronic diseases, including hypertension, heart disease, diabetes and cancer, as well as vision, hearing and dental impairments
Professional services	Four professional visits with the healthy person, once every five years—at about 40, 45, 50, and 55—with complete physical examination and medical history, tests for specific chronic conditions, appropriate immunizations and counseling regarding changing nutritional needs, physical activities, occupational, sex, marital and parental problems and use of cigarettes, alcohol, and drugs
	For those over 50, annual tests for hypertension, obesity and certain cancers
	Annual dental prophylaxis

(From Breslow, L. & Somers, A. The lifetime health monitoring program: a practical approach to preventive medicine. *New England Journal of Medicine,* 1977, *296*(11), 603–609, with permission.)

young American adults in the 25 to 34 age group and continue to cause many unnecessary deaths and permanent injuries throughout the middle adult years. An effective program for preventing accidents, as discussed in Chapter 8, must be successful in motivating individuals to take more protective measures as well as in effecting better control of hazards in the environment.

Nearly half of the deaths from accidental injuries in the adult years are caused by motor vehicle accidents. Although primary prevention strategies for such accidents have traditionally focused on driver education programs, environmental controls such as lower speeds limits, improved automobile and highway design, automobile safety devices, and motorcycle helmet laws have also been shown to be effective in reducing fatalities (DHEW, 1979).

The greatest risk factor for automobile fatalities is the driver's use of alcohol. Educational programs in the schools and over the media to increase public awareness and responsibility for drunk driving may help to reduce alcohol-related accidents, especially among young people. Legislated environmental sanctions, such as the higher drinking age and mandatory license suspension for repeated offenders of drunk driving, are also potentially effective, though as with other environmental controls they are difficult to enforce. The increasing public demand for stricter enforcement of drunk driving is a very positive sign because enforcement of legislation without public support is almost impossible.

Other accidents and violent acts that frequently result in homicide or suicide are also serious problems in the adult years. Firearms present an especially serious problem in young adulthood, as they are implicated in many accidental deaths and in most homicides and suicides. Preventive measures that could reduce the risk of firearm injuries range from encouraging safer storage to a complete ban on private ownership. Evidence from studies in England suggest that prohibiting posssession of handguns is effective in reducing firearm injuries in noncriminal assaults (DHEW, 1979). About 20 percent of the homicides in this country involve family members, close friends, or acquaintances (DHEW, 1979). Better firearm control would probably help to reduce the high incidence of homicides and accidental shooting deaths among young black males, and it might also curtail those impulsive suicides related to firearms that are prevalent among young white males.

Although firearm control could potentially contribute to the lowering of mortality from impulsive violent acts, it alone is not an adequate prevention strategy. In the white male population, the suicide rate remains high throughout the adult years, with 24.6 deaths per 100,000 in the 25 to 44 age group and 25.0 deaths per 100,000 in the 45 to 64 age group. Deaths from homicides and legal interventions are more prevalent among young black males 25 to 44 years of age (127.7 deaths per 100,000), but the suicide rate is also fairly high at 18.7 deaths per 100,000.

Primary prevention for acts of violence will necessitate a much stronger emphasis on correcting harmful social conditions that contribute to stress and loss of control, for example, unemployment and economic strain, overcrowded living conditions, too early and unprepared parenthood, and lack of opportunity to achieve personal goals. Although alcohol abuse definitely contributes to loss of control and violence, it is also a symptomatic warning of underlying stress and discontent. Though prevention of alcohol abuse is thus a very worthwhile goal, it should not be considered to be the major solution for violence. This is also true for emergency services such as crisis hotlines. Although such services have been very beneficial in preventing deaths, they cannot replace more ongoing education and support services or needed structural changes in society.

Mental Illness and Substance Abuse

Mental health problems cause much disability and suffering in adulthood and also substantially contribute to deaths from accidents, suicides, and homicides. Depression and manic depressive disorders are the most prevalent mental illnesses and they have the most serious consequences in terms of mortality. More than 80 percent of the suicides in the United States per year are believed to be precipitated by depressive episodes (DHEW, 1979). The psychoses, though less prevalent, are extremely destructive to individuals and families, and traditionally have necessitated long-term institutionalizations. Untreated acute psychoses can also be quite dangerous as they may precipitate acts of violence.

Although many of the biological determinants of mental illness are unknown, it is nevertheless possible to exert much control over acute illness episodes with well-organized and well-funded prevention programs. Persons who have experienced early childhood deprivation or abuse, those living under ongoing acute environmental stress, and those with a generational family history of mental illness are most vulnerable (Mohl, 1982). Prevention programs that are oriented toward identifying high-risk groups and offering acceptable supportive interventions may be most successful in preventing or controlling mental illness. Such interventions may include crisis counseling, organization or self-help support groups, stress management training, or ongoing institutional consultation. Early diagnosis and treatment can also be very effective in controlling the symptoms of most acute mental illnesses as well as in curtailing or postponing chronicity and its associated disabilities. The critical issue for mental health prevention efforts at present is the inadequate funding for community mental health. With financial cuts during the late 1970s and early 1980s, funding for prevention activities is very limited.

In addition to the major mental illnesses, substance abuse (particularly alcohol abuse) is a very serious health problem throughout the adult years. About 10 million Americans, or 7 percent of persons 18 years or older have been identified as alcoholics or problem drinkers. Alcohol abuse has been estimated to contribute to at least 10 percent of all deaths per year when deaths due to accidents, suicides, homicides, and chronic illnesses are considered (DHEW, 1979).

Furthermore, premature mortality associated with alcohol misuse is substantial. Years of potential life lost (YDLL) as a result of alcohol use is shown in Table 9–13. Deaths resulting from acute effects of alcohol account for relatively more mortality in younger persons. An average of 29.1 years of life was lost for each death associated with excessive blood alcohol levels, more common among younger persons, whereas the average for deaths caused by alcoholic cirrhosis was 14.4 years lost (MMWR, 1985).

Major preventive interventions for alcohol abuse include educational programs for youths and adults, various attempts to alter social mores and reduce individual and social stress factors, and law enforcement (DHEW, 1979). Preventive education programs that build on peer group counseling and support to resist drinking are generally more successful than programs that merely warn about the hazards of alcohol. Programs that use role playing and other behavioral techniques to teach problem-solving and coping skills are particularly helpful for assisting individuals to resist social pressure to experiment with alcohol or other drugs. Self-help groups such as Alcoholics Anonymous and Alanon are also very helpful for families who are already attempting to cope with alcoholism. Because chil-

TABLE 9-13. YEARS OF POTENTIAL LIFE LOST (YPLL) AND AVERAGE YPLL PER REPORTED DEATH, BY ALCOHOL-RELATED CAUSE OF MORTALITY—UNITED STATES, 1980

Cause of Death	No. of Deaths			YPLL			Average YPLL per Reported Death[a]
	Underlying Cause	Contributing Causes	Total	Underlying Cause	Contributing Causes	Total	
Alcohol dependence	3,436	10,340	13,776	52,831	154,228	207,059	15.0
Alcoholic cirrhosis	10,159	1,435	11,594	149,605	17,183	166,788	14.4
Alcohol abuse	797	3,395	4,192	17,368	83,738	101,106	24.1
Excessive blood alcohol	11	1,262	1,273	269	36,719	36,988	29.1
Alcoholic cardiomyopathy	518	96	614	7,782	1,420	9,202	15.0
Alcohol psychosis	344	205	549	5,683	2,993	8,676	15.8
Alcoholic gastritis	69	26	95	1,249	444	1,693	17.8
Alcohol polyneuropathy	3	6	9	9	43	52	5.8

[a]Average YPLL equals the total YPLL divided by the reported number of persons 1 year through 64 years old who died from each cause.
(From National Center for Health Statistics, Surveillance and assessment of alcohol-related mortality—United States, 1980. *Morbidity and Mortality Weekly Reports*, 1985, 34(12), 162.)

dren of alcoholics are at much greater risk for alcoholism than those in the wider population, their involvement in preventive programs such as Alanon is strongly encouraged.

The role of unmanageable social stress as a risk factor for mental illness and substance abuse, as well as for physical illness in adulthood, cannot be overemphasized. Preventive strategies that are directed toward reducing environmental stressors as well as those that focus on improving individuals' coping skills are needed (DHEW, 1979). Efforts to reduce social environmental stressors might include improving the work climate in institutional settings, strengthening neighborhood networks, creating better community support services, and fostering more healthy racial and ethnic attitudes. Because stressful events are not always preventable, individuals also must be better prepared to cope with stress at an early age. School-based educational programs that focus on teaching problem-solving coping skills for stressful situations would be helpful interventions as would more stress-management programs in work settings.

REFERENCES

Breslow, L. & Somers, A. R. The Lifetime Health Monitoring Program. *New England Journal of Medicine, 1977, 296* (11), 602–604.

Cypress, B. *Patients' reasons for visiting physicians: National ambulatory medical care survey, U.S. 1977–78.* DHHS Publication No. (PHS) 82–1717, series 13, No. 56. Hyattsville, Md.: National Center for Health Statistics, December 1981a.

DHEW. *Healthy people: The surgeon general's report on health promotion and disease prevention, 1979.* DHEW Publication No. (PHS) 79–55071. Washington, D.C.: U.S. Govt. Printing Office, 1979.

DHHS. *Smoking and health: A report of the Surgeon General.* DHHS Publication No. (PHS) 79–50066. Washington, D.C.: U.S. Government Printing Office, 1979.

Feller, B. Americans needing help to function at home. *Vital and Health Statistics,* Advance data No. 92. DHHS Publication No. (PHS) 83–1250; Washington, D.C.: National Center for Health Statistics, September 14, 1983.

Feller, B. *Prevalence of selected impairments, U.S. 1977.* DHHS Publication No. (PHS) 81–1562, Series 10, No. XX. Hyattsville, Md.: National Center for Health Statistics, February 1981.

Givens, J. *Current estimates from the health interview survey: U.S. 1978.* DHHS Publication No. (PHS) 80–1551, Series 10, No. 130. Hyattsville, Md.: Office of Health Research Statistics, November 1979.

Haupt, B. *Utilization of short-stay hospitals: Annual summary for the U.S., 1980.* DHHS Publication No. (PHS) 82–1721, Series 13, No. 64. Hyattsville Md.: National Center for Health Statistics, March 1982.

MMWR. Annual summary, 1980. Reported morbidity and mortality in the United States. *Morbidity and Mortality Weekly Reports,* 1981, *29*(54).

MMWR. Surveillance and assessment of alcohol-related mortality— United States, 1980. *Morbidity and Mortality Weekly Reports,* 1985, *34*(12), 161–163.

Madden, T., Turner, I., & Eckenfels, E. *The Health Almanac.* New York: Raven, 1982.

Mohl, P. C. Promoting mental health and reducing risk for mental illness. In M. Faber & A. Reinhaadt (Eds.), *Promoting health through risk-reduction.* New York: MacMillan, 1982.

National Center for Health Statistics. Advance Report of Final Mortality Statistics, 1981. *Monthly Vital Statistics Report, 33*(3, Suppl.). Washington, D.C.: Public Health Service, June 22, 1984.

National Center for Health Statistics. *Facts of life and death.* DHEW Publication No. (PHS) 79–1222. Hyattsville Md.: NCHS, 1978.

National Center for Health Statistics. *Health, United States 1981.* DHHS Publiction No. (PHS) 82–1232. Washington D.C.: U.S. Government Printing Office, December 1981.

National Center for Health Statistics. *Health, United States 1982.* DHHS Publication No. (PHS) 83–1232. Washington D.C.: U.S. Government Printing Office, December 1982a.

National Center for Health Statistics. *Health, United States and prevention profile, 1983.* DHHS Publication No. (PHS) 84–1232. Washington, D.C.: U.S. Government Printing Office, December, 1983a.

National Center for Health Statistics. *Physician visits: Volume and intervals since last visit, U.S. 1980.* DHHS Publication No. (PHS) 83–1572. *Vital and Health Statistics,* Series 10, No. 144. Washington, D.C.: U.S. Government printing Office, June 1983b.

National Center for Health Statistics. *The national ambulatory medical care survey, U.S. 1979 summary.* DHHS Publication No. (PHS) 82–1727. *Vital and Health Statistics,* Series 13, No. 66. Washington, D.C.: U.S. Government Printing Office, September 1982b.

National Center for Health Statistics. *Current estimates from the national health interview survey: United States, 1979.* DHHS Publication No. (PHS) 81–1564. *Vital and health statistics,* Series 10, No.

136. Washington, D.C.: U.S. Government Printing Office, 1981a.

Ries, P. *Americans assess their health: U.S. 1978.* DHHS Publication No. (PHS) 83–1570, Series 10, No. 142. Hyattsville, Md.: National Center for Health Statistics, March 1983.

Rudov, M. H. & Santangelo, N. *Health status of minorities and low-income groups.* U.S. Public Health Service. DHEW Pub. No. (HRA) 79–627. Washington, D.C.: U.S. Government Printing Office, 1979.

U.S. News and World Report. *World almanac and book of facts, 1984.* New York: Newspaper Interpress Association, 1984.

10

Patterns of Morbidity and Mortality over Age 65

Persons aged 65 and older represent a growing proportion of the total world population. This growth is particularly dramatic in developed countries. In the United States between 1960 and 1980, the proportion of the total population over 65 years of age grew from 9.2 to 11.3 percent. This represents an increase from 16.68 million persons in 1960 to 25.71 million in 1980. By the year 2000, it has been projected that there will be 31 million persons over 65 in the United States (Source Book on Aging, 1979).

As mentioned in Chapter 4, several major factors are contributing to this growth:

1. High birth rates. During the first decades of the 1900s, high birth rates were accompanied by lower infant, childhood, and young adult mortality rates so that large cohorts of births survived to old age (Source Book on Aging, 1979; White House Conference, 1961).
2. High immigration rates. Between 1880 and 1910, many immigrants, including many young children came to the United States. Additionally, young immigrant families had more children after their arrival. Both the young

immigrants and the children of young immigrants are now over or are approaching 65 years of age.

3. Improvements in public health, nutrition, disease prevention, and treatment. Better housing, sanitation, immunizations for communicable diseases, and other public health measures extended life so that a greater proportion of those born in the late 1800s and early 1900s lived to adulthood and old age than ever before. These cohorts of births are now over 65 years of age.

Among the older population, women outnumber men. Men over 65 (10.36 million) represented 9.4 percent of the U.S. male population in 1980, whereas women over 65 (15.35 million) represented 13.1 percent of the U.S. female population in the same year. The male to female ratio is thus 0.675. This excess of women is due to the longer life expectancies of women.

Life expectancy is increasing for both sexes. A man born in 1900 could expect to live 47.88 years, a woman 50.70 years. A man born in 1978 could expect to live 69.5 years, a woman 77.2 years. The differences in life expectancy between the sexes increased from 2.82 years in 1900 to 7.7 years in more recent times. A large proportion of this difference by sex in life expectancy is accounted for by excess deaths from accidents, suicide, and homicide among men under 35 years of age and by heart disease and lung cancer in the later age groups (Rice, 1981). These were discussed in Chapter 9. A white male who had reached age 65 in 1979 had an average expectation of 14.2 years of life remaining, a white female aged 65 in 1979 had an average expectation of 18.7 years of life remaining. The parallel figures for black males and females were 13.3 and 17.2 years, respectively.

Diseases in which older men show an excess over women predominate as causes of mortality, whereas diseases in which older women show an excess over men are predominately causes of morbidity. Women also have higher rates of disability when ill (Source Book on Aging, 1979). The divergence of mortality rates by sex is greater among whites than among nonwhites.

Overall, mortality rates for whites are substantially lower than those for nonwhites in the 65 to 69 and 70 to 74 age groups, although by 80 to 84 years of age, blacks appear to have lower mortality rates than do whites; these rates for the 80- to 84-year age group, however, are based on small numbers and may be subject to some reporting error (Source Book on Aging, 1979). Whites over 65 years of age represent 11.6 percent of the total white population in the U.S. in 1980. Nonwhites over 65 years constitute only 7.8 percent of the total nonwhite population.

Although there are many older adults who experience good health and freedom of activity, approximately 80 percent of adults over 65 years of age have at least one chronic health problem and half experience some limitation in activities of daily living (DHEW, 1979). In general, the population over 65 years of age is at higher risk of disease and death and is more likely to require medical services than are younger persons. In one study, persons 65 and older accounted for 15 percent of all visits to office-based physicians, 34 percent of all days utilized in short-stay hospitals, and 89 percent of all residents in nursing homes (Kovar, 1977). Older individuals make more visits per person to physicians and use hospital facilities more frequently than any younger age group (NCHS, 1982a). This older population also accounts for nearly one-third of monies spent on personal health care. Assisting older citizens to adapt to life with a chronic illness is a major nursing responsibility. Nurses have responsibility for the care of the elderly in a variety of health care settings. In order to plan the most effective and comprehensive nursing care for elderly patients, including primary, secondary, and tertiary prevention activities, nurses need to be familiar with the major health problems experienced by elderly persons, the effects of particular illnesses on function, and the relationship of specific illnesses to mortality.

This chapter first presents data on the major causes of mortality in the elderly. Subsequently, data describing patterns of acute and chronic disease are presented and related to limitation of activity. Finally, major approaches to prevention in the care of the elderly are discussed.

MAJOR CAUSES OF MORTALITY

The ten leading causes of death in the United States in 1982 for the 65 years and older age groups are shown in Table 10–1 and are compared with causes for the total U.S. population. Coronary heart disease is the leading cause of death for both sexes within the total U.S. population and in all the older age

TABLE 10–1. TEN LEADING CAUSES OF DEATH FOR TOTAL U.S. POPULATION AND SUBPOPULATION 65+ YEARS BY 10 YEAR AGE GROUPS, 1982

1982 Total U.S. Population	Age		
	65–74	75–84	85+
1. Heart disease	Heart disease	Heart disease	Heart disease
2. Malignant neoplasms	Malignant neoplasms	Malignant neoplasms	Cerebrovas- cular disease
3. Cerebrovas- cular disease	Cerebrovas- cular disease	Cerebrovas- cular disease	Malignant neoplasms
4. Accidents and adverse effects	Chronic lung disease	Chronic lung disease	Pneumonia and influenza
5. Chronic lung disease	Diabetes mellitus	Pneumonia and influenza	Atherosclerosis
6. Pneumonia and influenza	Accidents and adverse effects	Diabetes mellitus	Chronic lung disease
7. Diabetes mellitus	Pneumonia and influenza	Accidents and adverse effects	Accidents and adverse effects
8. Suicide	Chronic liver and cirrhosis	Atherosclerosis	Diabetes mellitus
9. Chronic liver and cirrhosis	Nephritis and nephrosis	Nephritis and nephrosis	Nephritis and nephrosis
10. Atherosclerosis	Atherosclerosis	Septicemia	Septicemia

(Compiled from National Center for Health Statistics. Advanced report of final mortality statistics, 1982. *Monthly Vital Statistics Report,* 1984, *33*(9, Suppl.), Tables 5, 7.)

subgroups. Coronary heart disease mortality rates tend to increase with age; the rate for the total U.S. population in 1982 was 326.0 per 100,000 persons. In the 65 to 74 age group, heart disease mortality rates were 1156.4 per 100,000. Rates for those age 75 to 84 years and 85 and over were 2801.4 and 7341.8, respectively. Deaths from heart disease accounted for 46.5 percent of deaths over 65 years of age (NCHS, 1984).

Malignant neoplasms are the second most frequent cause of death among older Americans, except in the 85 years and older group where it drops to third place, superseded by cerebrovascular disease, which was the third most frequent cause of death in both of the two younger age groups (65 to 74 and 75 to 84) and in the total U.S. population. Malignant neoplasms account for 15 percent of deaths over age 65; cerebrovascular disease accounts for 12 percent of deaths (NCHS, 1984).

Although six of the same causes of death appear among the fourth through tenth causes for the three age groups over 65, the order differs in the three age categories. For example, chronic lung disease is fourth as a cause of death in the 65- to 74-year and the 75- to 84-year age groups, but drops to number six in the 85-year and older group. Pneumonia and influenza, the fourth most frequent cause of death in those 85 and over, is seventh among deaths at ages 65 to 74 and fifth among deaths at ages 75 to 84. Chronic liver disease and cirrhosis, the eighth most frequent cause of death from 65 to 74 is not among the top ten causes in the other two age groups. It is replaced by septicemia.

Nephritis and nephrosis, the ninth most frequent cause of death in all three age categories over 65 years of age, is not among the ten leading causes for the U.S. population as a whole. It is replaced by suicide, the tenth leading cause of death among the total U.S. population; suicide is not among the top ten causes for those 65 years and older.

It should be noted that, except for accidents and adverse effects and for pneumonia and influenza, the remaining eight leading causes of death among the elderly all directly reflect the result of the aging process and long-term life-style patterns. Consider cardiovascular disease as an example. It has been documented that the effects of the common cardiovascular risk factors are approximately the same in all age groups (Shurtleff, 1974). Because the prevalence of most of these risk factors, including elevated blood pressure and elevated blood cholesterol, increase with age, the elderly are at high risk for mortality from cardiovascular disease. The one risk factor that may be of lower prevalence in the over 65 age group is cigarette smoking. It is generally too late for primary prevention of cardiovascular disease in this age group since most persons are well into the natural history stage of pathogenesis. It is possible, however, to intervene at the stage of secondary prevention. Early detection of risk factors and risk factor reduction through programs of supervised aerobic exercise regimes, modification of diet, and reduction or cessation of smoking is feasible. So is prompt treatment with medication or even surgery when indicated. Such measures can be lifesaving. Counseling elderly persons against sudden exertion, such as snow shoveling, can also be lifesaving. In colder parts of the country, heart attack deaths are higher during winter months.

Tertiary programs of rehabilitation for patients with existing cardiac disease can still improve the quality of life. For the eight chronic diseases that are among the ten leading causes of death in the over 65 age group, secondary and tertiary prevention must be the general focus of efforts at intervention.

In the case of accidents and adverse effects and of pneumonia and influenza, even primary prevention may be possible because these diseases generally represent sudden, acute events rather than a lifetime process. The high incidence of accidents may also be a result of the aging process in that a decrease in physical strength, flexibility or mobility, vision, hearing or other sensory deficits, poorer balance, and slower reflexes may all contribute to an increased probability of accident. Because of circumstances such as brittle bones, diabetes, or cardiovascular disease, the impact of an accident on the individual may be more severe in this age group. There is less ability to recover without complication. A higher rate of complication may be a factor in the higher case-fatality rate associated with accidents among the elderly. Similarly, immobility or limitation of activity due to chronic illness and already impaired lung function may contribute to higher mortality from influenza or pneumonia.

Rates for eight of the ten leading causes of death in the over 65-year age group decreased between 1968 and 1978 (Table 10–2). The decrease in diseases of the heart actually began in 1963. Although there is some question about why this decrease has occurred, national emphasis by the medical care system and by public education programs on risk factor intervention has probably had major impact on both incidence and mortality. Unfortunately, general population incidence data are unavailable (Blackburn & Gillum, 1980). Intervention efforts have been directed at diet modification to control fat, cholesterol, and calorie intake; regular exercise; stress reduction; hypertension control; weight control; and smoking cessation. Because all these were attacked more or less simultaneously, we may never know with certainty the relative contribution to the observed decline in U.S. mortality. Other simultaneous factors, that are likely to have affected mortality rates, are the development of emergency teams for dealing with heart attack victims before they get to the hospital, thus preventing many deaths from myocardial infarction, new drugs for treatment of heart disease, and possibly new surgical techniques.

TABLE 10–2. DEATH RATES PER 100,000 FOR 10 LEADING CAUSES BY 10-YEAR AGE GROUPS OVER 65 YEARS OF AGE, UNITED STATES, 1978

1978 Disease Rank Order for Total Group Over 65 Years	Age			
	Year	65–74	75–84	85+
1. Heart disease	1978	1275.1	2339.9	7084.3
	1968	1735.7	3952.3	9293.3
2. Malignant neoplasms	1978	818.5	1314.0	1450.5
	1968	783.4	1124.8	1477.6
3. Cerebrovascular disease	1978	256.2	966.2	2281.6
	1968	440.3	1386.2	3611.7
4. Chronic lung disease	1978	52.8	91.8	89.5
	1968	99.8	135.9	154.7
5. Pneumonia and influenza	1978	69.0	281.0	839.8
	1968	113.5	354.4	1169.7
6. Atherosclerosis	1978	26.0	156.9	638.4
	1968	44.5	241.6	1123.5
7. Accidents and adverse effects	1978	61.9	135.1	276.8
	1968	94.5	195.9	514.5
8. Diabetes mellitus	1978	66.7	150.0	211.9
	1968	102.2	189.1	258.3
9. Nephritis, nephrosis	1978	15.7	37.7	62.6
	1968	16.7	32.9	74.6
10. Chronic liver disease and cirrhosis	1978	41.2	29.9	18.0
	1968	41.3	27.9	22.8

(Compiled from National Center for Health Statistics. *Vital Statistics of the United States, 1978, Volume IIA, Mortality*. DHHS Publication No. (PHS) 83–1101. Washington, D.C.: Public Health Service, 1982, Tables 1–8, Section I.)

Some of the above efforts at primary and secondary prevention of heart disease could also have contributed to decreased mortality from cerebrovascular disease, atherosclerosis, cancer, and chronic lung disease because they share some common risk factors. For example, cigarette smoking is a risk factor not only for heart disease but also for lung cancer and chronic lung disease. A high fat diet is associated with heart disease, breast and colon cancer, and atherosclerosis. Improvements in detection and management of these other diseases may also have contributed to their decline.

Rates for the two causes that do not show a decrease in mortality, nephritis/nephrosis and chronic liver disease/cirrhosis, have changed little in this 10-year period. What change there has been has tended to be in the direction of higher rates, although this is not consistent in all age subcategories over 65. Nephritis/nephrosis, for instance, was lower in 1978 than in 1968 for the age groups 65 to 69 and 85 years and older, but was higher in 1978 than in 1968 for the other three age subcategories.

Very few renal diseases are preventable. The preventable renal diseases are associated with infections, drug- or chemical-induced disease (which could result from treatment of some other disease condition), obstructive or neurological causes, and stones. Although a huge medical care industry for care of renal failure has evolved, including dialysis and transplantation, access to these services is variable, always enormously expensive, and inconsistent as to effectiveness (Kunin, 1980).

Mortality by Sex and Race

In general, female mortality is lower than that for men. Differences between the sexes in rates of mortality from specific causes are observed. In 1978, heart disease mortality for women was less than half that for men at ages 65 to 69 (male rates, 1439.3 in 100,000; female, 606.3 in 100,000) although this difference gradually decreases in the older age groups. By 85 years of age, the rates were more similar, 7790.6 for men and 6673.5 for women (NCHS, 1982b). Lower rates of heart disease among women throughout early life have been attributed in part to protection by female hormones. After menopause, this protection ceases and rates begin the climb toward the levels of mortality present among men. In the past, however, women smoked less than men and are thought to have less stress since they did not work outside the home. A study is now being conducted to determine whether the picture is different among working women (Haynes et al., 1980). Similar patterns are seen for cerebrovascular disease and for atherosclerosis.

For malignant neoplasms, chronic pulmonary disease, pneumonia and influenza, and for accidents and adverse effects, mortality rates among women remain considerably lower than those for men throughout all ages over 65 years. Differences observed for the first three of these causes of death may relate to effects of smoking; among the current elderly, men smoked with much greater frequency than did women. Diabetes mellitus, although showing similar frequency of mortality for the sexes from age 65 through 74 years of age, increases more rapidly in women than in men above that age. Although reasons are unknown, it has been postulated that the higher percentage of body fat in women may be a factor.

Racial differences in mortality are also observed. For heart disease, malignant neoplasms, cerebrovascular disease, pneumonia and influenza, atherosclerosis, and accidents and adverse effects, nonwhites have higher mortality rates than do whites through age 79. Beginning with the 80- to 84-year age group, rates are higher for these causes of death among whites than among nonwhites. A similar pattern is observed for diabetes, except that the excess among whites does not appear until age 85 years and older. For chronic pulmonary disease and chronic liver disease/cirrhosis, nonwhites have lower mortality rates at all ages over 65 years, with the differences becoming more marked with age. Nonwhite mortality from nephritis and nephrosis is appreciably higher than white mortality at all ages over 65. However, all death rates for nonwhites in the oldest age groups must be viewed with caution as they are based on small numbers.

The higher mortality rates among nonwhites, particularly blacks, over 65 years of age is a continuation of higher rates for blacks at younger ages. Reasons for these differences have not been well investigated although studies of racial differences in cancer survival have shown that blacks are likely to be diagnosed at a later stage of the disease and are generally in poorer health at diagnosis than are whites. There have also been reports of histological differences in tumor type and racial differences in hormone receptor status; some histological types are more lethal than others and hormone receptor status relates to whether hormone treatments can be used effectively. Blacks and whites also vary in their rates of incidence for cancer of particular sites—whites have higher rates of breast and colorectal cancer, which are associated with good survival. Blacks have higher incidence of stomach and esophageal cancers, which have poorer survival. All these factors contribute to the overall differences in the mortality picture for cancer.

Similar racial differences in constitution or general health status could affect the other conditions for which nonwhites have higher mortality—heart disease, cerebrovascular disease, pneumonia and influenza, atherosclerosis, and accidents and adverse effects. Differences between the racial groups in promptness of seeking care, quality of care received, compliance with treatment, or quality of the home environment could also influence likelihood of mortality following onset of these conditions.

MAJOR CAUSES OF MORBIDITY

You will recall from previous chapters that acute conditions were defined by the National Center for Health Statistics as illness or injury of short duration, typically less than 3 months and involving either medical attention or 1 day or more of restricted activity. Of all the age groups, those over 65 years have the lowest incidence of such acute conditions, 111.0 per 100 persons per year in 1978 (Ries, 1983). On the other hand, this age group has the highest prevalence of chronic conditions. Largely because of these chronic conditions, the elderly experience more limitation in their activity and more days of disability. Some of these chronic conditions also contribute to high rates of injuries and accidents.

In general, the elderly view themselves as reasonably healthy despite the high frequency of chronic disorders; 69.7 percent of respondents over 65 years of age in a national survey of households rated their health as excellent or good. Only 8.5 percent rated their health as poor. Interestingly, the percentage of individuals rating themselves as fair or poor peaks at age 77 for women and at about age 83 for men, then drops; thus a higher percent of those who are the most elderly again rate themselves in good or excellent health. Perhaps these elderly persons hold a view that associates old age with debilitating illness and compare their own present health status with this view. Although a slightly higher proportion of men than women rate themselves in excellent health, a higher percentage of men also rate themselves as in poor health; women more often specify good or fair health (Ries, 1983). Whites generally rate their health more favorably than do nonwhites, particularly blacks. Such ratings are consistent with higher rates of morbidity and mortality among nonwhites.

Acute and Chronic Conditions

As in previous chapters, data presented here on acute conditions is based on published data from the National Health Survey. The principal diagnosis and principal reason for visits to physicians' offices probably reflect primarily acute illness, or acute episodes of chronic conditions, and are thus included in this discussion of acute conditions. Hospital discharges among the elderly probably relate more to chronic conditions or acute episodes of chronic conditions.

Upper respiratory conditions are the most frequent acute illness among persons over 65 years of age with an incidence of 46.5 per 100 population in 1969 for all respiratory conditions (Fig. 10–1). Of the upper respiratory conditions, influenza accounted for 22.4 cases per 100 population. Injuries were the other major cause of acute illness, with an incidence of 16.4 per 100. Both of these conditions show some seasonal fluctuation in rates with highest rates during the winter months. Winter is usually when influenza rates rise in the total U.S. population. Ice and snow increase the probability of injury both from falls and from automobile and pedestrian accidents.

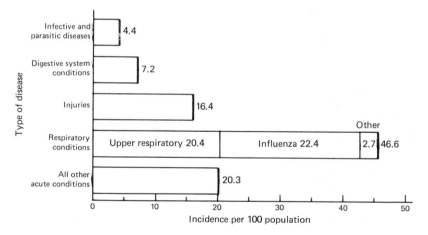

Figure 10–1. Incidence of acute conditions (medically attended) age 65 and over, United States, 1969. *(From NCHS. Acute conditions, incidence and associated disability. Vital and Health Statistics, Series 10, No. 77. DHEW Publication No. (HSM) 73–1503, 1973.)*

Elderly persons, not surprisingly, have more visits to physicians' offices than do younger persons. Results from the National Health Survey indicate that persons over 65 years of age averaged 4.1 office visits per year in 1977 compared to 3.3 for those in the next younger age group (45 to 64 years). Somewhat over half (55.6 percent) of visits by the elderly are symptom related. Another 22.7 percent comprise initiation and follow-up treatment for a particular disease condition. Diagnosis, screening, and preventive reasons account for another 17 percent of visits (Ezzati & McLemore, 1980).

As might be expected, the largest proportion of physicians' office visits were related to diseases of the circulatory system (26.5 percent). The distribution of office visits by principal diagnosis is shown in Table 10–3. Second were visits for diseases of the nervous system and sense organs (10.4 percent), followed closely by diseases of the musculoskeletal system (9.6 percent) and diseases of the respiratory system (7.9 percent). Hearing

TABLE 10–3. PERCENTAGE OF OFFICE VISITS BY PRINCIPAL DIAGNOSIS AT VISIT, PATIENTS 65 AND OLDER: UNITED STATES, JANUARY–DECEMBER 1977

Principal Diagnosis[a]	Percent Distribution
Infective and parasitic diseases	2.0
Neoplasms	4.9
Endocrine, nutritional and metabolic diseases	6.1
Mental disorders	1.8
Disease of nervous system and sense organs	10.4
Diseases of circulatory system	26.5
Diseases of respiratory system	7.9
Diseases of digestive system	4.5
Diseases of genitourinary system	5.4
Diseases of skin and subcutaneous tissue	3.4
Disease of musculoskeletal system	9.6
Symptoms and ill-defined conditions	4.3
Accidents, poisoning, and violence	4.1
Special conditions and examinations without sickness	6.6
All other diagnoses	2.7
Total	100.0

[a]Diagnostic groups are based on the eighth revision, International Classification of Diseases, adapted for use in the United States.
(Adapted from Ezzati, T. & McLemore, T. *The national ambulatory medical care survey, 1977 summary, U.S., January–December 1977.* DHHS Publication No. (PHS) 80–1795. Hyattsville, Md.: National Center for Health Statistics, 1980, Table 13.)

and vision impairments, fractures, sprains, arthritis, and upper respiratory infections account for most visits other than the circulatory system-related visits. The circulatory system visits probably reflect chronic rather than acute disease (Cypress, 1981).

All of these acute conditions have implications for the daily activities of the elderly. Nurses working in physician's offices, outpatient departments, and other settings where these older individuals are treated need to assess the patients' general functional ability and their living arrangements so they can assist these patients to plan modifications of their home environment to preserve safety of function and to obtain necessary services that they may be unable to perform for themselves.

As with physicians' office visits, the most frequent primary diagnosis associated with discharges from short-stay hospitals is circulatory disease, particularly heart disease; the rate of discharge over 65 years of age is 742.7 per 10,000 population in 1980. Digestive system disorders are the second most frequent primary discharge diagnosis, at 519.0 per 10,000 population, with major contributing disorders being ulcers, inguinal hernia, noninfectious enteritis and colitis, and cholelithiasis. In third place are neoplasms; malignant neoplasms account for 376.2 of the 425.0 per 10,000 rate for the total category. Close behind are the major respiratory system diseases, which rank fourth; 30.8 percent of these diagnoses are pneumonia (Haupt, 1982). These data and the frequency of discharges for other major systems are shown in Table 10–4.

If one looks at all listed diagnoses of hospitalized patients—a figure closer to a prevalence rate than to an incidence rate, and reflecting both acute and chronic illness—heart disease remains the leader at 2731.0 per 10,000 population. Digestive system disorders remain second and respiratory third. The category of endocrine, nutritional, metabolic and immune disorders is fourth; diabetes mellitus accounts for more than half of these. Close behind are diseases of the genitourinary system and diseases of the musculoskeletal system and connective tissue. Neoplasms rank seventh at 742.2 per 10,000 population.

Nurses, physicians, and other health care personnel working in hospital inpatient units may develop biased views of the elderly if they base their impressions of the health of the older population on the patients for whom they care. Practitioners in these settings see elderly persons who are generally sicker and

TABLE 10–4. RATE OF DISCHARGES (PER 10,000 POPULATION) FROM SHORT-STAY HOSPITALS FOR THE 10 MOST FREQUENT DISEASE CATEGORIES AND MAJOR SUBCATEGORIES, AND AVERAGE LENGTH OF STAY IN DAYS FOR PATIENTS 65 AND OLDER, UNITED STATES, 1980

Category of Diagnosis[a]	First Listed Diagnosis	All Listed Diagnoses	Average Days of Stay
1. Diseases of the circulatory system	1170.4	4311.2	11.2
Essential hypertension	(44.1)	(388.6)	(8.4)
Heart disease	(742.7)	(2731.0)	(10.5)
Cerebrovascular disease	(240.1)	(536.8)	(12.9)
2. Diseases of the digestive system	519.0	1228.9	9.4
3. Neoplasms	425.0	742.2	12.5
Malignant	(376.2)	(642.8)	(13.1)
Benign, in-situ, other	(48.8)	(99.4)	(8.2)
4. Diseases of the respiratory system	406.1	988.7	9.8
5. Diseases of the genitourinary system	284.5	820.3	8.8
6. Injury and Poisoning	288.8	526.6	13.2
Fractures, all sites	(154.1)	(209.9)	(16.2)
Sprains and strains of neck and back	(12.8)	(22.6)	(8.0)
Intracranial injury, lacerations and open wounds	(22.8)	(49.3)	(8.3)
7. Diseases of the nervous system and sense organs	248.7	616.1	6.2
8. Diseases of the musculoskeletal system and connective tissue	215.9	764.4	11.6
9. Endocrine, nutritional and metabolic diseases, and immunity disorders	170.7	897.1	11.9
Diabetes	(99.4)	(463.3)	(12.8)
10. Diseases of the skin and subcutaneous tissue	54.5	152.4	12.8

[a]Diagnostic categories are based on the ninth revision, International Classification Disease. (Compiled from *Current Estimates from the National Health Interview Survey: U.S. 1981.* DHHS Publication No. (PHS) 82–1569. Hyattsville, Md.: Public Health Service, 1982, pp. 32–33.)

more disabled than the elderly population as a whole. This population of hospitalized elderly may require careful discharge planning to enable them to function in the home and community and to obtain follow-up care after discharge.

Some of the discharge diagnoses could be iatrogenically caused during hospitalization. To avoid preventable iatrogenic disease, practitioners in hospital inpatient settings need to practice primary prevention. Effects of immobility, strange surroundings, new medications, and so on, may have serious consequences for individuals of older ages. They are at higher risk for muscle atrophy, impairment of joint mobility, development of decubitus ulcers, and pneumonia. Appropriate nursing care can prevent these conditions from developing. Mental confusion caused by the strange, perhaps fearful surroundings and new medications also is a risk. Efforts to orient these patients to surroundings and events can decrease the risk. Monitoring for mentation changes that could be drug-related may permit early detection of such effects so that dosage can be adjusted or the medication changed.

Quality of care has major impact on another measure, the length of hospital stay. This measure is used increasingly as a result of the recent DRG regulations passed by Congress. DRG stands for Diagnostic Related Group. Table 10–4 shows average length of hospital stay for common diagnoses. Fractures, with an average hospitalization of 16.2 days, contributes to placing the average length of stay for injuries and poisonings in first place, despite the relatively short stay associated with other diagnoses in the category. Neoplasms as a whole have the second longest average stay (12.5 days); malignant neoplasms average 13.1 days. Other categories with fairly long average hospital stays are circulatory system diseases; endocrine, nutritional, metabolic, and immune disorders; diseases of the musculoskeletal system and connective tissue; and diseases of the skin and subcutaneous tissue. Under the DRG system, hospitals are reimbursed for each patient based on a predetermined "usual and reasonable length of stay for patients in that category of diagnoses (e.g., fracture). These averages are determined from past data such as that shown in Table 10–4. If a patient stays less time than the usual and the care while hospitalized is less costly than that of the average patients used for determining a reimbursement figure, the hospital will make money; if a patient's costs are higher, then the hospital loses money. Quality of nursing care can have a major impact on how long a patient need stay. Prevention of complications is essential.

Differences in the ordering of acute and chronic conditions compared with the ranking of these same conditions as causes of mortality clearly reflects not only frequency of the disease, but also, case-fatality rates. Heart disease has both high incidence and high case-fatality rates. Neoplasms have a much lower incidence, but case-fatality varies widely by site. Some major sites, such as the lungs, have high case-fatality rates whereas others, such as the breast, have low case fatality. Although digestive diseases are common, they are rarely fatal. Thus neoplasms have a higher rank in mortality rates than in morbidity rates. Digestive diseases rank higher as a cause of morbidity than as a cause of mortality.

Nurses must help patients plan how best to adapt their lifestyle to accommodate and minimize the limitations imposed by these chronic causes of morbidity. For those conditions with high case-fatality rates, nurses have a responsibility not only to assist with medical care measures aimed at maintaining life but also to support the patient and the family in anticipating the possibility of death and helping them to cope with the related emotional, economic, and other consequences.

Limitation of Activity

An important reflection of the impact of disease in a population group is how much it interferes with normal activity. Table 10–5 shows activity limitations by sex for persons over 65 years of age living in the community in 1978. More men have general limitation of activity than do women; men also have more limitation of major activity such as ability to work or to keep house (43.2 percent) than do women (34.9 percent). The overall rate of 55 percent of elderly persons who have no activity limitation is contrary to the popular image of the incapacitated elderly person, although it should be noted that the 45 percent of persons over 65 years of age who do have such limitations does represent a substantial increase over the 23.6 percent of those 45 to 64 years of age who have activity limitation (Feller, 1981).

The 15 major chronic conditions accounting for activity restrictions are shown in Table 10–6. Although it would be

TABLE 10–5. PERCENT OF PERSONS OVER 65 YEARS OF AGE WITH LIMITATIONS OF ACTIVITY BY SEX, UNITED STATES, 1978

Gender	Activity Status		
	No Activity Limitation	*With Activity Limitation*	*With Limitation in Major Activity*[a]
Both Sexes	55.0	45.0	38.3
Men	51.8	48.2	43.2
Women	57.3	42.7	34.9

[a]Major activity refers to ability to work or keep house.
(Data abstracted from Givens, J. D. Current estimates from the health interview survey: U.S. 1978. *Vital and Health Statistics*, Series 10, No. 130. DHHS Publication No. (PHS) 80–1551. Hyattsville, Md.: National Center for Health Statistics, 1979, Table 14.)

informative to know what percentage of all older persons with a particular condition experience limitation of activity, the data are not available in that format. Rather, available data indicate what percentage of all persons over 65 report limitation in activity associated with a particular diagnosis (whether or not they have the diagnosis). Heart disease ranks number one as a cause of activity restriction, with 23.5 percent of those over 65 reporting limitation of activity due to heart conditions; men have slightly higher rates of activity limitation from this cause than do women (25.2 versus 22.2 percent). Women have a striking excess of activity limitation associated with the second-ranked chronic cause of activity limitations, arthritis and rheumatism. The percentage of women reporting activity limitation imposed by arthritis and rheumatism is nearly twice that of men (29.4 versus 15.6 percent). This is consistent with the higher prevalence of arthritis and rheumatism among women. Women also report somewhat higher rates of activity limitation due to visual impairments, hypertension (noncardiac), diabetes, musculoskeletal impairments and disorders, "other" conditions of the circulatory system, and mental and nervous conditions. Women have higher rates of fractures than do men, probably related to osteoporosis; this could contribute to the higher frequency of musculoskeletal-related limitation of activity. Among men, a higher percentage are affected by the other conditions listed, although, except for emphysema, the differences are not large (Givens, 1979).

TABLE 10–6. PERCENTAGE OF PERSONS OVER 65 YEARS OF AGE REPORTING LIMITATION OF ACTIVITY FROM THE 15 MOST FREQUENT CHRONIC CONDITIONS CAUSING LIMITATION, ACCORDING TO SEX, UNITED STATES, 1974

Selected Chronic Condition[a]	Both Sexes	Men	Women
1. Heart conditions	23.5	25.2	22.2
2. Arthritis and rheumatism	23.2	15.6	29.4
3. Musculoskeletal impairments and disorders (except paralysis)	13.4	12.1	14.6
4. Visual impairments	9.8	8.6	10.7
5. Hypertension without heart involvement	8.7	6.0	10.9
6. Diabetes	6.8	5.7	7.7
7. Other conditions of circulatory system	5.9	5.5	6.3
8. Peptic ulcer and other conditions of the digestive system	5.2	4.6	5.7
9. Cerebrovascular disease	4.9	5.8	4.3
10. Emphysema	4.4	7.9	1.6
11. Paralysis, complete or partial	3.6	4.2	3.2
12. Mental and nervous conditions	3.4	3.0	3.8
13. Hernia	2.8	3.2	2.4
14. Malignant neoplasms	2.2	2.8	1.8
15. Asthma, with or without hayfever	2.1	2.8	1.6

[a]A person can report more than one condition.
(Data exerpted from Wilder, C. S. *Limitations of activity due to chronic conditions in the U.S., 1974.* DHEW Publication No. (HRA) 77–1537, Series 10, No. 111. Hyattsville, Md.: NCHS, 1977.)

Because these data represent the percentage of the total population with impairment related to each condition, it may be assumed that the percentage of individuals with the disease who experience activity limitation may be much higher. Many older persons have several of these chronic conditions. It is probable that an individual who has multiple chronic conditions associated with limitation of activity is more likely to experience activity limitation than is an individual with only one condition. Nurses are most often the health care personnel who are in a position to assess the patient's life-style and resources and to plan adaptation of the environment and the individuals mode of functioning to minimize the impact of the illness on activities of daily living. Maintaining independent function is a high priority for most older persons.

Patients in Nursing Homes

Admission to a nursing home implies activity limitation requiring assistance in activities of daily living for at least a period of time. Among patients over 65 years of age who were residents in nursing homes in 1977, 43.8 percent had diseases of the circulatory system, including arteriosclerosis (23.1 percent), stroke (8.2 percent), congestive heart failure (4.6 percent), hypertension (3.9 percent), and heart attack or other ischemic heart disease (1.9 percent). Another 16.4 percent had mental disorders and senility without psychosis, 5.6 percent had diabetes, and 4.7 percent had arthritis and rheumatism (Hing, 1981). Among nursing home residents, prevalence rates of diabetes and major circulatory diseases other than arteriosclerosis did not show dramatic increases with increasing age. Women had the higher prevalence rate of hypertension and diabetes in all age subcategories over 65, whereas men had a consistently higher prevalence rate of chronic respiratory disease. Arthritis and rheumatism, arteriosclerosis, and senility did increase with age (Fig. 10–2). Women had a considerably higher prevalence rate of arthritis and rheumatism than did men, as well as higher rates of senility. Although the prevalence of atherosclerosis was higher among men at 65 to 74 years of age, the prevalence was higher among women after that age (Hing, 1981; Hing & Cypress, 1981).

Similar patterns are seen in discharges from nursing homes. Arteriosclerosis, heart disease, senility, stroke, and chronic brain syndrome are the five major diseases among nursing home discharges for both men and women although the order of stroke and senility is reversed for the sexes; senility is third for women and fourth for men, whereas stroke is third for men and fourth for women (Table 10–7). Hypertension and diabetes are the only two diagnoses found in common to both sexes among the sixth through tenth discharge diagnoses; hypertension is seventh for women and tenth for men. Diabetes is ninth for women and eighth for men. The other three in the top 10 for women are arthritis and rheumatism, hip fracture, and edema. For men, they are cancer, kidney disease, and chronic respiratory disease.

These discharge diagnoses are not directly comparable to the causes of activity limitation in Table 10–6 because each

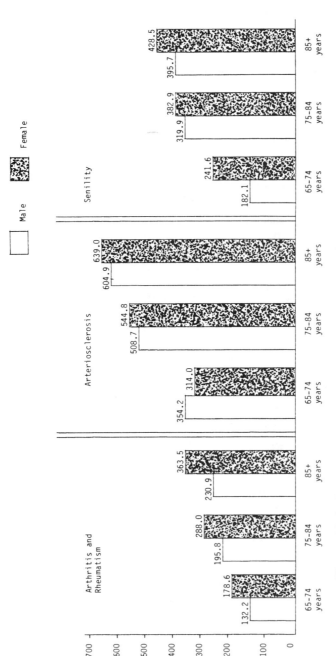

Figure 10–2. Prevalence rates per 1,000 nursing home residents for selected chronic conditions and impairments by age and sex: United States, 1977. (*Data from Hing, E. Characteristics of nursing home residents, health status, and care received, national nursing home survey, U.S. May–Dec. 1977. DHHS Publication No. (PHS) 81–1712. Hyattsville, Md., 1981, Figure 2.*)

TABLE 10-7. TEN MOST FREQUENT NURSING HOME DISCHARGE DIAGNOSES BY SEX, UNITED STATES, 1976

Order of Diagnosis	Women		Men	
	Diagnosis	Rate per 1,000 Patients Discharged	Diagnosis	Rate per 1,000 Patients Discharged
1	Arteriosclerosis	470.0	Arteriosclerosis	416.5
2	Heart trouble	379.4	Heart trouble	369.1
3	Senility	244.7	Stroke	252.1
4	Stroke	197.4	Senility	188.8
5	Chronic brain syndrome	196.5	Chronic brain syndrome	186.7
6	Arthritis and rheumatism	184.8	Cancer	149.5
7	Hypertension	169.5	Kidney trouble	148.1
8	Hip fracture	147.5	Diabetes	142.7
9	Diabetes	143.9	Chronic respiratory disease	133.5
10	Edema	101.5	Hypertension	127.8

(Data from Hing, E. & Cypress, B. *Use of health services by women 65 years of age and over, United States.* DHHS Publication (PHS) 81–1720, *Vital and Health Statistics,* Series 13, No. 59, Hyattsville, Md., 1981, Table 14.)

patient discharged receives a single discharge diagnosis whereas an individual can report simultaneous presence of multiple chronic conditions causing limitation and because different classification systems are used. Nonetheless, it is interesting to note that the vast majority of the ten major discharge diagnoses are also among the leading self-reported causes of activity limitation among the older population living in the community.

MAJOR FOCI OF PREVENTIVE EFFORTS

The leading causes of morbidity and mortality in the age groups over 65 years are, by and large, chronic diseases. In general, these develop over a long period of time either subsequent to a specific hazardous exposure, as with many cancers, or from long-term exposure to high-risk life-styles, as with heart disease.

The concept of health held by the elderly appears to be a functional one—if they are able to carry out activities of daily living, they are likely to perceive their health as good. If they are functionally impaired, they perceive their health as fair or poor. Seeking of health care is usually motivated by an actual or perceived dysfunction in health rather than preventive services, as evidenced by the 55.6 percent of office visits that are symptom related and the additional 15.4 percent of office visits related to initiation of treatment for a particular disease condition. This focus may result, in part, from a health care system that has had primarily a disease focus. Thus, interactions of persons in this age group with nurses, physicians, and other health care personnel are largely for purposes of treating acute symptoms, including acute exacerbations of chronic conditions, or for ongoing supervision and control of these conditions. Persons with worsening symptoms who have not previously been in the medical care system are likely to seek out necessary services to enable them to retain functional ability. Thus, the morbidity statistics for this age group largely reflect services for a tertiary level of intervention—diagnosis, treatment, and rehabilitation. Primary and secondary prevention receive much less emphasis.

This emphasis on illness care for the elderly is a function both of the aging process and of social circumstances. The elderly may wait longer to seek care, thinking that "nothing can be done," that they will be told they are terminally ill, that they can no longer live alone, or that it is too difficult or expensive to seek care unless the illness is serious. Also, health care professionals, who think of the aged as sick, are therefore less likely to think in terms of primary and secondary prevention when dealing with this age group. The all too frequently heard statements of nurses or physicians, "What do you expect at your age?" or "You're in pretty good shape considering your age," reflect an expectation that the old will be sick. This expectation is bound to affect the elderly and their perceptions of which illnesses and symptoms are worth bothering to treat. Thus, the statistical picture of morbidity among the elderly may be as much a reflection of effects of the distribution of services, what Medicare and Medicaid will pay for, and attitudes of health care practitioners and society toward health and illness in old age as it is a reflection of the health status and needs of the elderly. For these reasons, rather than focusing this discussion of prevention only on the diseases of high statistical frequency, the author has chosen to discuss preventive efforts by focusing on the aging process and the special needs that arise as a result of this process. It is hoped that this approach will alert care providers to the potential benefit of considering primary and secondary prevention for the older population.

Physiological Effects of Aging

In many ways, older persons are physiologically different from their younger counterparts. They have a decreased capability for adaptation to physiological and psychological challenges or stresses. Aging is associated with altered immune responses to specific antigens, altered physiological responses to exercise, to stress, to administration of hormones, drugs, nutrients, and so on (Adelman, 1980). Although age is useful as an index representing the processes that causally underlie the universal, progressing, and deleterious changes we call aging, it is at best a rough approximation; individuals may be physiologically and psychologically younger or older than their years in a variety of respects, showing a range of individual performance on age-related functions within any single age cohort. For purposes of research on aging, some more precise measure that classifies the psychophysiological level of function for each individual may be important and could potentially be developed. Costa and Adelman (1980) provide a good review of the various measures of functional age that have been developed. It currently appears that chronological age is still the best predictor of changes in physiological and functional status.

Because of the physiological differences of the elderly resulting from aging, it must be recognized in the process of assessment that the same definition for normality versus abnormality used in younger populations may not be applicable. The physiological differences of the elderly must be considered in decisions of whether to treat or not to treat and how to treat if treatment is given. The amount and kind of drugs appropriate for the elderly may be quite different from those for younger persons. Recently, it has been recognized, for example, that adult onset diabetes diagnosed in those over 65 most often can be satisfactorily treated without medication, solely by controlling the diet (West, 1978). Because the distribution of blood sugar values in the elderly population differs substantially from that in younger populations, question has arisen about the appropriate definition of normal—what values should be used to represent a diagnosis for diabetes. Blood sugars tend to increase as a normal part of the aging process. Is this increase in blood sugar at older ages associated with the same harmful effects as at younger ages? If not, then is treatment necessary? Such questions remain to be answered, but point up some of the special problems in managing disease in elderly patients.

Treatment with medication often can create new problems because of the high sensitivity of the elderly patient to drugs. Not only must physicians concern themselves with adjusting dose to account for this sensitivity, but both physicians and nurses must be alert to unexpected physiological or psychological changes in a patient that might reflect a drug response. Drug treatment should be considered as a source of sudden mentation changes in elderly patients.

Physiological changes of aging may also affect patterns of sleep and rest, elimination, and nutrition. Sensory function often decreases slowly but steadily; visual, auditory, taste, tactile, and temperature senses may all be affected. These changes, in turn, affect the individual's perceptions of the immediate environment, often leading to a sense of isolation or loss of control at a time when physical disability or disruptions in roles and relationships due to death or illness of spouse or friends interfere with existing social networks and availability of human resources to assist. If psychological adaptation is also impaired or decreased during the aging process, then ability to tolerate or cope with stress is impaired. Therefore, assessment of an older client must consider habitual patterns of functioning, methods of communicating, likes and dislikes, thoughts and feelings, beliefs and values, and resources so that any response to a new illness or disability helps the client comply with treatment and maintain as much as possible of what is important to him or her. Furthermore, such background factors are important baseline information in plans for primary and secondary intervention.

Accidents and the Elderly

The primary prevention activities with perhaps the greatest potential among the elderly relate to accident prevention. Accidents and injuries are among the 10 leading causes of mortality and are major causes of morbidity and disability for the 65 + age group. More than half of accidental deaths in this age group are due to falls that may occur in the place of residence. In fact, of all the 15.9 accidents per 100 persons over 65 years of age, 9.4 occurred in the home. Seventy-five percent of all injury deaths among the elderly are due to falls, fires and contact with hot substances, and vehicular crashes, including those involving pedestrians (Hogue, 1980). As Hogue points out in this excellent discussion of the epidemiology of injury in older ages, existing data indicate that accidents, like diseases, are not random events; thus they should be preventable if causes are known.

Physiological factors that are known to contribute to an increased risk of injury among the elderly are listed in Table 10–8 along with interventions that decrease the likelihood of accidental injury. Optimizing available sensory function is crucial. Any functional deficit can be compensated to some extent by adjustments in the physical environment that enable the individual to function safely with their handicap. Making such adjustments in the home environment is usually feasible. Making changes in the environment outside of the home is more difficult and probably requires intervention by public policy makers. Heavy traffic, bustling crowds in public places, and public transportation may all be difficult for a person with sensory or musculoskeletal impairments. It may be unsafe for some elderly

TABLE 10–8. SOME PHYSICAL FACTORS CONTRIBUTING TO AN INCREASED RISK OF INJURY AMONG THE ELDERLY AND POTENTIAL INTERVENTIONS

Physical Factor	Specific Considerations	Approaches to Prevention of Injury
Vision	Decreased visual acuity	Use of vision aids
	Increased sensitivity to light and glare	Homemaking adaptations like nonglare utensils; wearing of sunglasses, hats with brims to reduce glare outside.
	Slower adaptation to darkness	Use of nightlights; waiting for eyes to adjust before moving from place to place
	Blurring of contrast sensitivity	Use of contrasting colors to enhance visibility
	Alterations in visual field	Placement of objects at eye level; looking to sides before moving; colored tape on edges of steps
	Decreased spatial ability	Orientation instruction
Hearing	Decreased threshold sensitivity	Hearing aid
	Decreased loudness perception	Hearing aid; leaving car window open when driving so warning signals (e.g. sirens) can be heard
Sensory-motor function	Decreased reaction time	Anticipating events
	Loss of balance } Gait changes	Proper shoes; slower rate of walking with maximum width of base; lifting feet off the ground; nonslip floor surfaces; walking aids (e.g., cane)
	Coordination impairment	Larger handles on cooking utensiles, cannister lids, and other household implements
	Decreased tactile sensitivity	Use of bath thermometers to assess water temperature; daily assessment of extremities for undetected injuries

TABLE 10–8. (cont.)

Physical Factor	Specific Considerations	Approaches to Prevention of Injury
Musculoskeletal	Decreased muscle strength	Lighter cooking utensils and other household implements
	Decreased bone density	Avoiding falls by maintaining clear walkways; no throw rugs
	Decreased agility ⎫ Postural flexion ⎬	Structural changes, e.g., stall showers rather than step-over tubs, rubber mats, grab bars
	Decresed endurance	Frequent rest periods
	Joint deformity or change in range of motion	Long-handled implements; adjusting placement of objects
	Pain	Medication
Circulatory system	Altered cerebral function with tendency toward confusion	Avoiding change of environmental arrangements, e.g., furniture placement
	Orthostatic hypotension	Changing position slowly, e.g., sitting before standing when rising from recumbent position; avoiding sudden movements

persons to drive and it may be necessary periodically to screen elderly individuals for adequacy of vision, hearing, and reaction time for renewal of driver's licenses. Alternative sources of transportation may have to be provided to such elderly as a public service so they can maintain a degree of independence; many forms of public transportation currently available are physically challenging to the elderly. The high steps on buses and crowded vehicles that may require the elderly to stand are difficult for a young person with excellent balance, but almost impossible for many elderly persons. More readily available seating in public places where the elderly can rest would be helpful. Public education programs could sensitize the public to the special needs of the elderly.

Health care providers must also be aware of the likelihood that once an injury occurs, the effects on the older person are likely to be more serious than on a younger person. Because of osteoporosis, fractures are more likely to occur. Injuries resulting in breaks in the skin are more likely to produce infection because of decreased immune response. Activity restrictions imposed by the injury may contribute to permanent effects on physical mobility due to a loss of muscle tone, balance, and so on during the period of recuperation.

Fear of a future accident may also lead older persons to limit their future activity. Caregivers must plan ways to minimize these effects and to provide active rehabilitation once the initial injury has healed. This is particularly important in view of the tie of the older person's self-perception of health to functional ability. Furthermore, many of the chronic conditions associated with morbidity and mortality in the elderly may be exacerbated by the inactivity associated with accidental injury. Preexisting musculoskeletal conditions may be aggravated and the injury may produce a permanent musculoskeletal impairment. Cardiovascular function is enhanced by regular exercise; a lack of such activity may contribute to lower cardiopulmonary efficiency. Some gastrointestinal conditions may also be affected; inactivity may contribute to decreased motility of the intestines and can affect appetite and eating patterns. Older persons are more prone to respiratory infection as a result of decreased adaptive response of the immune system; inactivity may increase the risk. Because regular exercise also contributes to better oxygen uptake from the blood into the heart and skeletal muscle and increased glucose tolerance, such enforced inactivity may have implications for diabetic control (Source Book on Aging, 1979).

Chronic Illness in Older Persons

Heart disease, cerebrovascular disease, cancer, arthritis, and chronic dementia lead to much disability and often to institutionalization among the population over 65 years of age. Risk factors and causes of many of these conditions have been discussed in earlier chapters. By age 65, it is often too late for primary prevention of these diseases. Secondary prevention, particularly risk factor identification and treatment, may still be appropriate. The major need in this age group is to prevent disability from these diseases and to maintain maximum independence in the activities of life. This requires thorough evaluation and diagnosis, appropriate vigorous therapy of treatable conditions, and a comprehensive rehabilitative approach. Conditions such as thinning of bones in postmenopausal women, if detected early, can be treated by administration of additional estrogen and calcium. Vitamin supplements may be appropriate, particularly for those on limited or unbalanced diets because of restrictions ordered for certain diseases (e.g., cardiovascular or gastrointestinal disease) or because of dietary limitations imposed by dental problems.

Multiple chronic illnesses often lead to multiple physicians, each treating their own specialty disease. Patients may accumulate a wide spectrum of drugs over the years, some of which should not be taken in conjunction with others and some of which are outdated, but that the patient may still use as self-treatment of particular symptoms. Inappropriate use of drugs may exacerbate existing chronic conditions and precipitate new health problems. Mentation changes, cardiac irregularity, and dizziness are some of the problems that may arise. Periodic review of all drugs taken by older patients is useful.

Aging is accompanied by a decrease in lean body mass and an increase in the proportion of adipose tissue. Age-related degenerative changes in body composition also include a loss of muscle mass, motor function, and bone tissue, leading to fragile, easily fragmented bones. Whether such age-related decreases in muscle fiber and bone density can be prevented or stabilized by eating more food with amino acid, protein, and calcium is unknown (Source Book on Aging, 1979). We do know that other conditions of aging can be helped through appropriate dietary intervention. Common GI maladies of older persons, such as constipation, can be helped by high fiber diets and adequate hydration.

Maintaining adequate nutrition in the elderly poses a challenge. Many older persons report a loss of appetite. For many others, the dietary restrictions imposed for treatment of chronic conditions such as diabetes or heart disease make food less interesting; it is difficult to break eating habits of a lifetime. Many medications used in treating these diseases may have GI side effects. Dental disease may contribute to limited food intake. The depression of old age that may follow loss of a spouse or friends may lead to anorexia. Eating is often a social event and when one becomes isolated, whether because of deaths, physical incapacity, or limited economic resources, poor nutrition may follow. A well-balanced diet and adequate hydration, however, are essential to maintenance of health. Nurses must use their ingenuity in working with older patients to tempt finicky appetites and provide access to nourishing meals and social settings that facilitate maintenance of nutrition.

Regular exercise may contribute to maintaining physical as well as social and emotional health. Lederer (1978) reports improvement in social life, fewer physician visits, and fewer medications among those who undertake regular exercise. Exercise, with its cardiopulmonary benefits may also contribute to reducing the severity of effects in the event of respiratory infection.

Maintaining the older patient in familiar surroundings by adapting the environment to physical limitations can facilitate the maintenance of independence and can help prevent the depression and withdrawal that often accompany relocation. Involuntary relocation, in particular, often challenges the older person's adaptive abilities and may contribute to symptoms resembling senility. Illness often necessitates such relocation, whether to an acute care setting or to a long-tem care facility. Visual and verbal reminders to elderly patients of where they are and why as well as how they can obtain desired services (i.e., "press the call button if you need the nurse") may help. Appropriate architectural features to minimize barriers and hazards to independent function may also help prevent mental and emotional difficulties.

The goal of less dependency for the aged benefits both older citizens and society in general. Society benefits through reduced costs. Older citizens benefit from increased self-esteem and quality of life.

REFERENCES

Adelman, R. Definitions of biological aging. In S. Haynes & M. Feinleib (Eds.). *Second conference on the epidemiology of aging.* DHHS Publication No. (NIH) 80–969, July 1980, pp. 9–14.

Blackburn, H., & Gillum, R. Heart disease. In J. Last, (Ed.), *Maxcy-*

Rosenau public health and preventive medicine. Appleton-Century-Crofts, New York: 1980, pp. 1168–1201.

Costa, P., & Adelman, R. Functional age. In S. Haynes & M. Feinleib, (Eds.). *Second conference on the epidemiology of aging.* DHHS Publication No. (NIH) 80–969, July 1980, pp. 23–49.

Cypress, B. *Patients reasons for visiting physicians: National ambulatory medical care survey, U.S., 1977–78.* DHHS Publication No. (PHS) 82–1717, Series 13, No. 56. Hyattsville, Md.: National Center for Health Statistics, 1981.

Ezzati, T., & McLemore, T. *The national ambulatory medical care survey, 1977 summary, U.S., January–December 1977.* DHHS Publication No. (PHS) 80–1795, Series 13, No. 44, Hyattsville, Md.: National Center for Health Statistics, 1980.

Feller, B. *Prevalence of selected impairments, U.S. 1977.* DHHS Publication No. (PHS) 81–1562, Series 10, No. 134. Hyattsville, Md.: National Center for Health Statistics, 1981.

Givens, J. *Current estimates from the health interview survey: U.S., 1978.* DHHS Publication No. (PHS) 80–1551, Series 10, No. 130. Hyattsville, Md.: Public Health Service, 1979.

Haupt, B. *Utilization of short-stay hospitals: Annual summary for the U.S., 1980.* DHHS Publication No. (PHS) 82–1721, Series 13, No. 64. Hyattsville, Md.: National Center for Health Statistics, 1982.

Haynes, S., & Feinleib, M. *Women, work, and coronary heart disease: Prospective findings from the Framingham Heart Study. American Journal of Public Health,* 1980 70(2), 133–141.

Hing, E. *Characteristics of nursing home residents, health status, and care received, national nursing home survey, U.S., May–December, 1977.* DHHS Publication No. (PHS) 81–1712. Hyattsville, Md.: National Center for Health Statistics, 1981.

Hing, E., & Cypress, B. *Use of health services by women 65 years of age and over, U.S.* DHHS Publication No. (PHS) 81–1720, Series 13, No. 59. Hyattsville, Md.: National Center for Health Statistics, 1981.

Hogue, C. *Epidemiology of injury in older age.* Second Conference on the Epidemiology of Aging, March 28–29, 1977. DHHS (NIH) Publication No. 50–9691, July 1980.

Kovar, M. G. Health and the Health Care of the Elderly. *Public Health Reports,* 1977, *92,* 9–19.

Kovar, M. G. Morbidity and Health Care Utilization. In S. Haynes, & M. Feinleich (Eds.). *Second conference on the epidemiology of aging.* DHHS (NIH) Publication No. 80–969, July 1980, pp. 317–346.

Kunin, C. *Renal disease.* In J. Last (Ed.), *Maxcy-Rosenau public health and preventive medicine.* New York: Appleton-Century-Crofts, 1980, pp. 1228–1237.

Lederer, W. Get physically fit. *Parks and Recreation,* Oct. 1978.

National Center for Health Statistics. Advanced report of final mortality statistics, 1982. *Monthly Vital Statistics Report,* 1984 *33*(9, Suppl.).

National Center for Health Statistics. *Current estimates from the National Health Interview Survey, United States, 1981.* DHHS Publication No. (PHS) 82–1569, Series 10, No. 141. Hyattsville, Md., 1982a.

National Center for Health Statistics. *Vital statistics of the United States, 1978:* volume 11A, Mortality. DHHS Publication No. (PHS) 82–1101. Washington, D.C., U.S. Government Printing Office, 1982.

Rice, D. P. Sex Differences in Disease Risk. Handout at Symposium, *The changing risk of disease in women: An epidemiologic approach.* Oct. 22, 1981, Johns Hopkins University.

Ries, P. *Americans assess their health: U.S. 1978.* DHHS Publication No. (PHS) 83–1570, Series 10, No. 1420. Hyattsville, Md.: National Center for Health Statistics, 1983.

Shurtleff, D. Some characteristics related to the incidence of cardiovascular disease and death. *The Framingham Study.* Section 30. DHEW Publication No. (NIH) 74–599. Washington, D.C.: U.S. Government Printing Office, 1974.

Source Book on Aging (2nd ed.). Demographic aspects of aging and the older population in the United States. Chicago: Marquis Academic Media, 1979.

U.S. DHEW. *Healthy people: The Surgeon-General's report on health promotion and disease prevention.* DHEW Publication No. (PHS) 79–5507. Washington, D.C.: U.S. Government Printing Office, 1979.

West, K. M. *Epidemiology of diabetes and its vascular lesions.* New York: Elsevier, 1978.

White House Conference on Aging. *Aging in the states: A recent report of progress, concerns, goals.* Washington, D.C., January 1961, 22–24.

Section III

Applications of Epidemiology

Etiology and Natural History

As stated in Chapter 2, the natural history of a disease is the process by which diseases occur and progress in humans. Intervention in the disease process, ultimately, is aimed at halting, reversing or minimizing the process of pathological change. In general, the earlier in the disease process an intervention occurs, the easier it is to prevent or minimize damage. In order to plan interventions it is necessary to know the natural history of the target disease.

This chapter includes general concepts that are of importance in understanding the natural history of a disease. Applications of natural history are integrated throughout. The chapter also includes a description of the type of knowledge about the natural history of a specific disease that is needed by the practitioner and examples of how this knowledge can be used in patient management. The levels of prevention—primary, secondary and tertiary—were presented in Chapter 2 as they apply to each period or stage of a disease. Table 2–1 and the Prevention section of Chapter 2 should be reviewed before reading this chapter.

GENERAL CONCEPTS

The topics discussed here are included because they provide important concepts in understanding the remainder of the chapter, and these concepts have a significant impact on the choice of intervention. Understanding these concepts also should enable the health professional to review critically the literature on the natural history of a disease.

Natural History: A Continuum

As previously stated, there are two aspects to the natural history of a disease. One aspect is the process by which the disease occurs and the other is the process of disease progression. Webster defines a process as "a natural phenomenon marked by gradual changes that lead to a particular result." To describe the natural history is to describe the changes, that is the process, that leads from health to disease. Progression means to move forward, usually in a continuous, connected manner. To describe the progression of a disease, then, is to describe it's movement from one stage to another. The natural history may be conceived of as a continuum from where the individual is healthy—totally free of any abnormal or pathologic condition—to the opposite end of the continuum where frank pathology and clinical findings are present and death may occur. In order to understand the process, researchers attempt to identify significant phases along the continuum. These phases are divided into two periods subdivided into stages.

As discussed in Chapter 2, the first period prior to initiation of any changes at the cellular level is prepathogenesis. This period includes two stages, susceptibility and adaptation. Susceptibility represents a time of vulnerability when the ground work has been laid for development of disease through presence of factors favoring its occurrence. Susceptibility is followed by the stage of adaptation. Adaptation is the time when intra-cellular or intercellular reactions to some agent or stimulus may be occuring, but the reactions reflect the normal adaptation response of the cell or the functional system (e.g., the immune system). The second period is pathogenesis. The first stage in this period is early pathogenesis, a phase of sub-clinical cellular and tissue changes that represent the failure of the cell, tissue, or system to continue to adapt to or cope with the presence of a noxious agent or stimulus. The difference in response between prepathogenesis and early pathogenesis is determined by whether the response represents normal adaptation or a breakdown in the ability to adapt. A breakdown of normal adaptive response thus represents the beginning of the pathogenesis period, which extends from the earliest pathological changes to death. Latency, or induction, is the time between exposure to a disease-producing agent and presence of unequivocal disease. The period of latency includes prepathogenesis and at least part of the early pathogenesis stage.

Symptoms appear in some diseases during early pathogenesis, prior to when any available technology can identify the presence of early pathogenesis. For example altered emotional responses may occur in the early pathogenesis period for some brain tumors. In other instances, symptoms do not appear until late pathogenesis. A lump detectable by physical examination of the breast, nipple retraction, orange skin appearance of the breast, and nipple discharge are considered by most clinicians to be symptoms which are very late in the natural history of breast cancer. In such cases, the disease may sometimes be detectable by laboratory or other technological procedures. In the case of breast cancer, mamography can detect the disease prior to onset of symptoms.

Figure 11–1, which represents the natural history continuum as a straight line, illustrates the relationship of those stages to one another. At the left end of the line, points between a and b represent complete health with no abnormalities, even at the intracellular level. This is the period of prepathogenesis during which the individual may be susceptible but has not had

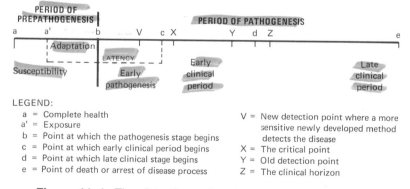

LEGEND:

a = Complete health
a' = Exposure
b = Point at which the pathogenesis stage begins
c = Point at which early clinical period begins
d = Point at which late clinical stage begins
e = Point of death or arrest of disease process

V = New detection point where a more sensitive newly developed method detects the disease
X = The critical point
Y = Old detection point
Z = The clinical horizon

Figure 11–1. The detection point, the critical point, and the natural history of a disease.

contact with the host. At the right end of the line is the worst stage of illness or death, point *e*. The period of intracellular changes occurs from *b* to *c*, beginning when an agent has contact with a susceptible host and the first intracellular changes occur. This is also the beginning of pathogenesis. Pathogenesis extends from *b* to *e*.

In many diseases it is only with the identification of substages within the stages of pathogenesis that it is possible to study and understand the onset of a disease and how and why the disease progresses. Cancer of the uterine cervix is one disease for which the natural history and its stages are reasonably well defined. The development of cervical cancer is believed to involve passage from normal cervical epithelial tissue to a dysplastic stage, to carcinoma in situ, to invasive carcinoma of the cervix, and then to death (Coppelson, 1967). Identification of these stages, which describe the process of the natural history, is the first step in understanding the progression of the disease. How or why it progresses through these stages may be studied once the stages are identified. Risk factors for the disease are important in determining how and why the process begins and progresses. Risk factors are discussed further in the following paragraphs.

Multifactorial Diseases and Stage-Specific Risk Factors

As stated in Chapter 2, multiple factors are generally involved in the onset and progression of a given disease. Several agents may interact in initiating the first stage of pathogenesis whereas others may promote the development of subsequent stages. Still others may affect the rate at which the stages of the disease progress. Cancer, for example, is now believed to result by a series of steps that include an initiation phase and a promotion phase (Pitot, 1981). One specific agent may produce an initial change in the DNA. A second factor may prevent or prolong the repair of DNA, producing multiple cells with abnormal DNA. A third agent may stimulate nucleic acid synthesis, which may lead to abnormal cells. Whether these abnormal cells are destroyed or whether they progress to malignancy may be dependent upon yet another factor. Whether the growth and multiplication of malignant cells continues unchecked may depend on still other factors. In this scenario, a cancer could be broken down into these stages: normal cellular DNA, abnormal cellular DNA, abnormal cells, malignant cells, malignant neoplasm, invasive malignant neoplasm.

After stages in the natural history have been identified, research focuses on identifying the factors associated with each stage of the natural history and how they relate to progression or transition between stages. Diabetes may serve as an example to further emphasize this point. Insulin dependent diabetes mellitus (IDDM) has been associated with a genetic predisposition (although there is a lack of good concordance between identical twins); environmental factors (beta cell cytotoxic virus and beta cell cytotoxic chemicals), presence of autoimmune phenomena in pancreatic Islets of Langerhans, seasonality, a temporal relationship to mumps, and the presence of neutralizing antibodies to Coxsackie B4 virus (Nerup, 1981). Attempts to understand what causes IDDM must consider logical relationships between these multiple factors, including potential biological mechanisms. A natural history that could be hypothesized as a sensible explanation for these associations is shown in Figure 11–2. The finding of genetic association that does not exhibit good twin concordance may reflect that only one twin was exposed to the viral agent and developed the infection. Seasonality and temporal associations may reflect the role of the viral agent in the disease; presence of viruses in the environment may fluctuate with time and by season, thus explaining the seasonality in the onset of IDDM. The presence of autoimmune phenomena and neutralizing antibodies may reflect beta cell destruction as a result of autoimmune processes or lack of regeneration after damage by the virus. Beta cell destruction may also occur as a direct result of viral infection in susceptible individuals (Nerup, 1981).

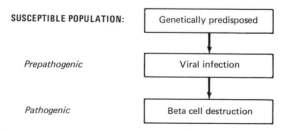

Figure 11–2. Hypothesized relationships in the natural history of insulin dependent diabetes mellitus.

Viral infection is a stage-specific risk factor in this hypothesized natural history of IDDM; it is not a risk factor in development of a genetic predisposition in the hypothesized natural history. That is, in the hypothesized natural history, a viral infection does not cause a genetic predisposition. Risk factors associated with only one stage in the natural history of a disease may be considered *stage-specific risk factors.*

Once the stages of a disease and the corresponding specific risk factors have been identified, methods of intervention at each stage may be studied. For IDDM, this may mean genetic manipulation (a method of primary prevention currently being investigated), immunization of genetically susceptible individuals (also primary prevention), medical treatment to eliminate or reduce beta cell destruction (secondary and tertiary prevention), or medical treatment with insulin to control hyperglycemia (tertiary prevention). It is not mandatory to prove that a factor causes a stage-specific reaction before doing a randomized trial to determine if an intervention method is effective. In fact, many hypothesized causal factors are verified as causal factors only through the process of a randomized intervention trial. For instance, if vaccination for Coxsackie B4 virus in genetically susceptible individuals was found in a randomized trial to eliminate the bulk of IDDM cases, then the hypothesized series of events is validated.

Unfortunately, many diseases are not understood well enough to identify stage-specific risk factors. Of course, the stages of a disease must be known or hypothesized before stage-specific risk factors may be studied. Fortunately, stages for most diseases are known or hypothesized; stage-specific risk factors may then be hypothesized from the risk factors known to be associated with the disease. Findings of research on stage-specific risk factors will have a major impact on intervention techniques utilized in the health care practice of the future.

Technology and Detection of Disease

The concept of the clinical horizon, which was first presented in Chapter 2, is a direct result of the status of research on stages of the natural history and is a function of available methods of detection. As previously stated, the clinical horizon is an imaginary line dividing the point where there are detectable signs and symptoms from where none are detectable. Detectable is the key word in this statement. Complete cell death or significant aberrant cellular changes are usually required to produce clinically recognizable disease. Although signs of early pathogenesis may be present, they are usually not measurable. Cell death and significant morphological cellular changes reflected in clinical disease are very, very late effects in the natural history of most diseases.

Scientists may be able to describe the mechanisms of prepathogenesis and pathogenesis of some diseases at the intracellular or tissue level. Stages of change in the cell thus may be known by research scientists. But until these changes can be detected by tests with proven predictive validity for clinical disease, early detection is not possible and diagnosis cannot be made until symptoms have been present for some time; until nonspecific symptoms become more specific to the particular disease in process, it cannot be diagnosed and treated.

An improvement in diagnostic technology will frequently change the stage of diagnosis related to the clinical horizon. Before x-rays were available, tumors were usually very large, causing severe symptoms before they were diagnosed. As the quality of x-rays improved and as computer enhancement was added, the ability to detect changes when symptoms are milder or absent, and thus to diagnose the disease earlier in the natural history, improves. This point is demonstrated graphically in Figure 11–1. In the past, cancer was detected between point d and e. The clinical horizon was very, very late. Now, cancers can be detected in the earlier clinical period of pathogenesis between c and d. The advent of electron microscopy, nuclear magnetic resonance, and other methods may move the clinical horizon further toward the left of the period of prepathogenesis, b to c, discussed above. Stages that precede the clinical horizon can only be hypothesized before more sensitive methods of detection are developed. Therefore, knowledge about the natural history of a disease is limited by our detection methods. To reiterate, the clinician should keep abreast of changes in diagnostic techniques and of how they affect our knowledge of the natural history of a disease. Such knowledge may have profound effects on application of secondary prevention activities and on the survival associated with a disease.

The Critical Point in Relation to the Detection Point

The critical point is a theoretical time in the natural history that is critical in determining whether there will be major or severe consequences of the disease. Examples of major consequences are serious disabilities, birth defects, coma, and death. If the point of detection is at point *Y* (Fig. 11–1) and the critical point is at point *X*, then no method of secondary prevention will be available. Cancer again serves as an example. Until very recently, a breast cancer of sufficient size to be detected by x-ray was considered to be in a late stage of pathogenesis; the neoplasm had existed for some time before detection and was often associated with metastasis. Treatment of breast tumors at this stage was not very successful. Let us say the detection point was at point *Y* during the invasive stage of pathogenesis. Since treatment of tumors (tertiary prevention) at this point was not very successful, the critical point was probably further to the left in the continuum, say point *X*. A new method of detection must be capable of detecting the tumor to the left of this critical point if survival from breast cancer is to be improved. Current methods of mammography appear to detect breast cancers prior to this critical point for women over age 50. Significant improvement in survival of such women with breast cancer has been found in a randomized trial (Shapiro, 1977). This increase in survival was not found for breast cancer in the younger women studied; presumably the type of breast cancer affecting young women has a critical point earlier in the natural history of the disease than does breast cancer past age 50 (this age difference may reflect premenopausal versus postmenopausal type breast cancer).

The improved detection techniques have moved the detection point toward the left to an earlier point in the natural history. If the detection point shifts to where it precedes the critical point, then significant opportunities for secondary prevention become available. Screening for breast cancer was not, until recently, an effective method of prevention for breast cancer because screening had no impact on survival. Now that the detection point has changed and appears to precede the critical point for most breast cancers in older women, screening is a efficacious method of secondary prevention method for women over age 50.

Efficacy and Survival Estimates

The question of whether a particular intervention actually minimizes or prevents damage is an important one; the answer requires knowledge about the natural history. Minimizing or preventing damage means that the natural history will be changed or altered in some way by the intervention. Changes or alterations considered beneficial are elimination of the disease, minimization of effect or disability, longer survival, and prevention of death. Longer survival may occur in two ways. In the first, the disease is totally eliminated by the treatment, for example, complete hysterectomy for carcinoma in situ. The second way is to slow down the length of time it takes for the disease to cause death. For example, an individual may survive for thirty years with diabetes instead of five years.

Efficacy is "the extent to which a specific intervention, procedure, regimen, or service produces a beneficial result under ideal conditions. Ideally, the determination of efficacy is based on the results of a randomized controlled trial" (Last, 1983). Prevention, intervention, or treatment may be considered synonomous terms here. Our objective is to minimize or prevent damage.

In evaluating the efficacy of a screening or diagnostic method for survival, the researcher and the clinician who reads research results must determine that appropriate analysis is used to evaluate survival. Figure 11–3, a modification of Figure 11–1, illustrates the difference between appropriate and inappropriate evaluation of survival associated with intervention.

Suppose that two women, Mary and Susan, develop a breast cancer that became pathogenic at the same point in time for each of them, point *a* in Figure 11–3, and each dies at age 35 from breast cancer, point *b*. Suppose Mary, at age 30, detected a lump in her breast, went to her physician, and following a biopsy was diagnosed and treated for breast cancer (point *K*). Susan, however, read about a local center that was screening for breast cancer using mammography. At the age of 25, point *L*, she had a mammogram that detected a lesion, was followed up by biopsy, and was diagnosed and treated for breast cancer. Mary survives until she is 35, 5 years since her diagnosis. Susan also survives until she is 35, which is 10 years after her diagnosis. Can it be concluded that screening improved survival? In

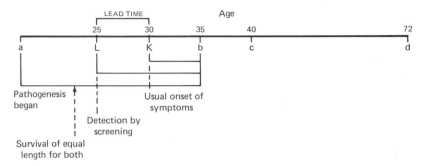

Figure 11–3. If two women develop a breast cancer at the same point in time (point *a*) and both die of breast cancer at age 35 (point *b*), then they have an equal survival. If survival is measured from point of diagnosis, point *L* for the woman whose lesion was discovered in screening and point *K* for the woman whose lesion was discovered at the usual onset of symptoms, then the survival of the two women would appear to be different, point *L* to point *b* for one woman (10 years) and point *K* to point *b* for the other woman (5 years). The interval between *L* and *K* is considered lead time and only reflects a difference in when awareness of the presence of disease existed. If the woman detected at point *L* had lived to be 40, then there would have been a true difference in survival, point *b* to point *c* a true difference of 5 years.

the past, most studies evaluating the effects of screening programs calculated survival for screened patients beginning with the time of diagnosis by screening and ended with their death. Patients diagnosed after seeking care for symptoms were used as the comparison group. Their survival time was measured from diagnosis (symptom onset) to death. If screening detects disease during early pathogenesis before symptoms are present, say point *L* rather than point *K* (Fig. 11–3), lead time is gained. Lead time is the extra time during which there is an awareness of the presence of disease, extra in the sense that it was recognized before symptoms were present. The lead time in this example is 5 years, the period in Figure 11–3 between points *L* and *K*. In the case of Mary and Susan, the five extra years for Susan merely reflects the lead time in detecting her disease. Presumably by detecting earlier, treatment will be more effective and the disease can be prevented from progressing. This is only true, however, if the screening method can detect the pathological change prior to the critical point. A false conclusion of increased survival may be made if comparisons of survival for patients detected by screening are made with the survival of those diagnosed because symptoms are present, unless lead time is subtracted out. Lack of control for this effect in such survival comparisons is called lead time bias. To be valid, survival comparisons must take account of lead times.

Case Definition

At this point, it should be apparent that the ability to determine who has a disease is an important aspect of studying and of treating a disease. Although diagnosing a disease may seem obvious, there can be multiple problems in identifying a person with a disease. A person who is identified as having a particular disease is called a *case* (Last, 1983). Identification of a person as a case requires a set of identification criteria that allow the clinician or researcher to clearly distinguish between a case and a noncase. A case may be identified by causative agent, by a symptom complex,, or by laboratory, x-ray or pathology findings. A combination of the above may also be used. Cancer is diagnosed by malignant findings from a biopsy; a case of squamous cell carcinoma must be differentiated from a case of oat cell carcinoma. Diagnosis of carbon monoxide poisoning is based on symptoms—headache, weakness, dizziness and a carboxyhemoglobin of 35 g/100 ml (Waldbott, 1978). Diabetes has no clear-cut case criteria. Some clinicians require a single finding of a specific level of fasting plasma glucose in order to diagnose diabetes. Some require this finding on more than one test, whereas others require a specific level of fasting plasma glucose and an abnormal glucose tolerance test. Other clinicians refuse to accept high plasma glucose as the sole criterion for diagnosis of diabetes. This reluctance is in part the result of a lack of conclusive evidence that correction of hyperglycemia prevents all of the pathological changes associated with diabetes (West, 1978).

The clinical manifestations of a disease are the result of factors common to the body's reaction to any stressor and factors unique to the specific disease. The unique factors are often more useful that the nonspecific factors in identification or diagnosis of a disease. The headache, weakness, and dizziness that are nonspecific characteristics of carbon monoxide (CO) poisoning do not alone provide sufficient information for diagnosing CO poisoning. When these symptoms are present with the specific findings of a carboxyhemoglobin of 35 g/ml, a factor specific to this disease, then CO poisoning may be diagnosed (Imbus, 1975).

Since multiple diseases may present similar symptom complexes, it is important to know the precise factor or factors that characterize the specific disease of interest. Although a nurse practitioner does not diagnose the disease, his or her plan of care requires knowledge of the precise disease under treatment. For example, health care and prevention activities necessarily differ for the ketosis prone diabetic and the ketosis resistant diabetic (West, 1978). While other criteria, such as presence or absence of an association with obesity, usual age at onset, and degree of abnormality of Islets of Langerhans, do vary for each, ketosis proneness or resistance is the critical criterion that differentiates them (Bonar, 1980). Both, however, are labeled as diabetes.

There is reason to believe that there may be several different types of diabetes with separate etiologies and natural histories, for example, diabetes induced by a beta cell cytotoxic virus and diabetes induced by obesity (West, 1978). Because the same pathological endpoint may be produced in different ways, it is important that the practitioner recognize different types or variants of a disease. Beta cell destruction can be caused in any number of ways, all resulting in a disease called diabetes (West, 1978). The significance to the practitioner is if different interventions and required or if the speed at which the disease develops in the different natural histories varies but each variant leads to a disease with the same name. In diabetes, weight control and modified diet may be utilized for an early stage of nonketosis prone adult onset diabetes. Oral hypoglycemic agents may be necessary in an individual with a later stage of nonketosis prone adult onset diabetes, and insulin therapy may be necessary in even later stages. A ketosis prone juvenile onset diabetic will most likely need insulin therapy at the point of detection.

Similarly, it is necessary to know with precision the natural history of specific types of cancer. Cancer of the breast and of the lung have different etiologies, different risk factors, and different patterns of progression even though both share the label of cancer. Even within the site-specific label of being cancer, specification by cell type may be important in the natural history. For instance, oat cell carcinoma of the lung and squamous cell carcinoma of the lung may have different etiologies. They do progress at different rates and they vary in their responsiveness to treatment.

THE STUDY OF DISEASE AS A PROCESS

The process of studying a disease is discussed to facilitate understanding of the current status of knowledge about the natural history of a disease. The phases (Table 11–1) are given for ease of discussion and to roughly parallel the order of occurrence of research on the natural history of a disease. For any specific disease, we commonly have more knowledge from the research or activities of the types listed in Phase I and less from Phase II type activities. Epidemiological researchers, however, do not currently proceed in an orderly fashion through these phases.

TABLE 11–1. THE EPIDEMIOLOGICAL PROCESS FOR STUDYING THE NATURAL HISTORY OF A DISEASE

Phase I

    Clinician recognition of an undiagnosable and unusual complex of symptoms and clinical findings

    Formulation of case definition for the first recognized cases

    Case finding

    Determination of incidence and prevalence rates and the duration or survival associated with the disease

    Determination of factors associated with the disease

    Formulation and testing of preliminary hypotheses

Phase II

    Revision of case definition

    Literature review

    Hypothesis generation

    Formulation of stage specific case definitions

    Determination of stage specific incidence and prevalence rates

    Determination of average duration in a stage

    Confirmation of stages in the natural history

    Determination of alternate pathways in the natural history

    Determination of risk factors in the natural history

    Experimentation

Although the first case reports on a new disease may generate basic research on biochemical, metabolic, or other pathologic processes that are responsible for the disease manifestation, the bulk of the research that follows usually will be epidemiological in nature. Epidemiological methods may be applied to determination of etiologic factors, determination of the natural history of the disease, and determination of the efficacy of various screening, diagnosis and treatment procedures. One epidemiological research project may address one or more of these purposes at the same time.

Phase I

A new or previously unrecognized disease or syndrome has to be identified in some way. Legionnaire's Disease was first recognized as a distinct disease after an outbreak of pneumonia among legionnaires attending a state convention in Philadelphia. (MMWR, 1976) After the U.S. Centers for Disease Control (CDC) did an in-depth investigation of the Legionnaire's outbreak, a specific causative agent was found (MMWR, 1977a). Subsequent to the identification of this organism, the CDC found that several pneumonia outbreaks prior to the 1977 Philadelphia Legionnaire's Convention had been caused by the same organism (MMWR, 1977a,b). In other words, the disease had existed prior to its identification, or recognition, as a specific disease. In this case, recognition occurred because of the cluster of cases at the Legionnaire's Convention that were of unexplained etiology and because there was a high mortality rate associated with the problem.

A disease is new when clinicians are unable to label the problem; i.e., there is no known specific diagnosis for the problem. Usually, recognition of new diseases requires awareness of several cases by one clinician or practice group. In addition to knowledge of several cases, recognition usually occurs because the cases have a severe or serious health outcome, such as paralysis, infertility, severe birth defects or death. This means that most of the cases of the new disease are at the late clinical stage. Occasionally, an early clinical case may be encountered, but generally the first cases represent the worst clinical cases, that is the late pathological stage.

A clinician who cannot locate any specific disease diagnosis that matches the complex of symptoms and clinical findings observed will have several options: to do nothing with the information, to report the findings to a government agency such as CDC, or to report on the case series in a publication. A published report on the cases may be the most common response although there is no way of determining how many diseases have gone unrecognized because of clinician inaction.

A published report on a case series will be descriptive in nature and for each case will describe age, sex, symptoms, significant history, clinical findings, treatment, and outcome. The clinician will report what he or she thinks is important or what he or she thinks may be risk factors for the disease. Presence of more than one case in the same family will be noted. If several cases have factors in common, such as excessive alcohol consumption, then that is often reported.

Once there is awareness of a possible new disease or syndrome, additional case data will be accumulated. Clinicians traditionally will report a series of cases. These case series reports provide information similar to that provided in the first report on a new disease but they will also expand on the initial information. For example, if the original report described abnormal SGOT levels, secondary reports may include findings for a whole panel of liver function tests. Or if the original report described the failure of particular treatment regimens, the secondary reports may describe successful treatment regimens. Any potential causative factors described in the first report will usually be reported as present or absent in secondary reports. Factors not previously described that may be of importance in disease etiology will also be included in secondary reports. Once case reports begin to accumulate, epidemiologists usually begin to study the new disease.

Before beginning the study of a new disease, researchers must be reasonably certain that the syndrome in question really constitutes "a unique new disease or syndrome". To be considered such, it must have a unique complex of characteristics that together result in a specific pathological condition. This represents the case definition. The *most* precise and specific case definition would be formulated from a number of cases after clinicians have identified *all* the findings associated with the disease or syndrome for each case including symptoms and the findings from hematology, blood chemistry, x-ray, NMR, histology, and pathology. Since such detailed and comprehensive information is seldom available for the majority of the initially reported cases, a case definition formulated at this point must be considered preliminary and should be revised as more information becomes available.

Once a preliminary case definition has been formulated, case finding, a concerted effort to find cases, must follow. Most often, case finding is done by clinicians and epidemiologists at major medical centers or state or federal government health agencies. Efforts are made through a variety of channels to request case referrals from the medical community.

State or federal agencies may publish preliminary information on the cases in state health publications or in the Morbidity and Mortality Weekly Report (MMWR) of CDC. Such reports will be largely descriptive, providing background information on the problem and the case definition. Incidence, prevalence, or attack rates or frequencies will be given. The outcomes or sequalae, such as permanent pathology and chronic illness or death, will be reported. (The second report in the MMWR related to Karposi's sarcoma and *Pneumocysts* pneumonia, which were later found to occur in persons with acquired immune deficiency syndrome (AIDS), recently recognized as a new disease, is given in the appendix to this chapter as an example of such a report.)

At this point in Phase I, epidemiologists would investigate factors reported present in cases to determine which ones are associated with the disease and may play an etiologic role for the disease. Hypotheses may be generated and tested for various risk factors suggested by primary and secondary case series reports. At this point in the research on AIDS, for example, it was determined that there was a strong association between AIDS and homosexuality (although it was not known if this was a reporting phenomenon) (MMWR, 1981a, b). For toxic shock syndrome, it was recognized that the cases were adult females in whom onset appeared to be associated with menses (MMWR, 1980). For Reyes syndrome, it was recognized that the cases were children in whom onset appeared to be associated temporally to a recent infection (Hattwick, 1979). Such information may provide a basis on which to formulate etiological hypotheses. If there is no basis for a hypothesis, then research will generally be directed to various host, agent, or environmental factors

including age, sex, race, smoking, alcohol, drug use, sexual preference, occupation, hobbies, infection history, general medical
history, family medical history, and nutrition. This has been
called a fishing expedition, because the researcher is fishing and
does not know what might be caught (in terms of causative
agents). Such studies are necessary to look for leads on causation when no reasonable hypothesis exists.

Phase II

As further data become available, serious consideration must be
given to refining the case definition for the disease as the preliminary case definition was based on a limited number of predominately late clinical cases and a limited amount of information about the cases. Publicity about the new disease may lead
to earlier diagnosis of cases. Using the same methods utilized in
formulating the preliminary definition, decisions based on more
cases and more detailed information will be made to determine
if revisions are needed. The most specific case definition would
be based on *all* of the findings associated with the disease or
syndrome, including symptoms, hematology, blood chemistry,
serology, immunology, x-ray, histology, and pathology. A complete set of such information should be collected for each organ
or system of the body that may be affected by the disease. *The
same information and test results should be gathered for every
individual* who is believed to suffer from this disease. Testing
procedures and test interpretation should be similar for all persons evaluated so that a standard definition of a case can be
used to asesmble cases for study. Lack of such comprehensive
and consistent testing of the original or secondary cases frequently results in case definitions that are not as precise or specific as is desirable. Table 11–2 provides a list of minimum criteria needed for developing an adequate definition.

The next step is to decide which hypothesis of the natural
history will be studied. A literature review of studies from laboratory and clinical disciplines may aid in choosing the most
biologically plausible natural history hypothesis.

Epidemiological research on the hypothesized natural history of a disease may be seen as directed to answering a number
of questions. These questions include: What are potentially
causal factors? What are the identifiable stages of the natural

TABLE 11–2. MINIMUM CRITERIA FOR THE MOST PRECISE AND SPECIFIC CASE DEFINITION[a]

Descriptive factors: Age, sex, race, socioeconomic status, occupation

Significant medical/family history

Estimated date of onset

Estimated date of exposure, if relevant

Symptoms

Diagnostic test findings

  A standard comprehensive set should be used for all suspected cases. Similar methodology and interpretation should be used for each test.

  Preferably these should be available for every organ or system that may be involved in the condition

Treatment

Outcome

Date of death or recovery, if recovered

[a]This information must be uniformly available for a reasonable number of cases to make it meaningful. Usually 20 or more would be required.

history? What are the stage specific incidence and prevalence rates? What are the average durations for each stage? In what ways, other than through progression to the next stage, might an individual leave a stage in the natural history? What risk factors are associated with each stage? What factors influence the stage-specific incidence rates? What factors are associated with how fast the natural history progresses? The whole array of epidemiological methods discussed in previous chapters is used in attempts to answer these questions. Confirmation of findings from cross-sectional and retrospective studies by prospective designs is often desirable.

Sometimes, however, ethical considerations make it impossible to do anything other than cross-sectional or retrospective research. For instance, a study of a factor that affects the rate at which those with carcinoma in situ develop invasive cervical cancer could not, ethically, be done prospectively. That is, one would not purposely withhold treatment from women with in situ cervical cancer just to see how a factor influences their development of invasive cancer.

Risk factors must be considered separately for each stage of the disease. The important question is what factors influence the development of each stage or the movement between stages. For instance, are age, race, age at first pregnancy, and number of sexual partners risk factors for developing dysplasia? A risk factor may affect only one stage or may affect all stages. A risk factor that affects an early stage may not show an affect on a late stage, and a risk factor for a late stage may not be a risk factor for an early stage. The factors mentioned for dysplasia are risk factors for cervical cancer (Cramer, 1982). They may not be risk factors for more than one stage. That is, they may not be risk factors for dysplasia but may be risk factors for carcinoma in situ of the cervix. If a factor is associated with a specific stage, the question may be asked, how does the factor influence the stage-specific incidence rate (negatively or positively, i.e., does the rate increase or decrease) and to what degree does it influence the rate (quantitative assessment on degree of influence becomes necessary)? A risk factor may also influence the stage-specific incidence in time. The next stage might develop more rapidly or more slowly because of a particular risk factor. Age seems to be a major factor in the rate at which the natural history occurs or progresses for many diseases and conditions. The question as to what factors are associated with staying in a stage versus moving to the next stage (or regressing back to an earlier stage) is also considered.

A systems model or a sophisticated mathematical technique may be necessary to understand all of the stage-specific risk factors, the process and the progress of the natural history of a disease. A tremendous amount of information is generated from the work described above for Phase II. Frequently, the only way to understand the natural history as a whole is to design a systems model to study and interpret the findings. The good news is that it is not vital to the practitioner to understand anything other than the stages, the sequence of stages, the time of regression for any stage, stage-specific risk factors, and efficacious intervention methods by stage. Knowledge of stage-specific incidence and prevalence rates and average durations in each stage will also be needed. The planning of intervention strategies for any one stage or level of prevention is greatly improved as a result of the findings associated with the stages and their risk factors.

Experimentation

The stages in the natural history and the factors affecting each stage can be conclusively determined only by experimental evidence from experiments or randomized controlled trials. Such research is designed to determine whether control or minimization of a stage or a factor will eliminate the disease, reduce the disease, lessen the severity of the disease, or prolong the time in a stage. A study of whether immunization of those genetically susceptible to Coxsackie B4 virus will have an impact on the incidence rate of IDDM is one example. Another example is to determine if reduction or elimination of exposure to a particular substance associated with a change from a latent stage to an active stage affects the natural history. For instance, if a substance or a factor is associated with dysplasia changing to a carcinoma, a trial may be done to determine the effect of eliminating or reducing the exposure. Computer simulations may assist in suggesting the most vulnerable, most effective factor or stage at which to intervene. Whenever feasible, intervention before clinical illness is preferable.

USING INFORMATION ON NATURAL HISTORY IN CLINICAL PRACTICE

The epidemiological process for studying the natural history of a disease provides a basis for critical examination of the related literature and provides a mechanism for assessing the extent of available knowledge. In order to halt, reverse or minimize the process of pathogenesis, the clinician requires a basic knowledge of disease progression and the factors that contribute to or cause the diseases of concern in his or her practice area.

Prevention at any stage may not require a full understanding of the natural history of a disease. Banning asbestos or imposing stringent restrictions on asbestos exposure may eliminate mesotheliomas. Stopping smoking may drastically reduce lung cancer and heart disease. Immunizations of high-risk individuals may greatly reduce IDDM. Elimination of aspirin use in childhood infections may eliminate Reyes syndrome. In each example, primary prevention is possible based on information on risk factors that were identified by epidemiological methods. For each, very little is known about the natural history, particularly the stage-specific risk factors, of the diseases. It is apparent that this lack of knowledge may not prevent the development of an effective intervention strategy. But what about all those individuals who never had any of the risk factors and still developed the disease? We all know of such people. Others who have all the risk factors never develop the disease. Only in understanding the entire natural history and the stage-specific risk factors will we be able to answer these questions.

The other side of the coin is the diseases for which we not only know little or nothing about stage-specific risk factors but also have not identified risk factors that can be effectively eliminated. Late age at first pregnancy, nulliparity, and obesity have all been linked to breast cancer (Chamberlain, 1982). Preventing obesity is unlikely to be an effective method of preventing breast cancer. Having children is not always a choice (never-married women and infertile women). And, while having children at a younger age may reduce breast cancer risk, it increases risk for cervical cancer. We do not know enough about the natural history and stage-specific risk factors of breast cancer to plan primary prevention strategies. Secondary prevention through the use of mammography screening of women over fifty years of age, however, is now a possibility. The prevalent therapy of radical mastectomy, though prolonging life, was a severe price to pay for the inadequate knowledge on the progression of the disease and the possibility of using less radical treatment procedures. Emerging knowledge has finally proved the safety of alternative treatment procedures at early stages.

The inability to offer effective primary or secondary prevention alternatives means that tertiary prevention is the only choice for many diseases and conditions. Arthritis is a disease in this category. Primary and secondary prevention strategies are unavailable for many diseases because we know too little about their natural histories and the factors influencing it. Medical costs in dollars, in disability, and in deaths illustrate the tremendous burden of a health care system directed to tertiary prevention. We have no choice but to concentrate our efforts largely on tertiary prevention when we do not know enough about the natural history of diseases and the stage-specific risk factors associated with them.

The other aspect of prevention today is that most primary and secondary intervention methods are dependent upon an individual choosing to reduce his or her risks. When an individual chooses not to reduce risk, the person will frequently state "anything can kill you" or "Uncle Joe smoked and drank and was overweight and an obsessive worker and he was run over by a drunk driver at 90 years of age." If we could explain the chain of events (the stages) that lead to a disease outcome and the factors that influence the outcome of each stage to individuals who are nonbelievers, a greater willingness to change may occur. When we can tell someone what will happen, in what order, how and why and when it will happen or not happen at each stage, and the probability of it happening, it will have a much greater impact than telling someone they have a risk factor that may lead to a problem in 5, 10, 15 or 20 years. One of the keys to such information likely possessing sufficient motivational power to cause change is our ability to provide information that indicates a very high probability of disease. For instance, if we could tell someone that because of their characteristics they will have a 95 percent likelihood of dying from a given disease, it is far more likely that they will be motivated to change. There always will be individuals who will end up in the tertiary level of health care. For them, we must know the best intervention methods to halt, minimize or reduce their pathological process. The clinical stages of the natural history and the factors that influence them then become crucial in planning effective tertiary care. Recognition of the role of estrogen and estrogen receptors in the clinical prognosis of breast cancer is an example of how such information may be valuable in planning treatment (DeSombre, 1984).

A list of the types of knowledge that are helpful to the clinician has been provided in Table 11–3. The clinician must consider which diseases, conditions, or syndromes are most prevalent in his or her practice area. For these conditions, the clinician should have up-to-date information on the natural history. If the clinician is unfamiliar with some of these, a reasonable way of updating knowledge is to prioritize study by the disease prevalence rate. That is, learn about the most prevalent conditions first.

After gaining a basic, or general, knowledge about the relevant diseases and conditions, the clinician should consider the appropriate level of prevention for his or her practice area. Hospital staff see patients and diseases predominantly at the tertiary level of prevention, although they might identify risk factors among family members that require intervention. Clinic and public health nurses see patients with problems that could be classified at all three levels of prevention. The type of clinic setting or specialty may affect where most patients are classified. Planned Parenthood clinics see patients at the primary

TABLE 11–3. HELPFUL KNOWLEDGE FOR THE PRACTITIONER ON THE NATURAL HISTORY OF A DISEASE

General information

    General description of disease

    Classifications and types of disease that may come under a general classification such as cancer or diabetes

    Basic pathology for the disease

    Methods of diagnosis: accuracy, sensitivity, and specificity of each

    Treatment for the disease

    Stages of the disease

    Risk factors associated with the disease

Tertiary prevention

    Clinical stages of the disease

    Description of characteristics of the disease at each clinical stage (i.e., stage-specific case definitions)

    Treatment methods by stage

    Factors which influence prognosis

    Secondary conditions or disease that may be associated with the primary disease

    Factors that influence or are associated with the development of a secondary condition

    Side effects of treatment

    Factors associated with side effects

    Average duration of each clinical stage with and without treatment

    Outcome (e.g., death, disability, sterility, paralysis)

Secondary prevention

    Prepathogenic or presymptomatic stages of the disease

    Description of the characteristics of each secondary stage (stage-specific case definitions)

    Intervention strategies and their efficacy

    Stage-specific risk factors for the secondary stages and the first tertiary stage

    Stage-specific incidence and prevalence rates (planners and administrators only)

    Average durations by stage

    Alternate pathways and direction of change between stages

    Competing risks

Primary prevention

    Description of stages and sequence of stages if more than one stage

    Factors associated with the stages or with likelihood of change to another stage

    Directions of change between stages

    Intervention methods and their efficacy

    Average time in a stage (i.e., prepathogenic latency or induction period)

level. A venereal disease clinic and a gynecological screening clinic see patients at the secondary and tertiary levels. The public health nurse may see clientele predominately at the primary level whereas the visiting nurse may see them largely at the tertiary level.

Information about disease natural history may be sought by level of prevention or for the whole natural history. Although practitioners should be familiar with disease stages and risk factors, it is only in planning and implementing intervention strategies by level of prevention that it becomes necessary to have information about all details listed in Table 11–3.

Intervention and prevention strategies do vary by stage. Primary prevention strategies include such activities as health education, counseling, immunization, personal or environmental exposure control (e.g., use of respirators or special ventilation when working with asbestos), isolation, restrictive laws (e.g., drunk driving laws) and medication (e.g., oral contraceptives). Secondary prevention strategies include screening, selective examinations, high-risk questionnaires with selective examinations, and abortion. Tertiary prevention is centered around medical treatment. The type of activities utilized at the primary level may also be utilized at the secondary and tertiary level. For example, if an obese woman has gall bladder disease, she should receive health education or counseling related to weight reduction. The practitioner knowledgeable about risk factors for gall bladder disease will also know that estrogens and oral contraceptives are a risk factor (Connell, 1978). Documentation of estrogen use or contraceptive needs and use would therefore be important to this patient's care.

Tertiary Prevention

Tertiary prevention predominantly involves medical treatment. The epidemiological data most useful at this stage include knowledge of the types of classification systems used for the disease, the case definition for each type, the clinical stages of the disease, the clinical definitions for an individual in each stage, the intervention and treatment methods for each clinical stage, and any factors that influence the clinical stages or survival. Age almost always plays a role, as does general state of health. Attitude and psychological factors generally affect most diseases at the clinical level by influencing the pathological progression of diseases. Specific factors such as estrogen and estrogen receptors in breast cancer were already mentioned. Side effects of treatment may affect the health of the individual or attitude towards continuing care. The negative or undesirable effects of chemotherapeutic agents and radiation are examples where the health of the individual may be worse because of the treatment than because of the disease. Death from infections caused by chemotherapy-induced neutropenia is not uncommon in cancer patients (Inagaki, 1974).

In another aspect of tertiary prevention, a second disease or condition is caused by, or associated with, a primary condition or by treatment for the primary condition. Knowledge of risk factors that may lead to a second disease are of particular importance. For instance, transplant patients tend to have cancer rates well above those of the general population. This is believed to be a consequence of immunosuppressive therapy rather than the primary condition that led to the need for the transplant (Hoover, 1973, 1977; Kinlen; 1979). Therefore, the practitioner may counsel transplant patients about the importance of avoiding risks known to be associated with cancer. Risk factors such as smoking, heavy alcohol consumption, workplace exposure to carcinogens, and poor nutrition should all be avoided. A former burn patient with scarring is at increased risk for skin cancer and should be cautioned against sunning or unnecessary sun exposure (Cobb, 1967).

The nurse at the administrative level needs to be familiar with incidence and prevalence rates and the average durations for disease in planning staff needs. If responsible for planning prevention programs, the nurse has to be knowledgeable about the entire natural history of the disease for which the programs are planned. Bed assignments may need to be altered depending upon the disease natural histories and the risk factors associated with their treatment. For instance, an infectious disease with a short period of communicability prior to diagnosis (that is, not diagnosable during its period of communicability) would not require isolation and therefore would not require a private room for the infected patient. The individual could be safely put in a ward. A community that has had several cases of AIDS can be expected to have an increasing need for hospital isolation beds. Development of policy and procedures for the protection of staff and patients is also a responsibility of the nurse administrator that is dependent upon knowledge of the risk factors and the natural history of a disease.

Secondary Prevention

Secondary prevention techniques are directed to the identification of individuals who are in the early pathogenic or very early clinical phases of a disease's natural history. Screening for early disease is the technique utilized most often. To screen for a disease, the practitioner must know the stage-specific case definition for early pathogenic or early clinical cases. That is, the practitioner must know the differences that characterize an individual who is clinically ill from one who is in an early pathological stage. The practitioner must also know the difference between an individual who is in the susceptible or prepathological stages and one in the early pathogenic or early clinical stage. Males in their thirties or forties who have a family history of heart disease, have high cholesterol levels, are overweight, smoke, lead sedentary lives, and have hypertension and abnormal exercise tolerance tests may be considered in the early pathological stages of heart disease. This could be a stage-specific case definition for early pathogenic heart disease. They may not be considered early clinical cases until angina is present upon exertion. These stages could be differentiated from later clinical stages by the lack of any demonstrable artery disease or cardiac pathology. In this example, although the diagnosis is stage dependent, there is no definitive way to differentiate the stages without doing a complete set of diagnostic tests. A man who reports never having had angina or heart disease may develop angina with the administration of an exercise tolerance test, part of the necessary workup for determining if a man is in an prepathological stage, an early pathogenesis stage, or in a early clinical stage. A history of heart disease may be denied, but resting electrocardiograms and the results of laboratory or other tests may suggest otherwise. Therefore, it is necessary to do a full set of tests whenever there is any doubt as to an individual's stage of disease.

The difference in treatment between the early pathogenic and the early clinical stages for the above example would be the utilization of sublingual nitroglycerin as needed for angina. Both groups would receive education and counseling on diet, smoking, alcohol, and weight reduction. And, both groups would be encouraged to participate in or provided with supervised exercise programs. Because of the abnormal exercise tolerance test, unsupervised exercise should be discouraged in men with early clinical disease. Both groups would also be treated with antihypertensive drugs. Periodic reassessment is necessary to determine if the individuals are still in these stages or if they have reverted to an earlier stage. Although some individuals always require antihypertensive agents and may continue to show abnormal exercise tolerance tests, others may no longer require drugs or have an abnormal exercise tolerance test.

The practitioner utilizes information on the average duration of the early pathogenic and the early clinical stage in planning the aggressiveness and frequency of application of intervention methods. A short stage of early pathology or a short early clinical stage means that there is little time for treatment and that identification methods or screening tests must be performed more frequently.

Breast cancer may serve as an example to illustrate this point further. With breast cancer it is likely that the same stages are present in all breast cancer cases but that in younger women the duration in a stage is greatly reduced. This would mean that the disease progresses more quickly through its natural history when younger women are affected. The previously discussed lack of efficacy for breast cancer screening in the under-50 age group could thus have been due to insufficient frequency of screening, rather than differences in the critical point.

Information on stage-specific incidence and prevalence rates assists the practitioner in planning and evaluating screening and intervention programs and in educating and counseling the individual. The practitioner may discuss with the individual how long he or she is likely to have the condition before it progresses, in the event changes are not made. At the same time, the individual may be told the probability with which certain actions are likely to result in reversal of the process, a slowing of the process, or halting of the process at its current stage. A clinician who is not knowledgeable about the natural history of the disease will not be in a position to provide such information and will thus be a less effective counselor or educator.

As in tertiary prevention, the administrative nurse uses information on stage-specific incidence, prevalence, and duration in planning and evaluating secondary prevention programs.

Surveillance programs may be necessary to detect drug side effects such as megaloblastic anemia in epileptic patients receiving anticonvulsants (several of the anticonvulsants are antifolate compounds). Monitoring oncology nurses for cytogenetic changes may be necessary if it is suspected that ventilation and personal protective devices provide inadequate protection when preparing chemotherapeutic agents and additional controls are not feasible under the current hospital administration. (Adequate ventilation and protective devises would be considered primary prevention.) Policy development, then, must also consider secondary prevention.

Primary Prevention

For most diseases and conditions the bulk of the public may be in the stage of susceptibility. Exceptions include individuals who already have some later stage of the disease, persons who are immune, or persons who are no longer at risk because of removal of the involved organ. For example, women who have had a complete or radical hysterectomy are no longer at risk or susceptible to uterine or cervical cancer. Diseases confined to one sex, race, or ethnic background also limit the susceptible population.

The prepathological stage, however, specifically represents a group at high risk of developing the disease because they have a set of risk factors that indicate a greater probability of developing the disease. Again, the practitioner must be knowledgeable of the set of risk factors or criteria that make the individual at high risk or defined as in the prepathological stage. Ordinarily, this definition will be based entirely on risk factors and not on any laboratory, x-ray, or clinical evidence of a problem. By definition, they are in a stage that precedes the presence of any such findings. For heart disease the definition might be a man age 25 to 70, overweight, sedentary, who has high cholesterol levels, smokes, and has a family history of heart disease. Exercise tolerance tests, electrocardiograms, blood pressure, and other cardiac tests should all be normal. For breast cancer, the definition might be age 35 to 70, slightly to greatly overweight, with a family history of breast cancer, first child born after age 25 or without children, and early first menses. Some clinicians would include fibrocystic breast disease as part of a prepatho-

logical stage for breast cancer. Others would argue that fibrocystic breast disease is an early pathological stage.

An individual in the incubation period of a communicable
disease may be in a prepathological stage, but it is extremely
important for the practitioner to be aware that the infectious
agent may be highly communicable at this point. Therefore, isolation may be called for even though the individual is not clinically ill. And, at the same time, the individual may need to be
closely monitored for changes to a clinical stage if the disease is
rapidly progressive or produces severe consequences such as
paralysis, coma, or death.

The type of primary prevention that is planned, then,
requires a knowledge of the characteristics of individuals which
would make them at high risk, that is susceptible to the disease
or health problem. It also requires a knowledge of the health
problem or disease in the community. See Chapter 15 for further
discussion on community analysis. Again, a knowledge of the
average duration and the stage-specific incidence and prevalence rates is necessary in understanding and planning intervention strategies and in providing education and counseling.

Many primary prevention activities are instigated by legislation or administrative decisions made at the community or
institutional level. Clinicians are instrumental in assisting with
such programs, including immunizations, health education, and
occupational safety programs. Moreover, clinicians have numerous opportunities to engage in primary prevention as part of
their daily practice. Knowledge of risk factors for various preventable diseases leads to identification of individuals who may
be more susceptible to a particular condition. Once identified,
health education aimed at reducing susceptibility of high-risk
individuals can be initiated. A patient in the hospital for eye
surgery needs education regarding how to maximize safety at
home to prevent accidents. This same patient may have a family
history of heart disease, a sedentary life style, and a diet high
in saturated fats. Education directed at changing exercise and
diet habits in order to prevent heart disease is also appropriate
primary prevention. Sometimes opportunities arise to engage in
such primary prevention with a patient's family—the smoking
son of an MI patient, the overweight daughter of a diabetic
patient. Knowledge of the natural history stages provides a
framework for explaining risks to family members and what can
be done to reduce risks. Anticipatory guidance for new parents,

counseling in preparation for retirement, or counseling the wife of a terminally ill patient are all forms of primary prevention for which need may arise in daily practice.

Administrators also engage quite regularly in primary prevention activities based on knowledge of disease natural history. Development of policies and procedures to prevent the spread of communicable disease to other patients and staff—for example, covering care of equipment and linens of infectious patients, handwashing procedures, staff immunization requirements—builds on such knowledge. Needs may vary by unit. Awareness of potential hazards in the institution is needed together with knowledge of probable effects of exposure. Musculoskeletal injuries, effects of exposure to radiation, anesthetic gases, ethylene oxide sterilizers, chemotherapeutic drugs, and infectious agents are among the hazards to be addressed through development of policies, procedures, and staff education programs.

REFERENCES

Bonar, J. R. *Diabetes* (2nd ed.). New York: Medical Examination Publishing, 1980.

Chamberlain, J. Carcinoma of the female breast. In D. L. Miller & R. D. T. Farmer (EDs.). *Epidemiology of diseases.* Boston: Blackwell Scientific publications, 1982.

Cobb, L. M. Trauma: experimental aspects In R. W. Raven & F. C. J. Roe (Eds.). New York: Appleton-Century-Crofts, 1967.

Connell, E. B. The pill: Risks and benefits. In M. C. Diamond & C. C. Korenbrot (Eds.). *Hormonal contraceptives: Estrogens and human welfare.* New York: Academic Press, 1978.

Coppleson, M., Reid, B., & Pixley, E. *Preclinical carcinoma of the cervix uteri: Its nature, origin and management.* New York: Pergamon Press, 1967.

Cramer, D. W. Uterine cervix. In D. Schottenfeld & J. F. Fraumeni, Jr. (Eds.). *Cancer epidemiology and prevention.* Philadelphia: W. B. Saunders, 1982.

Davis, J. *Personal communication.* Wisconsin Division of Health, 1980.

De Sombre, E. R., Greene, G. L., King, W. J., & Jensen, E. V. Estrogen receptors, antibodies and hormone-dependent cancer. In E. Gurpide, R. Calandra, C. Levy, & R. J. Soto (Eds.), *Hormones and cancer.* New York: Alan R. Liss, Inc., 1984.

Hattwick, M. A. W., & Sayetta, R. B. Time trends of Reyes syndrome based on national statistics. In J. F. S. Cocker (Ed.). *Reyes Syndrome II.* New York: Grune & Stratton, 1979.

Hayes, W. J., Neal, R. A., & Sanstead, H. H. Role of body stores in environmentally induced disease: DDT & lead. In D. H. K. Less & P. Kotin (Eds.). *Multiple factors in the causation of environmentally induced diseases.* New York: Academic Press, 1972.

Hoover, R., & Fraumeni, J. F. Risk of cancer in renal transplant recipients. *Lancet, 2,* 55.

Hoover, R. Effects of drugs—immunosuppression. In H. H. Hiatt, J. D. Watson, & J. A. Winsten (Eds.). *Origins of Human Cancer.* New York: Cold Spring Harbor Laboratory, 1977.

Imbus, Harold R. Clinical aspects of occupational medicine. In *Occupational Medicine: Principles and practical applications.* Chicago: Year Book Med. Pub., 1975.

Kase, N. Estrogen replacement therapy for the menopause. In M. C. Diamond & C. C. Korenbrot (Eds.). *Hormonal contraceptives estrogens and human welfare.* New York: Academic Press, 1978.

Kinlen, L. J., Sheil, A. G. R., Peto, J., & Doll, R. A collaborative UK–Australasian study of cancer patients treated with immunosuppressive drugs. British Medical Journal, 1979, *2,* 1461.

Last, J. M. (Ed.). *A dictionary of epidemiology.* New York: Oxford University Press, 1983.

MMWR. Respiratory infection—Pennsylvania. *Morbidity and Mortality Weekly Reports,* 1976, *25*(30), 244.

MMWR. Follow-up respiratory illness—Philadelphia. *Morbidity and Mortality Weekly Reports,* 1977a, *26*(2), 9.

MMWR. Follow-up respiratory illness—Philadelphia. *Morbidity and Mortality Weekly Reports,* 1977b, *26*(6), 43.

MMWR. Toxic shock syndrome—United States. *Morbidity and Mortality Weekly Reports,* 1980, *29*(20), 229.

MMWR. *Pneumocystis* pneumonia—Los Angeles. *Morbidity and Mortality Weekly Reports,* 1981a, *30*(21), 250.

MMWR. Kaposi's sarcoma and *Pneumocystis* pneumonia among homosexual men—New York City and California. *Morbidity and Mortality Weekly Reports,* 1981b, *30*(25), 306.

Nerup, J. Etiology and pathogenesis of insulin-dependent diabetes mellitus: Present views and future developments. In J. M. Martin, R. M. Ehrlich, & F. J. Holland (Eds.). *Etiology and pathogenesis of insulin-dependent diabetes mellitus.* New York: Raven Press, 1981.

Oakley, W. G., Pyke, D. A., Taylor, K. W. *Diabetes and its management.* Melbourne: Blackwell Scientific Publications, 1973.

Pedoe, H. Tunstall, Coronary heart disease. In D. L. Miller & R. D. T. Farmer (Eds.). *Epidemiology of diseases.* Boston: Blackwell Scientific Publications, 1982.

Pitot, Henry C. *Fundamentals of oncology* (2nd ed.). New York: Marcel Dekker, Inc., 1981.

Preuss, O. P. Beryllium and its compounds. In C. Zenz (Ed.). *Metals and Mettaloids in Occupational Medicine: Principles and Practical Applications.* Chicago: Year Book Med. Pub., 1975.

Shapiro, S. Evidence on screening for breast cancer from a randomized trial. *Cancer,* 1977, *39,* 2772–2782.

Waldbott, G. L. *Health effects of environmental pollutants* (2nd ed.). St. Louis: C V Mosby Co., 1978.

Webster's seventh new collegiate dictionary. Springfield, Mass.: G. & C. Merriam Company, 1965.

West, K. M. *Epidemiology of diabetes and its vascular lesions.* New York: Elsevier, 1978.

APPENDIX: Kaposi's Sarcoma and *Pneumocystis* Pneumonia Among Homosexual Men—New York City and California

During the past 30 months, Kaposi's sarcoma (KS), an uncommonly reported malignancy in the United States, has been diagnosed in 26 homosexual men (20 in New York City [NYC]; 6 in California). The 26 patients range in age from 26–51 years (mean 39 years). Eight of these patients died (7 in NYC, 1 in California)—all 8 within 24 months after KS was diagnosed. The diagnoses in all 26 cases were based on histopathological examination of skin lesions, lymph nodes, or tumor in other organs. Twenty-five of the 26 patients were white, 1 was black. Presenting complaints from 20 of these patients are shown in Table 1.

Skin or mucous membrane lesions, often dark blue to violaceous plaques or nodules, were present in most of the patients on their initial physician visit. However, these lesions were not always present and often were considered benign by the patient and his physician.

A review of the New York University Coordinated Cancer Registry for KS in men under age 50 revealed no cases from 1970–1979 at Bellevue Hospital and 3 cases in this age group at the New York University Hospital from 1961–1979.

Seven KS patients had serious infections diagnosed after their initial physician visit. Six patients had pneumonia (4

Reprinted from *Morbidity and Mortality Weekly Reports*, 1981, *30*(25), 305–307.

TABLE 1. PRESENTING COMPLAINTS IN 20 PATIENTS WITH KAPOSI'S SARCOMA

Presenting Complaint	Number (Percentage) of Patients
Skin lesion(s) only	10 (50%)
Skin lesions plus lymphadenopathy	4 (20%)
Oral mucosal lesion only	1 (5%)
Inguinal adenopathy plus perirectal abscess	1 (5%)
Weight loss and fever	2 (10%)
Weight loss, fever, and pneumonia (one due to *Pneumocystis carinii*)	2 (10%)

biopsy confirmed as due to *Pneumocystic carinii* [PC]), and one had necrotizing toxoplasmosis of the central nervous system. One of the patients with *Pneumocystis* pneumonia also experienced severe, recurrent, herpes simplex infection; extensive candidiasis; an cryptococcal meningitis. The results of tests for cytomegalovirus (CMV) infection were available for 12 patients. All 12 had serological evidence of past or present CMV infection. In 3 patients for whom culture results were available, CMV was isolated from blood, urine and/or lung of all 3. Past infections with amebiasis and hepatitis were commonly reported.

Since the previous report of 5 cases of *Pneumocystis* pneumonia in homosexual men from Los Angeles, 10 additional cases (4 in Los Angeles and 6 in San Francisco Bay area) of biopsy-confirmed PC pneumonia have been identified in homosexual men in the state. Two of the 10 patients also have KS. This brings the total number of *Pneumocystis* cases among homosexual men in California to 15 since September 1979. Patients range in age from 25 to 46 years.

Editorial Note: KS is a malignant neoplasm manifested primarily by multiple vascular nodules in the skin and other organs. The disease is multifocal, with a course ranging from indolent, with only skin manifestations, to fulminant, with extensive visceral involvement.

Accurate incidence and mortality rates for KS are not available for the United States, but the annual incidence has been estimated between 0.02–0.06 per 100,000; it affects primarily elderly males. In a series of 92 patients treated between 1949 and 1975 at the Memorial Sloan-Kettering Cancer Institute in

NYC, 76% were male, and the mean age was 63 years (range 23–90 years) at the time of diagnosis.

The disease in elderly men is usually manifested by skin lesions and a chronic clinical course (mean survival time is 8–13 years). Two exceptions to this epidemiologic pattern have been noted previously. The first occurs in an endemic belt across equatorial Africa, where KS commonly affects children and young adults and accounts for up to 9% of all cancers. Secondly, the disease appears to have a higher incidence in renal transplant recipients and in others receiving immunosuppressive therapy.

The occurrence of this number of KS cases during a 30-month period among young, homosexual men is considered highly unusual. No previous association between KS and sexual preference has been reported. The fulminant clinical course reported in many of these patients also differs from that classically described for elderly persons.

The histopathologic diagnosis of KS may be difficult for 2 reasons. Changes in some lesions may be interpreted as nonspecific, and other cutaneous and soft tissue sarcomas, such as angiosarcoma of the skin, may be confused with KS.

That 10 new cases of *Pneumocystis* pneumonia have been identified in homosexual men suggests that the 5 previously reported cases were not an isolated phenomenon. In addition, CDC has a report of 4 homosexual men in NYC who developed severe, progressive, perianal herpes simplex infections and had evidence of cellular immunodeficiencies. Three died, 1 with systemic CMV infection. The fourth patient is currently undergoing therapy. It is not clear if or how the clustering of KS, pneumocystis, and other serious diseases in homosexual men is related. What is known is that the patients with *Pneumocystis* pneumonia described in the previous report showed evidence of impaired cellular immunity and previous or current CMV infection. Furthermore, serologic evidence of past CMV infection and active shedding of CMV have been shown to be much more common among homosexual men than heterosexual men attending a sexually transmitted disease clinic. A specific serologic association with CMV infection has been demonstrated among American and European patients with KS and herpes-type virus particles have been demonstrated in tissue culture cell lines from African cases of KS.

It has been hypothesized that activation of oncogenic virus during periods of immunosuppression may result in the development of KS. Although immunosuppression often results in CMV infection, it is not yet clear whether CMV infection precedes or follows the above-mentioned disorders.

Although it is not certain that the increase in KS and PC pneumonia is restricted to homosexual men, the vast majority of recent cases have been reported from this group. Physicians should be alert for Kaposi's sarcoma, PC pneumonia, and other opportunistic infections associated with immunosuppression in homosexual men.

12

Disease Control and Surveillance

Although nursing practice encompasses the health of individuals, families, and communities, the major focus of nursing education and practice has traditionally been the individual. Health of the family has probably gained the most attention in community nursing practice. Although community health and community assessment are discussed in many texts, they generally receive lower priority in nursing education and practice, even in community health nursing, than does the health of the individual. This is somewhat ironic because the general health of a community may have impact on the health of individuals within that community. Certainly, monitoring health events in a community is crucial to early detection of disease outbreaks so that prompt intervention with control measures can prevent the spread and limit the incidence of disease. The greatest impact on the health of individuals may be made through control activities directed at high-risk groups that have been identified through surveillance or research. If one's objective is to improve the health of the individual, therefore, at least a portion of one's attention must be focused on the community group.

A community need not be conceptualized as a large geopolitically defined area such as a neighborhood, city, or county. For health professionals working in an institution such as a hospital, the community that affects individual health can be conceptualized as a micro-community composed of the hospital patient and staff populations. The health status of this community can be assessed and monitored for occurrence of unusual health events using the same methods applied to the geopolitical community. Institution of control measures, once causes of unusual events have been identified, can contribute to maintaining the health of individuals within this hospital community.

The appropriate target group or community depends on the practice setting and the types of health care problems that are encountered. To a public health nurse, the community or population of interest may be infants born in a particular county. Neonatal death rates may have been observed, through a review of death certificates, to be much higher in the city than in the rest of the county. The practitioner may then wish to determine whether this difference is a result of differences in prenatal care, delivery practices, or other factors that *vary* between the city and the rest of the county. Such a study may lead to recognition that in the city there is an increase in live deliveries of infants weighing less than 500 grams. Because infants weighing less than 500 grams do not generally survive, these live deliveries lead to an increase in the reported neonatal mortality. This increase requires no control activities as it results from medical care changes and reporting practices and there is presently no control activity known that could save these infants.

A nurse supervisor will be interested in the inpatient population of his or her hospital. A hospital patient surveillance system may have suggested a sudden increase in hepatitis cases and the supervisor wishes to quickly determine if the cases are predominantly in one unit (e.g., dialysis), one diagnostic group (e.g., leukemics), or in particular types of units (e.g., surgical). It may be determined that a new nurse had hepatitis when hired and spread the disease to all units where she worked as a float nurse. Control measures would include assuring that this nurse does not work again until treatment is instituted and the nurse is no longer contagious, that all identified cases are isolated and treated, and that all immediate contacts are treated with gamma globulin.

A staff nurse working in cardiovascular medicine is concerned with the health of patients in the intensive care unit and hypothesizes that the group of patients with frequent visitors do worse than those without frequent visitors. The nurse may initiate a study to investigate this question. If they are found to do worse, the unit may change its visiting policy. As illustrated in these examples, groups or populations to which surveillance and control methods are applied may be defined according to the interests of the practitioner.

This chapter addresses surveillance, investigation, and control of diseases as one aspect of group health care. _Surveillance may be defined as_ "ongoing scrutiny, generally using methods distinguished by their practicality, uniformity, and frequently their rapidity, rather than by complete accuracy. Its main purpose is to detect changes in trend or distribution in order to initiate investigative or control measures" (Last, 1983). The surveillance of a particular disease or health problem encompasses all aspects of the natural history of disease occurrence and spread pertinent to effective control. A surveillance system may also be considered a reporting system, that is, a system by which reports are made for some purpose. Another term sometimes used interchangeably with reporting system is registry. In epidemiology, the term *register* refers to "a file of data concerning all cases of a particular disease or other health-relevant condition in a defined population such that the cases can be related to a population base. With this information, incidence rates can be calculated" (Last, 1983). Some authors, myself included, differentiate between a reporting system and a registry by including in the latter the regular following of cases to determine case status, i.e., deceased, in remission, and so on. Date of diagnosis and case status may then be used to determine prevalence and survival rates. "The register is the actual document, and the *registry* is the system of ongoing registration" (Last, 1983). By these definitions, the pattern of cancer in the community may be monitored by a reporting system (reports of first diagnosis only) or by a registry (reports include stage at diagnosis, treatment, and ongoing reports of status). Birth defects are usually under surveillance through initial reporting only, although high-risk infants may be followed on a registry. Cancer surveillance, in contrast, is usually ongoing.

SURVEILLANCE

Surveillance of a disease or health problem may be carried out for several purposes. Information from a surveillance system may stimulate thought and increase awareness of health/disease patterns. Ultimately, however, the purpose is to spot new or developing problems quickly and bring them under control. A secondary purpose is to evaluate the effectiveness of control measures. For both purposes, the ultimate goal is to reduce or eliminate unnecessary suffering and disease. Reasons for surveillance are listed in Table 12–1.

Surveillance is a tool by which practitioners can quickly become aware of a potential problem (in terms of who, what, when, where, and how much). Investigation of the potential problem is the next step. Investigation naturally follows surveillance for there is little or no value in awareness if it is not determined why a sudden change in frequency of disease (a potential epidemic) has occurred or why there has been a steady increase or decrease. During investigation it is determined whether a problem really exists and, if so, it is then described more fully. Investigation also includes delineation of a probable cause of the problem. In many cases, once a probable cause is identified, control efforts will then be developed and applied. The hepatitis outbreak mentioned earlier in this chapter is one example of immediate development and application of control measures. In other instances, investigation and delineation of a possible cause may lead to in-depth research to document the cause. This occurred with toxic shock syndrome; although tampons were implicated early on as a probable cause, no reasonable action could be taken without further information on whether all tampons were involved, whether certain circumstances of use were involved and so forth.

Many surveillance systems exist today. The U.S. Centers for Disease Control (CDC) have monitored many infectious dis-

TABLE 12–1. VALUE OF SURVEILLANCE

Defines problem
Permits quick awareness of potential problem
Permits quick investigation and control
Reduces lost work time, workmen's compensation and insurance costs
Affords legal protection
Supports later research
Allows evaluation of control measures
Stimulates thought and increases awareness
Reduces cost of ad hoc morbidity and mortality studies

eases for years. Many states, as well as the World Health Organization (WHO), have surveillance programs with mandatory reporting of communicable diseases. Health professionals should familiarize themselves with local, state, and federal reporting requirements. Information may usually be obtained from local public health agencies. *Universally mandatory reportable diseases,* which also require quarantine, include plague, cholera, yellow fever, and smallpox. Louse-borne typhus fever and relapsing fever, paralytic poliomyelitis, malaria, and viral influenza are also reportable under WHO (22nd World Health Assembly). These illnesses are usually reportable first by telephone or telegraph followed by a written report. Rapidity of report is vital to containment of a widespread outbreak. For practical reasons, the American Public Health Association divides reportable communicable diseases into five classifications. The first class of case reports, which are universally required, has already been discussed. The second classification of *regularly reportable* diseases has two subclasses; one includes those needing rapid reporting to the local health authority followed by weekly reports mailed to next superior agency (e.g., state health department). Typhoid fever and diphtheria are examples. The second subclass includes collective weekly reports to local health agency of such disases as brucellosis or leprosy. The third major classification is *selectively reportable* diseases in endemic areas. This class has been subdivided into three categories based on speed of reporting needed (telephone; most practical means; and weekly collective report by mail). Examples are tularemia, coccidioidomycosis, and clonorchiasis. Food poisoning, infectious keratoconjunctivitis, and others come under the fourth major class, *obligatory report of epidemic—no case report required.* Outbreaks of such problems should be rapidly reported (telephone) to the local health department. Class five, *official report not ordinarily justifiable,* includes diseases that are usually sporadic and uncommon or where the report is of information value but of no practical value. *Control of Communicable Diseases in Man* (1985) is a handy and practical guide to the likelihood of reporting being mandatory. Because local and state laws vary, it is best to consult this guide or the local health department to be sure that compliance is maintained. Table 12–2 provides a general list of reportable health problems.

More recently, Legionnaire's disease, toxic shock, and acquired immune deficiency syndrome (AIDS) have been added

TABLE 12–2. GENERALLY REPORTABLE DISEASES

Acute respiratory diseases, viral
Anthrax
Botulism
Chancroid
Cholera
Conjunctivitis, inclusion (of the
  newborn)
Diarrhea of the newborn (epidemic)
Diphtheria
Encephalitis, infectious
Gonorrhea
Hepatitis A
Hepatitis B
Histoplasmosis
Influenza
Keratoconjunctivitis
Legionellosis
Leprosy
Leptospirosis
Listeriosis
Malaria
Measles (rubeola)
Meningococcic meningitis,
  meningococcemia

Mumps
Paratyphoid fever
Pertussis (whooping cough)
Plague
Pneumonia
Poliomyelitis
Psittacosis (ornithosis)
Q fever
Rabies
Rat-bite fever
Relapsing fever
Rubella (German measles)
Salmonellosis (typhoid and paratyphoid
  fevers, enteritis)
Shigellosis (bacillary dysentery)
Smallpox (variola)
Syphilis
Tetanus
Tuberculosis
  Pulmonary
  Other than pulmonary
Typhoid fever
Typhus fever (endemic flea borne,
  louse borne)
Yersiniosis

Other communicable diseases that may be reportable in some areas:

Actinomycosis
Amebiasis (amebic dysentery)
Choriomeningitis, lymphocytic
Coccidioidomycosis (coccidioidal
  granuloma, "valley fever")
Conjunctivitis, acute bacterial
Conjunctivitis, epidemic hemorrhagic
Granuloma inguinale (donovanosis)
Hemorrhagic jaundice
  (icterohemorrhagic spirochetosis,
  Weil's disease)
Impetigo contagiosa
Kawasaki disease
Lymphogranuloma venereum
  (lymphogranuloma, inguinale, climatic
  bubo)

Mumps
Pediculosis (lousiness)
Pneumonia, bacterial and mycoplasmal
Q fever
Reye's syndrome
Ringworm (favus)
Rocky Mountain spotted fever
Scabies
Staphylococcal infections
Streptococcal infections, hemolytic,
  including puerperal fever
Toxic shock syndrome
Trachoma
Tularemia

(Compiled from Benenson, A. S. (Ed.). *Control of communicable disease in man* (14th ed.).
Washington, D.C.: American Public Health Association, 1985.)

to the CDC list of reportable diseases. CDC also has a birth defects surveillance system for selected hospitals. Some state health departments, such as Wisconsin, have sudden infant death surveillance systems. Influenza surveillance is common in many states. Cancer surveillance systems or registries exist in several states including Connecticut, Iowa, Wisconsin, and New Mexico. State health departments should be consulted for a list of these and other notifiable diseases.

The American Hospital Association sets requirements for surveillance of infectious diseases in hospitals. Surveillance systems exist in some states for farm accidents, acute pesticide poisonings, birth defects, occupational accidents, and others. Death certificates are frequently used as surveillance tools for infant mortality, occupational accidents and diseases, cancer, heart disease, diabetes, accidents, suicide, and other purposes. Workmen's compensation data is used for surveillance of occupational accidents and diseases by many states.

Nurses have designed some of these surveillance systems. Nurses also serve as investigators and analysts in many of these systems. Nurses may also be involved in these systems as initial reporters to the system.

A surveillance and control system, whether for hospital infections (e.g., *Staphylococcus aureus*), community infectious diseases (e.g., measles), chronic diseases (e.g., cervical cancer), untoward effects of drugs (e.g., nausea, birth defects), or untoward effects of medical procedures (e.g., pain, bladder infections) can be broken down into several steps.

1. Planning the surveillance system
2. Collecting the data
3. Analyzing the data
4. Interpreting the data
5. Investigation (when indicated)
6. Control (when required)
7. Evaluation

PLANNING A SURVEILLANCE SYSTEM

Before planning a surveillance system the practitioner should have a reasonably well defined and specific purpose for the surveillance system. Answering the questions listed in the following section will be useful in developing a clear statement of purpose. The success of the surveillance system is dependent on clear and specific goals or purposes.

Planning of the surveillance system may be viewed as a series of questions (Table 12–3) that the practitioner must raise and answer before a system can be implemented. Before addressing these questions, however, the practitioner should review any surveillance systems with similar purposes that have been developed previously. Such a review should include an examination of purposes of the system, reporting forms utilized in each system, source of the reports, frequency of reporting, and adequacy (effectiveness) of the system. A review of this type will prove helpful in the design of the new system.

What is to be reported? A decision must be made as to what specifically is to be reported. Is one looking for all infectious diseases regardless of level of confirmation or severity? If one is interested in community surveillance of herpes, should reports be made of any recurrent genital lesion not diagnosed as syphilis, gonorrhea, or venereal warts or is laboratory verification of herpes necessary? Should both children and adults be reported if oral or ophthalomological herpetic lesions are suspected? Should a sexual partner of a genital herpes case be reported if this partner does not have a lesion and reports never having had a lesion but is the only potential source of infection for the *index case,* "the first case in a family or other defined group to come to the attention of the investigator" (Last, 1983)? Are all potential contacts to be reported? It can be seen from these questions that instituting a herpes surveillance system is not quite as simple as saying all herpes cases must be reported. In defining what is to be reported, a specific definition of what

TABLE 12–3. SUMMARY OF BASIC QUESTIONS IN SURVEILLANCE

How is a case to be defined and what is to be reported?
Where is the information to come from?
Who reports it?
Who is responsible for it?
How frequently is it to be reported/analyzed?
What is to be done with the raw data once it is in hand?
How is it to be evaluated?
Who needs the information?
Who will evaluate the generated information?

constitutes a case must be delinated. The following items should be considered in any delineation of what is to be reported:

1. Specific name of disease or health problem, e.g., not kidney disease but glomerular nephritis (Existing coding systems should be utilized where available)
2. Any laboratory tests or confirmation requested or required to be reported as a case, e.g., positive breast biopsy required for a report of breast cancer; a radiologic finding would not be acceptable)
3. Date of onset
4. Precipitating factor, e.g., verification of drug utilization may be necessary to define a case associated with side effects of drugs
5. Date or dates of likely contact or exposure to a precipitating factor, e.g., in infectious disease, environmentally- or occupationally-induced disease
6. Symptoms or symptom complex (which may be used to define a case)
7. Time period (duration) of symptoms, if relevant
8. Age of case if age criteria is required to define a case, e.g., a case of toxic shock was defined as being in women over 12 years of age

In summary, it is necessary to provide a specific definition of how broadly or how narrowly a case is to be defined in order that an individual be reported as a case.

Then a decision must be made as to what other information to collect about each case. The following items relevant to the natural history may be of interest.

Demographic data
Site of problem, e.g., vagina, eye, bladder, skin, postoperative wound
Date of onset
Date of probable contact (infectious)
Potential contacts (infectious)
Laboratory or other tests done
Date of tests
Types of symptoms
Symptom duration and severity
Treatment

Current status
Sequence of events (accidents, infections)
Source of report and date of report
Instruments or procedures possibly or probably contributing
   to or causing this problem
Where acquired or happened
Agent or likely agent
Protective measures utilized or not
Alcohol or drug use (accidents, birth defects, etc.)

Before a decision is made on the items to include in the report, the practitioner should consider a number of questions that are essential to planning the surveillance system.

The first of these questions addresses *where the information is to be obtained*. Table 12–4 lists some sources of information that may be utilized in a surveillance system. An occupational health surveillance system may utilize several sources. In a hospital infection surveillance system, all units in the hospital may be asked to report; a state cancer surveillance system may utilize the medical records department of each hospital in the state as the sole source of information. In making a decision about the source or sources to utilize, the planner should consider likely compliance with the request to report, whether reports will be reliable and on time, completeness of information available at a

TABLE 12–4. SOURCES OF INFORMATION FOR SURVEILLANCE

Medical records
Preemployment physicals
Patient or employee (questionnaires, interviews)
Spouse
Absentee reports
Hospital records
Medical insurance
Life insurance
Workmen's compensation records
Other clinical records (in house)
Local clinic, emergency room, or other hospital records
Discharge physical (from company)
Union records
Personnel records

given source, comparability between sources (if several sources are utilized), and cost factors.

The next question that may be asked is, *Who will complete the written report and in what order?* The patient, the unit clerk, the physician, the nurse, the medical records department librarian, the hospital administrator, the local health officer, the pharmacist, the school nurse, the insurance company clerk, the clinic nurse, and the pathologist could be used to report. In making a decision about who should report, consideration must be given to the level of accuracy needed, the likely completeness of the report (i.e., who provides more complete information), the timeliness required (time may be vital), and the likelihood that a report would be submitted. The Wisconsin health department found that switching from a physician-based to a hospital–medical records librarian-based cancer reporting system increased reports from around 30 per cent to over 90 per cent of cases. If there are several tiers in the reporting chain, the individuals who are responsible at each level must be identified. For example, a case of salmonellosis may be reported by a physician to the local health officer (at the local health department), who then reports to the regional or state health department epidemiologist, who then reports it to the U.S. Centers for Disease Control. The type of individual (secretary, unit clerk, nurse, physician, pharmacist, medical records librarian, pathologist, etc.) must be specified at each level of the reporting system and then the names, addresses, and telephone numbers of those individuals should be obtained. In conjunction with this delineation of who reports and the chain or order of reporting, one individual should be ultimately responsible for seeing that reports are made. If responsibility is not clearly placed and delineated to those in the reporting system, the system will likely be of little value and eventually collapse.

It is often helpful to have people who will participate in the reporting system help with the design of the system and find out how best to meet their needs through the system. A system that they see as beneficial and that meets their needs is more likely to be a system that works and meets your needs. For example, physicians reporting cancer cases may report more completely and more accurately if a meeting is held with representative doctors to determine what type of information may be of help in planning treatment and frequency of follow-up of their cases. They may wish to compare survival rates for their hospital with other similar types of hospitals in the state. If they see that their rates are lower or higher, they may wish to determine what is different about their cases, treatment, or frequency of follow-up visits. Such planning will contribute ideas, clarification, and identification of problems. Going through all the steps in designing the system jointly with the principal system designer will help the physicians, nurses, or other individuals doing the reporting to understand the decisions that are made and will lead to a personal interest in the quality of the system. At the same time, the principal designer will obtain a more complete and accurate system.

The next two questions to address in designing a surveillance system are: *How frequently are data to be reported?* and *How frequently are data to be analyzed?* A case may be reported as soon as it occurs, or cases may be reported daily, weekly, monthly, or yearly. The frequency of reporting depends on the nature of the disease or health problem and the specific purposes of the surveillance system. For example, hepatitis should be reported daily, carbon monoxide poisoning should be reported immediately, and cancer should be reported at least monthly. Analysis may also be done daily, weekly or monthly. Again the frequency depends on the nature of the disease or health problem, and the purposes of the surveillance system. Generally analysis is done with the same frequency as reporting. That is, if daily reports are required these reports should be analyzed daily, weekly reports analyzed weekly, and so on. Exceptions do occur. In the case of acquired immune deficiency syndrome (AIDS) it may be necessary to report cases immediately so that sexual contacts can be located and further contacts eliminated or reduced; here frequency of reporting is necessitated by the control measures that are needed. Analysis of AIDS surveillance data may be necessary only on a monthly basis, however. In the case of birth defects, annual analysis may be sufficiently frequent.

Reporting may be required more frequently than analysis if those who report are likely to forget to report because of the time interval. For instance, a nurse is more likely to report a drug side effect if he or she has to complete a report form at the time the effect occurs rather than completing the reports once a month. Frequency is also dependent on time and staff resources. The nurse who must care for a full unit with little help is not very likely to spend much time completing forms. There is little value in frequent reporting and analyses if the system staff do not have the time to monitor and investigate the data that is produced from frequent monitoring.

The final questions to address in planning a surveillance system are: *What are you going to do with the raw data once you have it? Who needs the information provided by the system? How is the information to be evaluated?* and *How is the surveillance system itself to be evaluated?* As the definition of surveillance indicates, a surveillance system is meant to provide information. Rare case reports only become information when they are considered in relation to other case reports, i.e., epidemiological analyses. At the minimum, general frequency counts and rates are determined. Frequency counts and rates may also be examined within categories of place, time, and age. In producing this data the practitioner seeks to determine if the incidence or prevalence rate is unusual (suggesting an epidemic) or if there is a trend that would indicate that a problem may be developing. The decision whether both frequency counts and rates are to be generated or if only frequency counts are to be studied must be based on a determination of whether the counts are of sufficient size to make rates meaningful in view of the size of the population denominator to be utilized. In general, rates are usually preferable. Extremely rare diseases, however, are usually reported in surveillance system reports as frequency counts because the number of events in the numerator is too small relative to the denominator to detect changes in rates.

Breaking down the surveillance data by place, time, and age allows for consideration of unusual changes or trends. If an incidence rate is unusual in a particular part of the hospital, a particular school, a particular community, a particular age group, or in a particular period of time, it can provide useful clues as to what may be contributing to an increase or trend. Another reason for such analyses is that sometimes a change in rates may not be apparent at the general population level but becomes readily apparent with more detailed analyses (a dilution type effect). The following theoretical example may make this clearer. Analysis of hospital infections determines that 14 cases of staff needle punctures per month is the usual number for the hospital. The latest analysis has determined that there are 15 cases during the current month. Fifteen cases are no more than would be within the expected range for the hospital. If the hospital has a staff of 1000; the needle puncture rate would be 15 in 1000 or 1.5 per 100 staff. One staff member suggests that it is possible that the needle sticks are much more frequent than 1.5 per 100 staff in her unit. A more detailed analysis is then done by determining the rate of needle sticks for each unit. Table 12–5 presents the findings.

After detailed analysis it is apparent that unit six has a much higher rate than that which is generally the case for the other hospital units. General analysis would have missed this finding. Investigation is now required to determine why this unit has such a high rate.

In general, the information generated by a surveillance system should result in a regular and periodic summary report of results of analyses. This report is then distributed to the providers of the data and to others who need or wish to have the information. As previously indicated, determination of the needs of the providers and meeting those needs in the report are vital links in a good surveillance system. An example of such an effort is a cancer registry reporting back to a local hospital how it's treatment and survival patterns compare to other hospitals in the registry. Summary reports may also include reports of investigations done as a result of the generated information. The CDC, for example, routinely report such investigations based on their surveillance data in the *Morbidity and Mortality*

TABLE 12–5. HYPOTHETICAL DATA ON NEEDLE PUNCTURES BY HOSPITAL UNIT

Unit	Frequency	Staff Size	Rate (per 100 staff)
1	1	65	1.54
2	1	55	1.82
3	1	50	2.00
4	2	200	1.00
5	1	110	0.91
6	5	80	6.25
7	0	100	—
8	1	90	1.11
9	1	50	2.00
10	2	200	1.00
Total	15	1000	1.50

Weekly Report (MMWR). Such a CDC report may describe an investigation of a giardia outbreak in a rural Colorado town or an investigation of health complaints associated with a particular baby food.

As previously stated, to determine if a potential problem is to be investigated, some evaluation of the information generated (the frequency counts and rates) must be done. The presence of data alone does not guarantee that a problem will be recognized. Someone must organize and evaluate the data. The limited time of an individual or scarce staff resources of an agency for review of data can often be utilized most efficiently by using a computer. Where computer resources are unavailable, hand tabulation and review are required. If no evaluation is done, it is not worth the time, money, and effort to collect the raw data.

An informal evaluation may consist merely of someone looking at the information generated (without additional analysis) for possible epidemics or serious upward trends. For example, the nurse epidemiologist may look at the data in the needle puncture example and decide to investigate the cause of the excess in unit 6. Or, a statistical test may routinely be done to determine if the current rate is significantly different from that for some previous period of time. Although the statistical test to be utilized depends on the characteristics of the data, the chi square test of differences is used most frequently. The rapid increase in computer utilization may contribute to routine use of statistical tests. Although the latter should not entirely replace the informal procedure, it does have the advantage of extremely rapid evaluation of large amounts of information. This would mean that the reviewers would have to spend time considering only likely problems, not all the data. In other words, a lot of data may be reduced to a more manageable work load. It also avoids the problem of tired, overworked individuals missing important information because they have had too large a volume of data to review. The thalidomide tragedy is one example where the increase in severe birth defects should have been readily recognizable, but simply was not recognized until a large number of children had been affected (Taussig, 1962). In another case, 70 per cent of the workers in one plant manufacturing a particular substance developed severe bladder problems, most requiring surgery, before anyone noticed (Joint NIOSH/OSHA, 1978). The most important thing to remember is that the ultimate purpose of a surveillance system is to spot new or developing problems quickly before needless suffering occurs. To accomplish this purpose, the data must be effectively reviewed and evaluated.

Once all of the above questions have been resolved, attention should be given to development of an evaluation plan for the surveillance system as a whole. It should address such questions as: Was the purpose of the system met? For instance, were there any investigations carried out? Did these investigations lead to the identification of a problem that was subsequently controlled or eliminated? What proportion of investigations led to control or elimination? Other system evaluation questions might include whether a problem was identified earlier than it would have been without the system. How much earlier? Did the reduction in time to recognition have an impact on the rate of suffering? Administrative- or process-related questions that may be addressed in a system evaluation are quality of reporting, timeliness of reporting (late reports are of little value if there are so many that the epidemic is over before it is even recognized), adequacy of the reporting frequency (the system requested frequency), completeness of reporting (i.e., what proportion of all cases are actually reported), timeliness of summary reports, and how well needs of report providers are being met. Table 12–6 summarizes system evaluation questions.

TABLE 12–6. SYSTEM EVALUATION QUESTIONS

Questions related to system goals

Was the purpose of the system met?
  Were there any investigations carried out?
  Did these investigations lead to identification of a problem that was subsequently controlled or eliminated?
  What proportion of investigations led to control or elimination?
Was a problem identified earlier than it would have been without a system? How much earlier?

Administrative and process questions

How high is the quality of the reporting?
How timely are the reports?
Is the reporting frequency adequate?
How complete is the reporting?

DATA COLLECTION

Most of the issues related to data collection have been addressed in the previous discussion of planning a surveillance system. In making the final determination of which pieces of raw data are to be collected, it must be recognized that the success of the system will be, in part, dependent upon collecting the minimum amount of information necessary, yet sufficient for analysis and interpretation and to determine whether more information is needed, that is, whether an investigation is needed. Completeness of reports, compliance with reporting schedules, and cooperation of personnel are often a function of how much data are to be collected. As a result, the value of the entire reporting system may be dependent on the length and ease of completing the report forms.

During the regular operation of the surveillance system, periodic review of the data collection process should be carried out. This periodic review should consider the process-related items already discussed, i.e., quality of reporting, timeliness of reporting, completeness of reporting, and adequacy of reporting frequency. During the first phase following implementation of a surveillance system, consideration should also be directed to the appropriateness of the original choice for the sources to be utilized and for the individuals responsible for reporting. The periodic review of the data collection process is intended to determine if the data collection process is working. Regular review and elimination of problems should avoid a late realization that the purpose of the surveillance system was not met because of problems in the data collection process.

DATA ANALYSIS AND INTERPRETATION

As indicated previously, both the items on the report that are to be analyzed and the analytic procedures should be selected during the planning phase. Then, at the time analysis is carried out, data necessary for analytic procedures such as case counts, incidence or prevalence rate calculations, graph preparation, and other descriptive procedures to be utilized will be in place. Statistical tests of differences or of trends may also have been

selected. Such statistical tests usually test the current situation
against some previous situation. For example, an infection control nurse might wish to determine if there is a statistically significant increase in the hepatitis case rate for one month (or
week) when compared to the previous month (or week). With
some health problems, such changes are obvious from descriptive data and tests of significance are unnecessary.

Statistical tests of differences or of trends may also compare
one group to another (e.g., one surgical unit compared to
another one or one county compared to another county). Comparison of groups, however, as in the latter case is usually done
only after initial analysis and interpretation rather than as a
routine procedure. The intent of all such analysis is the determination of whether an epidemic exists. An epidemic is defined
as "the occurrence in a community or geographical region of
cases of an illness, a specific health-related behavior, or other
health-related events clearly in excess of normal expectancy"
(Last, 1983). To determine if this definition is met, it is necessary to know what is normally expected. Normal expectations
can most easily be obtained from a previous period of time or
from a similar comparison population. (See Chapter 3 for discussion of selection of comparison groups.) With a surveillance system, previous data from a comparable time period are generally
available and can be utilized. The definition of an epidemic also
includes the phrase "clearly in excess." When a hospital unit
that normally only has two *nosocomial* (arising while patient is
in a hospital or as a result of being in a hospital) hepatitis cases
in a month has ten cases in 1 week, it has a clear excess and
thus an epidemic. With many diseases and health problems such
a clear excess is not always present. This situation leads to the
utilization of statistical tests of differences to distinguish
between the normal or usual situation for an equivalent time
period and the current situation. When the difference in frequency is a statistically significant difference (i.e., not likely due
to chance), it is considered in clear excess.

The time periods being compared must be equivalent. The
case rate for 1 previous week must be compared to the case rate
for the current week; the number of cases for today must be
compared to the number of cases for a previous day. Which day
or week or year is utilized for comparison purposes depends
upon factors such as whether a seasonal variation exists, which
most recent time periods may be part of the epidemic, and the

quality of the data available during different time periods. Sometimes current data are compared individually against several equivalent time periods or against an average for several equivalent periods (e.g., the average weekly rate for the same season in previous years).

Some epidemics may or may not be recognized as epidemics because of the comparison time period that is utilized. Ideally, if seasonal variations in rates normally exist, then comparisons should be made between similar seasons. If reporting quality or completeness has changed substantially over time, presence of an epidemic could be masked or, conversely, appear to be present when it is not. There is little value in doing tests of differences if quality or completeness has changed substantially (never assume reporting changes are responsible, rather investigate and verify). If it is believed that an epidemic has developed over a period of time, it may be advisable to do a statistical test of trend or to use several earlier time periods to provide a comparison.

When a trend develops over a long period of time, an awareness problem arises. If the time from the first exposure to a causative factor until onset of an epidemic is short, a problem may be recognized relatively easily. Conversely, a long latent period accompanied by a slow increase in the rate of exposure to a causative agent may make it impossible to label an apparent problem as an epidemic. This would be true, for example, in the case of a carcinogen such as asbestos, which has a 20- to 40-year latency period from exposure to onset of disease symptoms leading to diagnoses of mesothelioma. Diagnosed cases resulting from a single site of occupational exposure to asbestos (e.g., one shipyard) may be scattered throughout many years and geographical locations and therefore not be identifiable as related to the prior common exposure. Similarly, new drugs or medical procedures are often introduced slowly over a period of time; even with a short latency period between exposure and onset of the associated disease, new cases may be scattered in time and place and thus be difficult to relate to the common exposure (the drug or the medical procedure). Oral contraceptives are a case in point. It was several years after use of the pill began before anyone recognized the association between the pill and strokes, myocardial infarctions, and thromboembolisms in women over 35 (Ory, 1980).

Interactions of the disease, population at risk, and medical practice dynamics may also mask presence of an epidemic. For example, the frequency with which hysterectomy was performed for conditions other than cancer of the uterine cervix (e.g., fibroids) varied widely over time (Woodbury, 1977). Thus, the number of women at risk of developing cancer of the uterine cervix varies according to the number of women in the population who have a uterus and a cervix. Surveillance of cervical cancer rates must adjust for changes in the number of women at risk in order to interpret rates. Concurrent with these variations there was a dramatic change in sexual habits, a behavioral factor highly associated with occurrence of such cancers (Cramer, 1982; Zelnick & Kantner, 1977). These changes in sexual behavior, in turn, affect likelihood of exposure to the causal agent for cancer of the uterine cervix. This advent of increased sexual activity among women, which resulted after introduction of the pill, occurred concurrently with the decrease in number of women at risk that resulted from the high rate of hysterectomies. A real increase in cancer of the uterine cervix from increased sexual activity could have been masked by this decrease in size of the population at risk if the reduction was not considered in analysis of surveillance data.

Trends over a prolonged period of time are frequently documented by surveillance systems. Unfortunately, little has been done to investigate such trends within the context of concurrent routine surveillance system investigations. In addition to looking for sudden significant changes, analysis for trends must also be routine. In the past, if work was done to study such trends, it was more often done by outside parties who became interested in the phenomena. Surveillance systems have thus been criticized as insensitive methods of recognizing or becoming aware of potential problems. Were the appropriate analyses routinely conducted, however, such criticisms could be shown to be unjustified. Many trends are obvious when rates are simply graphed over time. At other times it may be necessary to do a statistical test of trend. The need for statistical tests should not be viewed as a major concern because biostatistical consultants may be called upon for assistance.

Interpretation of the data, thus, is basically focused on the question of whether there is evidence that an epidemic exists or that a problem is developing. Remember, a surveillance system is not designed to give answers; it is meant to alert the practitioner to potential problems. In some cases the answer may be clear cut. When there is a question as to whether a problem exists, issues of staff availability, time, and cost can play a vital role in the type of interpretation that is made or whether any interpretation is done. For example, in a hospital with several nurse epidemiologists, a borderline increase in rates will likely be detected as a suspect epidemic and investigated. With only one nurse epidemiologist on the staff, such a borderline increase may be overlooked or ignored, particularly if the epidemiologist is already busy with investigating a previously identified problem. In still other cases, a decision may be made on the basis of a hunch. One investigator may usually have time to investigate what appears to be a potential epidemic, but if the surveillance system simultaneously suggests potential epidemics of pneumonia, staphylococcal infection, and salmonella, the increase in salmonella cases may be ignored. At the same time, a stimulus such as a press report of a small nonepidemic increase of some problem (e.g., infants born with ductus arteriosus) may lead administrators to decide to divert resources to investigate this problem.

When the surveillance system is designed to include periodic interpretation of the data, any lack of interpretation may be suspicious. An interpretation that a potential problem exists means that an investigation should be done. If an investigation is not done and as a result an existent problem is not identified, then the system has not fulfilled its purpose. Such a circumstance puts both the health professional and the organization in the rather precarious legal position of having ignored what was known to be a possible problem.

INVESTIGATION

Investigation may be divided into two phases. The preliminary phase may be defined as the time during which some additional information is collected. The investigator may wish to do a literature review related to diagnosis of this problem or to previously identified epidemiological features (natural history, latency period, susceptible age groups, time trends, suspected or known etiological agents, and so on). Whether such a review is necessary depends on the investigator's level of knowledge about this problem. Regardless of whether a literature review is needed, the investigator should first consider the simplest explanations for the apparent problem. A new, young, and aggressive physician who reports religiously may have a drastic impact on the number of cases reported. Introduction of a new diagnostic technique may mean that previously unrecognized cases are reported. Reporting changes as a result of staff changes or new diagnostic tools are the most likely simple explanations for what may appear to be a problem. If such explanations are eliminated the second phase is entered.

The investigation then encompasses the following: determination of what additional information needs to be collected, review of case definition with modifications of definition as necessary, verification of case status (i.e., meets case definition), delineation of an appropriate comparison group, additional case ascertainment (previously unreported), collection of new data, analysis of new data, interpretation, and statement of conclusions. The investigator must make sure that the case and comparison groups are subject to the same data collection procedures and to the same depth of ascertainment for all data. Failure to do so may result in faulty interpretation and conclusions. The investigation should be carried out with the same rigor and standards that would be applied to any epidemiological research project.

As with any epidemiological research project, the goal of the investigation is to determine if a problem exists (an epidemic or upward trend over time) and to delineate potential or actual etiological agents. Most infectious etiological agents can be identified. For many chronic diseases of noninfectious etiology, however, it may be possible only to suggest potential etiological agents. As a result, control efforts for chronic diseases may have to be postponed until research can be done to determine the causative factors. Control efforts may, however, be applied in the absence of verification of causative factors. For example, AIDS was, through its epidemiological features, highly suspected to be related to homosexual activity with multiple partners. Even though the specific causative agent was unknown, control efforts could be directed at reducing homosexual contacts. Utilization of the Pap smear to reduce cervical cancer mortality through early detection is another example of control efforts in the absence of a known cause for the disease.

During the course of an investigation it may become apparent that assistance (more manpower or knowledge) may be needed. Whenever an investigation is beyond the scope or ability of the immediate investigator, assistance may be sought from the local health department, which may request, if necessary, assistance from the state health agency, which may then request assistance from the CDC. Such assistance is readily available from CDC. It is usually necessary to pursue a request for assistance through the hierarchy: local agency first, district or state second, then CDC. In some cases, however, it may be necessary to go directly to CDC in order to stimulate state or local interest. A state health department may have insufficient staff, insufficient funds, or administrators who do not want to get involved in major public issues such as a possible epidemic of anencephaly in families living near a pesticide plant. Such factors may lead to a local agency or hospital receiving an avoidance type response from a state health agency when a request for assistance is made. A phone call to CDC that describes the situation may lead to development of a method by which CDC can call and offer help either overtly or by more covert means. For instance, a scenario might be set up where an "old buddy, how are you doing" call is made, then the conversation is shifted by the CDC staff member to a discussion of difficult problems, then eventually to what problems currently exist, and so forth. Sometimes it is easier or more appropriate for CDC to call and say "Hey, I got this call today from Racine County about an excess of anencephaly around a pesticide plant. Do you need any assistance in looking into this problem?" Most often CDC staff are personally acquainted with state epidemiologists and they usually know how best to approach them. CDC now offers assistance for investigation of communicable diseases, suspected environmentally-induced problems, and investigation of unusual cancer or birth defect clusters.

CONTROL OF DISEASES AND OTHER HEALTH PROBLEMS

Control measures should be implemented whenever possible. Control measures are those activities that will reduce or eliminate the epidemic or the problem that has been identified. Control measures may include:

Quarantine

Immunizations

Preventive therapy, e.g., administration of gamma globulin to an individual who has been exposed to hepatitis

Eradication or reduction of host vector, e.g., rats or mosquitos

Medical treatment of individuals who may spread the disease, e.g., syphillus

Early diagnosis, e.g., cervical cancer or contacts of VD cases

Reduction or removal from exposure, e.g., environmental or occupational exposure to asbestos

Market ban or selective restriction of an agent, e.g., pesticides or drugs not to be given during pregnancy

Nutritional supplements, e.g., iron or folate for anemia

Other medical treatment—Product modifications, e.g., child proof safety caps

Which control measure or measures are utilized depends upon the problem identified, what caused the problem, and the likelihood for success of a given measure. The simplest, most effective, most practical, and least resource consumptive method or methods represent the best choice. The reader should refer to Chapter 5 for a discussion of control measures related to infectious diseases and Chapter 6 for discussion of control measures related to diseases of noninfectious etiology.

During the development of a control plan, the practitioner must consider several aspects of the situation. The target population at whom the control measures are directed is a major concern. The best control effort may be to apply control efforts selectively to a certain segment of the population. This was done with the international control of smallpox; immediate contacts of known cases were isolated and vaccinated first, then entire population groups were vaccinated. The location for control efforts must also be considered. For example, will only a single unit in the hospital or in a particular school be the target or does adequate control necessitate measures to be applied in the whole hospital, in all classes at one school, or in all schools in the community? The final factors to consider are the period of time during which control efforts will be required and the planned start-up and completion dates for the control effort.

Data collection must continue during and after control efforts so that the effectiveness of control measures may be evaluated. Implementation of control measures may have little or no effect if the wrong or inadequate measures are taken or if they are implemented after the epidemic. Inability or failure to implement control efforts effectively eliminates the value of a surveillance system.

EVALUATION

Evaluation has been discussed earlier in this chapter and is discussed further in Chapter 15, Health Planning and Evaluation. It cannot be emphasized enough that evaluation must be carried out as a routine component of surveillance and disease control programs, with system revisions made as necessary. A surveillance system that never generates potential problems and has never been evaluated may be a totally worthless system. Insensitive systems that have been evaluated, modified, and evaluated again but that still remain insensitive after a few rounds of modification should, in most cases, be eliminated. Occasionally a system may be kept in operation for purely informational purposes despite recognized insensitivity. The usual rationale is the need for baseline data and the potential for occurrence of just one major epidemic entailing large societal costs. One may argue whether the health care establishment can afford such systems. In the interest of controlling costs of health care, the need for surveillance systems must be clearly delineated and goals established. Evaluation of the system can then focus on how well goals are met. Assuming that the original goals were well conceived to meet community health needs, such an evaluation will provide a reasonable basis for evaluating the costs and benefits of the surveillance system.

REFERENCES

Benenson, A. S. (Ed.). *Control of communicable disease in man (14th ed.)*. Washington, D.C.: American Public Health Assoc., 1985.

Cramer, D. W. Uterine cervix. In D. Schottenfeld & J. F. Fraumeni, Jr. (Eds.), *Cancer epidemiology and prevention.* Philadelphia: W. B. Saunders, 1982.

International health regulations (1969), 2nd annotated ed. Geneva: WHO, 1974.

Joint NIOSH/OSHA Current Intelligence Bulletin. *NIAX Catalyst ESN, U.S.D.H.E.W., U.S.O.S.H.A. Current Intelligence Bulletin, 26,* May 22, 1978.

Last, J. M. (Ed.). *A dictionary of epidemiology.* New York: Oxford University Press, 1983.

MMWR. A cluster of Kaposi's sarcoma and *Pneumocystic carinii* pneumonia among homosexual male residents of Los Angeles and Orange Counties, California. *Morbidity and Mortality Weekly Reports,* 1982, *31*(23); 305.

Ory, H. W., Rosenfeld, A., & Landman, L. C. The pill at 20: An assessment. *Family Planning Perspectives,* 1980, *12*(6), 178.

Taussig, H. B. A study of the German outbreak of Phocomelia. *JAMA,* 1962, *180*(13); 80.

Woodbury, M. A. *A Systems approach to understanding hysterectomy patterns and the natural history of carcinoma of the cervix uteri.* Master's Thesis, Emory University, 1977.

Zelnik, M. & Kantner, J. F. Sexual and contraceptive experience of young unmarried women in the United States, 1976 and 1971. *Family Planning Perspectives,* 1977, *9*(2); 55.

Screening

A major strategy for secondary prevention of disease is screening. Screening is defined as the presumptive identification of unrecognized disease or defect by the application of tests, examinations, or other procedures that can be applied rapidly and inexpensively to populations. Its purpose is to distinguish among apparently well persons, those who probably have a disease from those who probably do not. Screening is not intended to be diagnostic; persons with positive results on a screening test require additional diagnostic tests and examinations in order to establish a definitive diagnosis. Screening procedures may include cytological tests, blood tests, x-rays, urinalysis, amniocentesis, examination for scoliosis, and a variety of other procedures.

Screening tests may be applied unselectively to an entire population, for example, blood pressure screening of all persons attending a health fair, or may be applied selectively to certain groups of persons known to have a high risk for a disease. Examples of selective application to high-risk population groups are screening workers exposed to bladder carcinogens by cytological analysis of urine for bladder cancer, using mammograms to screen women with family history of breast cancer, or doing tuberculin tests on children in inner city schools. Such applications of screening tests, whether unselectively to entire populations or selectively to high-risk groups, are examples of *mass screening*.

Screening may also be used as part of periodic health examinations in a private physician's office or a health maintenance clinic. Pap smears, for example, are often included as a part of the routine examination for women, and electrocardiograms are standard for middle-aged men. Regular height, weight, hearing, and vision measures of children are taken in pediatricians' offices or well-child clinics, or on home visits by nurses in order to detect early lags in growth and development or early impairment of hearing and vision. This type of screening, where clinicians use screening tests to search for disease among their own patients who have come in for a general check-up or for consultation regarding unrelated symptoms, is called *case-finding*. With case-finding, the clinician has an explicit responsibility to follow up any abnormal results. In mass screening, follow-up is usually limited to referring those individuals who test positive to their private physician or to a facility with follow-up capability.

Multiphasic screening, the use of a variety of screening tests on the same occasion, is another application of screening. Recent advances in technology have led to automated, sophisticated test techniques that permit mny tests to be run on a single blood sample. These procedures have been used for a variety of purposes including (1) establishing baseline data and classifying persons entering care at a particular health care facility, (2) periodic surveillance of persons with established disease, (3) hospital preadmission and preoperative examinations, (4) health evaluations for employment and life insurance, (5) as adjuncts to sickness consultations or periodic health examinations, and (6) risk factor appraisal.

Questions have been raised about such uses of multiphasic screening. Part of the concern arises from the fact that the basic definition of normal versus abnormal is based on the customary normal curve, a statistical concept, rather than a clinical one. Abnormalities are defined as laboratory values that lie outside some specified range, usually two standard deviations from the mean. On this curve there will always be normal persons who are defined as abnormal.

In any general population resembling the normal population from which the laboratory derived its normal range, one could expect one person in 20 to have an abnormality. In the case of multiphasic screening where many tests are done simultaneously, the probability of a falsely abnormal result is considerably increased, yet a clinician feels obligated to follow up abnormal results because failure to do so could be hazardous.

Because abnormal values on many of the clinical laboratory tests could be a sign of any of a variety of disease conditions, the patient may be thrown into what Schneiderman (1981) has called the subspeciality loop (Fig. 13–1) in an attempt to rule out systematically each of the conditions that potentially explain the elevated value.

As a way of minimizing this problem, Elvebach (1972) proposed using age- and sex-specific percentiles rather than standard deviations to define abnormality. This approach overcomes dependence on the normal curve (dependence is inappropriate because many biochemical values are not normally distributed), deals with the problem that a value normal for one group (e.g., older women) may be highly abnormal for another group (e.g., young men), and recognizes that health and disease represent a continuum on which separation of one from the other by a simple cutoff is quite arbitrary.

Mass screening, case-finding, and multiphasic screening are all examples of prescriptive screening, screening done for the purpose of better controlling disease through early detection in presumptively healthy individuals. Screening is also used by

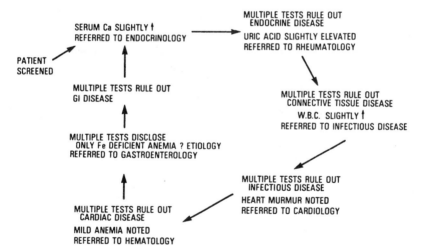

Figure 13–1. As patients are referred from one specialty to another in pursuit of the ubiquitous laboratory "abnormality," they may fall victim to an endless circle, the Subspecialty Loop. *(From Schneiderman, L.* The practice of preventive health care. *Menlo Park, Calif.: Addison-Wesley, 1981, p. 6.)*

epidemiologists for research purposes. Screening of a population may be done to estimate prevalence of disease. Furthermore, these screened populations may be followed over time, using periodic screens to identify new cases of the disease to determine incidence rates.

CHARACTERISTICS OF SCREENING TESTS

How do screening tests differ from diagnostic tests? Diagnostic tests are generally used on patients who have come to a treatment center seeking an explanation for symptoms they are experiencing. Diagnostic tests are ordered by a physician, require specialized equipment or expertise to administer, are generally expensive, often time consuming, and may incur a degree of discomfort, pain, or risk for the patient. Results of diagnostic tests are usually of sufficient accuracy to establish a definitive diagnosis; they can thus be used as a basis for initiating treatment.

In contrast to diagnostic tests, screening tests are generally offered to apparently healthy populations as a way of determining whether it is probable that they have a disease; it is presumed that identifying probable disease before symptoms appear permits early initiation of treatment and, therefore, will affect the prognosis for the patient. The scientific basis for establishing the validity of this presumption was discussed in Chapter 11. The accuracy of screening tests is insufficient as a basis for initiating treatment; follow-up diagnostic testing of individuals with abnormal results on the screening test must be done. Although the initial cost of doing a screening test may be low because these tests are generally inexpensive and can be administered by an individual with minimal training, the economic cost of the follow-up testing of those screened as abnormal can be considerable. If the yield of confirmed cases of disease is high among those screening abnormal and the test can identify the majority of diseased persons in the screened population, then the cost of screening and follow-up can be justified. If the yield of confirmed cases is low relative to the number of positives on the screening test who are confirmed healthy, then screening becomes harder to justify.

The particular characteristics of screening tests that need to be considered are shown in Table 13–1 and are compared for screening and diagnostic tests. As mentioned previously, screening tests are generally simpler, less accurate, less expensive, less risky, and more acceptable to a presumably well population than are diagnostic tests. These characteristics make mass screening programs feasible. To induce participation, an ideal screening test should take only a few minutes to perform, require minimal preparation by the patient, and require no special appointments. Tests requiring special diets, for example, fasting blood sugar, are not feasible for mass screening. Neither are tests that involve special appointments, discomfort, or risk; for example, proctoscopy carries risk of bowel perforation. Tuberculin testing as a screening procedure is feasible only if the screening population is "captive," for example, children in a school, because a follow-up reading is required. Quick and simple examinations such as blood pressure determinations or the Snellen eye chart for vision screening are ideal screening tests from the standpoint of acceptibility.

The cost of the test is a function of both the cost of the procedure itself and of the cost of subsequent evaluations performed on patients with positive test results. The need for follow-up testing is a function of the accuracy of the test. Accuracy is dependent on two characteristics, the validity and the reliability of the test. Reliability involves the repeatability or replicability of the results—the ability of a test to give consistent results in repeated applications. Reliability is dependent both upon the precision of the test—how much variation is present in the test itself—and upon variation introduced by different persons

TABLE 13–1. CHARACTERISTICS OF SCREENING AND DIAGNOSTIC TESTS

Characteristic	Rating of Screening Test	Rating of Diagnostic Test
Accuracy	Low–moderate	High
Simplicity	High	Moderate–low
Cost	Low	Moderate–high
Safety	High	High–low
Acceptability	High	Moderate–low

applying the test. Variability in the result of a test procedure administered at two different times to the same sample by the same tester (for example, a split sample of blood) could be a function of variability in how the procedure was performed or interpreted by the tester (intra- and interindividual variability), or a function of variability in the test conditions, such as the effects of change in room temperature upon the chemical reagent used or the age and storage conditions of the reagent. Variability inherent in the test is called test–retest reliability and is obtained by doing the test two or more times on the same sample and calculating the statistical correlation of results across a number of samples. The measure of variability introduced by different persons applying the test is usually tested by examining the correlation of the results when two or more persons administer the test separately to the same individual or sample. This correlation is known as interrater reliability. Another correlative measure, intrarater reliability, assesses the consistency of a single individual at doing the test and interpreting the results.

Validity indicates how well a test result represents reality. In the case of screening tests, validity is assessed by the frequency with which the result of the test is confirmed by more vigorous diagnostic procedures. Validity is measured by the sensitivity, specificity, and predictive values of the test. *Sensitivity* is the frequency with which persons who have the disease test positive, i.e., the probability of the test correctly identifying a case. *Specificity* is the frequency with which persons who do not have the disease test negative, i.e., the probability of correctly identifying noncases. These measures are illustrated in Table 13–2. The distribution of a population with respect to disease status and screening test results, which are used as the basis for these measures, are shown in Table 13–3. Those persons with the disease (reading down in Table 13–3) can have two test results, true positives or false negatives. Sensitivity then is the percentage of all those with the disease (true positives plus false negatives) who test positive. Thus, the formula for sensitivity, as shown in Table 13–2, is

$$\text{Sensitivity} = \frac{\text{True positives}}{\text{True positives} + \text{False negatives}} \times 100$$

Persons without the disease may have false-positive results on the screening test or true-negative results (Table 13–3). Spec-

TABLE 13–2. MEASURE OF RELIABILITY AND VALIDITY OF SCREENING TESTS

Characteristic	Measures	How Calculated
Validity	Sensitivity	$\dfrac{\text{True positives}}{\text{True positives} + \text{False negatives}} \times 100$
	Specificity	$\dfrac{\text{True negatives}}{\text{True negatives} + \text{False positives}} \times 100$
	Predictive value positive test	$\dfrac{\text{True positives}}{\text{True positives} + \text{False positives}} \times 100$
	Predictive value negative test	$\dfrac{\text{True negatives}}{\text{True negatives} + \text{False negatives}} \times 100$
Reliability	Test–retest reliability	Correlation of results on two tests on same samples
	Interrater reliability	Correlation of results on same samples done by two or more evaluators
	Intrarater reliability	Correlation of results on same samples done several times by a single evaluator

ificity is based on the percentage of these two test results that are true negatives (Table 13–2).

Sensitivity and specificity for a new test are determined by applying the test to a population for which disease status is known. These values are independent of disease prevalence. They are reciprocal to some degree, however, in that increasing sensitivity inevitably causes some decrease in specificity. Conversely, increasing specificity decreases sensitivity.

TABLE 13–3. DISTRIBUTION OF DISEASE STATUS AND SCREENING TEST RESULTS IN A POPULATION

Screening Test Result	True Diagnosis		
	Diseased	*Not Diseased*	*Total*
Positive	True positives	False positives	True positives + False positives
Negative	False negatives	True negatives	False negatives + True negatives
Total	True positives + False negatives	False positives + True negatives	True positives + False positives + False negatives + True negatives

This is particularly true for tests based on a continuous distribution of test values. A level, called the screening level, must be chosen somewhat arbitrarily to represent abnormality. Because there is an overlap in the distribution of test values for individuals with and without the disease at any cutoff level defining abnormality, some individuals will be misclassified. In blood pressure measurement, for example, 140 mm Hg and 90 mm Hg, respectively, are frequently used as cutoffs for systolic and diastolic pressures for declaring a person positive for hypertension in a screening program. A significant number of persons testing positive on the screen may be false positives whose pressure was temporarily elevated because of anxiety over having their pressure taken or because of some stressful event on the way to the screening site, for example, a near accident in the parking lot. This cutoff, although likely to correctly classify as probable hypertensives all those who truly have hypertension, will also misclassify as probable hypertensives many who are not. Sensitivity is excellent, but specificity is low. Using a cutoff of 160 mm Hg and 100 mm Hg may misclassify some true hypertensives as normal but is less likely to misclassify individuals without hypertension as abnormal; at this level, sensitivity is lower, but specificity is higher than in the previous example.

Consider the following example: Phenylketonuria (PKU) is an inborn metabolic defect affecting metabolism of protein. This condition can be detected by a blood test for phenylalanine levels. Nearly three-fifths of the 50 states require or recommend testing newborn infants for this condition before hospital discharge. In a population without PKU, blood levels of phenylalanine may vary from 0 to 12 mg %. In a population with the disease, phenylalanine levels may range from 6 to more than 50 mg %. Levels in an individual may vary from time to time depending upon factors such as recency of ingesting protein foods, which metabolize to produce phenylalanine, and the amount of such foods ingested. Levels also vary by age. Thus, the distribution of phenylalanine values in infants with and without PKU may resemble that shown in Figure 13–2. Between 6 and 12 mg % there is overlap in the distribution, with many healthy children and some children with PKU. Some value must be chosen to serve as the cutoff level for declaring normal versus abnormal. In the diagram shown, declaring 6 mg % as the cutoff (screening level) would represent 100 percent sensitivity—all

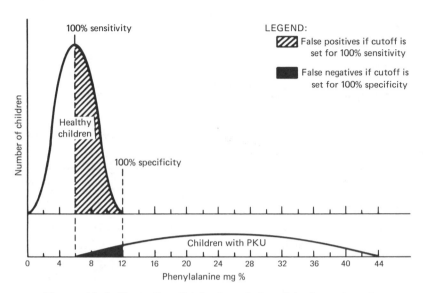

Figure 13–2. Illustrative distribution of phenylalanine values in normal children and children with PKU.

diseased children would be correctly screened as positive; there would be no false negatives. This would produce a large number of false positives, however, (Fig. 13–2). Using 12 mg % as the cutoff for declaring normal versus abnormal would produce a test that is 100 percent specific; this would, however, produce a substantial number of false negatives. Therefore, to maximize sensitivity and specificity of the test, an intermediate value such as 9 to 10 mg % represents an acceptable compromise, maintaining reasonably high sensitivity and reasonable specificity.

Predictive values of a screening test, unlike sensitivity and specificity, are measures dependent on the prevalence of disease in the population to which the test is applied. Predictive values describe the frequency with which test results represent correct identification of disease status among those screened. The predictive value of a positive test is the proportion of those testing positive who have the disease. The predictive value of a negative test is the proportion of those testing negative who do not have the disease. These are usually expressed as percentage of positives or percentage of negatives who were correctly identified (see Table 13–2).

Because predictive values vary with the prevalence of disease in the screened population, they are useful in deciding whether or not to use a particular test in a given population. For a test with a fixed sensitivity and specificity, increasing the prevalence rate of the disease in the population to be screened increases the predictive value of a positive test. Because groups at high risk of developing a disease are likely to have a higher prevalence of that disease than a general population, screening of high-risk populations can improve the predictive value of a positive test. This means fewer false positives to be followed up for diagnoses relative to true positives (Table 13–4).

Returning to the previous example of PKU, let us examine the effects of disease prevalence on predictive values in two hypothetical population distributions of disease and phenylalanine levels. In a general population, the prevalence of PKU among white births is 9.6 in 100,000 and among nonwhite births 4.6 in 100,000 (National Research Council, 1975). Suppose that sensitivity and specificity of the test have been determined to be 94 and 90 percent, respectively. Applying these approximate values in a screen of 100,000 white newborns would produce the values shown in Table 13–5A. Nine of the ten infants with PKU would be correctly diagnosed, and one would have a false negative test. Among the 99,990 infants without PKU, 4999 would have false-positive test results and require a

TABLE 13–4. PREDICTIVE VALUE OF A POSITIVE TEST AS A FUNCTION OF DISEASE PREVALENCE FOR A LABORATORY TEST WITH 95% SENSITIVITY AND 95% SPECIFICITY

Prevalence of Disease in Screened Population (%)	Predictive Value of Positive Test (%)
1	16.1
5	50.0
10	67.9
20	82.6
50	95.0

(Adapted from Galen, R. S. Selection of appropriate laboratory tests. In D. S. Young (Ed.), *Clinician and chemist.* Washington, D.C.: The American Association for Clinical Chemistry, 1979, p. 76.)

TABLE 13–5. RESULTS OF HYPOTHETICAL SCREENING FOR PKU

A. Test Result	PKU Present	PKU Absent	Total
Positive test	9	4999	5,008
Negative test	1	94,991	94,992
Total	10	99,990	100,000

Prevalence = 10/100,000
Sensitivity = 90%
Specificity = 95%

Predictive value positive test = $\dfrac{9}{5008}$ = 0.180%

Predictive value negative test = $\dfrac{94,991}{94,992}$ = 99.999%

B. Test Result	PKU Present	PKU Absent	Total
Positive test	900	4,950	5,850
Negative test	100	94,050	94,150
Total	1,000	99,000	100,000

Prevalence = 10/1000
Sensitivity = 90%
Specificity = 95%

Predictive value positive test = $\dfrac{900}{94,150}$ = 15.385%

Predictive value negative test = $\dfrac{94,050}{94,150}$ = 99.894%

diagnostic workup to determine that they do not have PKU. The predictive value of the postive test is a dismal 0.180 percent; 555.4 subjects with false-positive tests must be given a diagnostic workup for every case detected (4999 divided by 9). Predictive value of a negative test is excellent at 99.999 percent.

Unfortunately, to date no high-risk group for PKU has been identified. Let us suppose, however, for illustrative purposes that some high-risk group were identifiable. Further, let us assume that the likely prevalence of disease among this high-risk population is 10 in 100. Using the same screening test with the same sensitivity and specificity to screen this high-risk population produces the results shown in Table 13–5B. Predictive value of a positive test has increased to 15.385 percent; only about 6.5 subjects with false-positive results must be followed for every case detected. Predictive value of the negative test shows only a negligible change.

CRITERIA FOR SCREENING PROGRAMS

Because screening procedures are applied to well persons and because of the potential economic and psychological costs incurred by misclassification of disease status, a benefit should accrue to the individual screenees as a result of the program in addition to the cost–benefit to society accruing from earlier detection and treatment of the disease.

Consider the four possible outcomes of a screening test: (1) true positive, (2) true negative, (3) false positive, and (4) false negative. Individuals with accurate results, the true positives and true negatives, can benefit from screening. Individuals with true negative results benefit from the peace of mind that comes from knowing they are disease free. Those screenees with true positive results, however, will benefit from the detection of their disease only if three conditions are met: (1) the screening test has detected their condition at an earlier stage of disease than would have the presence of symptoms; (2) earlier detection can lead to improving their prognosis because an effective treatment is available; and (3) the available treatment is acceptable to the patient and the physician. If these conditions are not met, then there is no benefit to individuals with true positive results. For example, sickle cell screening has been criticized on the grounds that no benefit accrues to the diseased individual because no effective treatment is available to change the prognosis; the patient merely lives longer with anxiety about having sickle cell disease. Neither has benefit accrued to those with sickle cell trait. The hypothetical benefit is that identification of trait, accompanied by counseling, would change the childbearing patterns of couples at risk of conceiving a child with the disease; evidence from at least one study shows no difference in childbearing patterns of counseled couples (Holroyd et al., 1982). If the three conditions are met, then the economic cost of treating the condition is likely to be lower than it would be without screening, both because of less complicated initial treatment and because of the decreased probability of disability.

Those individuals with false positive results are likely to be somewhat unhappy with the screening program. First, they experience a period of time when they must worry about whether they have the disease. Second, they must undergo a series of diagnostic tests that, at the very least, take time away from work, home, friends; these tests may be uncomfortable and painful, and involve unpleasant side effects or some degree of risk. Finally, someone must pay for these tests; if health insurance pays, such costs eventually will be reflected in higher premiums. Individuals who do not have health insurance must pay the costs out of their own pockets. Although individuals will be relieved to learn that they do not have the disease, they are likely to resent the unnecessary economic and psychological costs. Follow-up testing also imposes a burden on the health care system. If the positive predictive value of a screening test is low, then large numbers of false positives must be processed through diagnostic procedures. Time, facilities, and personnel must be available, and a good referral program must be in place.

Finally, there is the individual with the false negative test. This individual also may be harmed as a result of the screening program. Although it could be argued that this individual is no worse off than would be the case if not screened, such is not always the case. Major harm would arise if, when symptoms appear, the individual recognizes them as early signs of the disease for which he or she was recently screened negative and therefore ignores them rather than seeking medical attention. As a result, the cost of treating the condition may be higher than otherwise would be the case, and the patient's prognosis may be negatively affected. Legal action could ensue. As a precaution, some health education about signs and symptoms and the possibility that these could develop in the future despite negative screening results might be usefully included in the screening program.

The criteria that should be met by a good screening program are listed in Table 13–6. These criteria address the scientific, social, and ethical issues relevant to screening. They imply careful selection of tests based on accuracy, good epidemiological description of the natural history of the disease, evidence of the efficacy of earlier treatment (see discussion of lead time bias, Chapter 11), and a positive cost–benefit to society. The criteria for screening programs also imply careful selection of the population to be screened and inclusion of plans for program evaluation. The principals of planning and evaluation described in Chapter 15 are readily applicable to screening programs. Both general measures of community health, such as changes in morbidity or mortality related to the disease, and specific demographic and follow-up data on screenees to evaluate rates of

TABLE 13–6. CRITERIA FOR A SCREENING PROGRAM

1. Test has high sensitivity and specificity.
2. Test meets acceptable standards of simplicity, cost, safety, and patient acceptability.
3. Disease that is focus of screening should be sufficiently serious in terms of incidence, mortality, disability, discomfort, and financial cost.
4. Evidence suggests that the test procedure detects the disease at a significantly earlier stage in its natural history than it would present with symptoms.
5. A generally accepted treatment that is easier or more effective than treatment administered at the usual time of symptom presentation must be available.
6. The available treatment is acceptable to patients as established by studies on compliance with treatment.
7. Prevalence of the target disease should be high in the population to be screened.
8. Follow-up diagnostic and treatment service must be available and accompanied by an adequate notification and referral service for those positive on screening.

diagnostic follow-up and the predictive values of positive and negative results should be included in evaluation protocols. An example of the importance of such monitoring is a program in the inner city area of an Eastern city that screened for cervical cancer. Although substantial numbers of women were screened, the predictive value of the positive test was low; very few cases of cervical cancer were detected. Review of the intake records revealed that the majority of participants were middle-income married women rather than the lower-income single women at high risk of developing cervical cancer who were the target population of the screening program.

Planning and evaluation of screening programs on the basis of criteria relies on epidemiological data. The following facts about each disease must be sought:

1. Incidence, prevalence, and mortality from the disease, preferably age- and sex-specific
2. Progression of the disease with and without treatment at various stages, to include morbidity, mortality, and length of the early asymptomatic period (latency)
3. Risk factors associated with development of the disease
4. Availability of screening tests, their safety, sensitivity, and specificity in the early stages of the disease, and their unit cost

PRACTICE GUIDELINES

Although a variety of published protocols provide primary health care practitioners with guidelines for use of screening procedures in preventive health practice, there is far from unanimous agreement on screening protocols. For example, there is disagreement among the Canadian Task Force on Periodic Health Examinations, the American Cancer Society, and the American College of Obstetrics and Gynecologists regarding the circumstances appropriate to screening for cervical cancer using the Pap smear (Schneideman, 1981). Also, as new studies are completed it is frequently necessary to reevaluate recommendations about a specific screening protocol. The American Cancer Society in 1980 changed its position regarding the use of chest x-rays for lung cancer screening based on reevaluation of the evidence (American Cancer Society, 1980).

Each clinician must evaluate the proposed screening program in terms of the criteria in Table 13–6 and in terms of the actual dollar cost relative to the health benefits to individuals and society. There is an extensive literature quantifying cost–benefit, but this is beyond the scope of this chapter. Administrators will need to attach dollar figures to various programs and relate this cost to benefit for purposes of obtaining funding. They will need to demonstrate the benefit of their preferred program relative to others competing for the same pot of funds and to present convincing scientific arguments for their recommendations. Clinicians must be able to evaluate the cost of case-findng to their practice and their patients, weighing the harm versus benefit of using a particular test, the impact of using the test on cost of health services and use of resources within his or her own practice setting, the burden of suffering associated with the condition both for individuals (patient and family) and for society, and the risk status of the particular patient. The clinician is in a position to collect the information necessary to establish likely risk—a thorough health and behavioral history is invaluable. If the clinician is familiar with the epidemiological evidence regarding risk factors, he or she is in a position to identify patients at high risk for specific diseases. Use of screening tests selectively on high-risk patients rather than on all patients in a broad category is likely to be most effective. For example, a cytological analysis of urine for a patient occupation-

TABLE 13–7. RECOMMENDED SCREENING TESTS FOR EARLY DETECTION BY MASS SCREENING OR SCREENING OF HIGH-RISK GROUPS

Test for General Population and High-Risk Groups	Disease	Applicable Population
Serological testing	Syphilis	Pregnant women before 16th week
Thyroxine testing	Neonatal hypothyroidism	All neonates
Microbiological inhibition and fluorometric tests	Phenylketonuria	All neonates
Maternal serum alpha-feto protein testing	Neural tube defects	Pregnant women
Visual acuity testing	Refractive vision defects	School children
Blood pressure measurement	Hypertension	General population
Mammography	Breast cancer	Women over 45[a]
Papanicolaou smear	Cancer of the cervix	All sexually active women
Blood group and antibody tests	Blood group incompatibility in pregnancy	Pregnant women
Microbiological examination of urine	Bacteriuria in pregnancy	Pregnant women
Cervical and urethral smears	Gonorrhea	Pregnant women
Iontophoresis sweat test	Cystic fibrosis	Siblings of cystic fibrosis patients
Serum creatinine phosphokinase determination	Duchenne muscular dystrophy (DMD)	Female relative of DMD patients
Resistance of serum hexosamine to heat inactivation	Tay-Sachs disease	Ashkenazi Jews and other high-risk groups
Amniocentesis	Down's syndrome	Parents with translocation of chromosome 21 or family history of Down's; pregnant women over 35 years of age
Serological testing for *Toxoplasma gondi*	Toxoplasmosis	Nonimmune pregnant women who keep a cat or who eat raw meat

TABLE 13–7. *(cont.)*

Test for General Population and High-Risk Groups	Disease	Applicable Population
Cervical and urethral smears	Gonorrhea	Persons with history of multiple sexual partners
Blood tests	Syphilis	Persons with history of multiple sexual partners
Blood hemoglobin concentration	Iron deficiency anemia	Premature babies; babies of multiple pregnancy or an iron-deficient woman; persons of low socioeconomic circumstances
Stool test for occult blood	Cancer of colon and rectum	Persons with history of colitis, familial polyporis or villous adenomas, or family history of cancer of the colon
Cytological analysis of urine	Cancer of the bladder	Workers occupationally exposed to bladder carcinogens; smokers
Urine testing for glucose	Diabetes mellitus	Family history of diabetes; abnormalities associated with pregnancy; physical abnormalities such as circulatory dysfunction and hand vascular impairment
Tuberculin test	Tuberculosis	Family of tuberculosis patients; children living in high prevalence areas (generally lower socioeconomic conditions); elderly in high prevalence areas

[a]Canadian Task Force recommends women 50–59; American Cancer Society recommends women over 40 years. Frame and Carlson recommend it for women over 50 with large fatty breasts.

ally exposed to bladder carcinogens who is also a heavy smoker makes some sense, but routine cytological analysis on all adults does not. Electrocardiographic testing of a overweight, hypertensive middle-aged man who smokes and has a family history of heart disease may be useful, but to routinely screen all middle-aged men is probably of little use (Canadian Task Force, 1979).

With these issues in mind, the Canadian Task Force on the Periodic Health Examination developed a set of recommendations for periodic health examinations, including appropriate screening tests and screening examinations. Tables 13–7 and 13–8, list the screening tests and examinations recommended by this group respectively. The procedures included in these Tables received a rating of A or B from the Task Force as to use with the specified population. A recommendation of A means that there is good evidence to support the use of a periodic health examination; a recommendation of B is supported by fair evidence. Procedures with ratings of C through E, reflecting poor evidence to support their use, were not included in the Tables. The reader is referred to this report and to a four-part review of screening tests by Frame and Carlson (1975), which is mostly consistent with the Canadian recommendations. The Frame and Carlson articles are particularly helpful in detailing the rationale behind each recommendation.

The reader will note that some tests that are widely used or frequently proposed for use are not included, for example, mass screening with hemocult tests for colon cancer, self-testicle examination, and breast self-examination (BSE). We shall consider the issue of BSE as an example of how to think through the screening issues.

It has been suggested that BSE be taught to high school girls as a form of screening for breast cancer. It is hypothesized that habits established at an early age, in this case monthly practice of BSE, are more likely to become routine behaviors and if all women were thus to develop the habit of monthly BSE, early detection of breast cancer would lead to early treatment and substantial reductions in mortality. In fact, self-examination by the patient is the way in which 90 percent of breast malignancies in one study were detected (Thiessen, 1971), whether or not the patient had been instructed in systematic, periodic breast examination. In a study of women receiving annual physician examinations, 38 percent of all breast tumors

TABLE 13–8. RECOMMENDED CLINICAL EXAMINATIONS FOR EARLY DETECTION OF DISEASE

Examination	Disease	Applicable Population
Flexion, abduction, and Ortolani maneuver	Congenital hip dislocation	Newborns
Height, weight and anthropometric measurements	Malnutrition Obesity Problems of physical growth (hormonal)	High-risk groups: Infants and young children, adolescent girls, pregnant women, those nursing unusually long, food faddists
Inspection and cover–uncover test	Strabismus	Children
History-taking and clinical examination	Hearing impariment	Infants whose parents suspect a defect, who fail to react to unusual noise outside of their field of vision or who manifest decreased or absent of babbling Children with retarded or defective speech development Adults reporting hearing difficulty or who fail to respond to the normal spoken voice
Inspection	Cancer of the skin	Outdoor workers and those in contact with polycyclic aromatic hydrocarbons
Oral examination	Orthodontic conditions	General population, particularly children
Physical inspection	Scoliosis	School children
Physical palpation of breast	Breast cancer	Women over 50 (Canadian Task Force) All adult women over 20 (Frame & Carlson)

were discovered by the patients between physician examination (Venet et al., 1971). Because women seem to be so successful at finding tumors and because BSE is inexpensive and can be done frequently without much investment of health care resources, this recommendation seems more than reasonable at first glance, particularly since establishing the habit early should overcome the patient compliance problem. The Thiessen study found that only 30 to 35 percent of women with breast tumors discovered them by doing routine BSE. Some additional problems that have not been considered in this recommendation follow:

1. Studies have documented time lags ranging from 6 to 18 months between the time women detect a lesion and the first physician contact.

2. It has been demonstrated that it is difficult for women with large, pendulous, or fatty breasts to detect lumps (Thiessen, 1971). These same women may have a higher risk of developing breast cancer.

3. No increase in survival has been demonstrated among women under 50 who are screened by a combination of mammography plus palpation (Venet et al., 1971), let alone by BSE. Although there is little question that treatment of Stage I breast cancer is associated with dramatically longer survival than either untreated Stage I cancer or cancer diagnosed at later stages, it has never been demonstrated that BSE more frequently detects Stage I cancer.

4. Although breast cancer is the leading cause of death due to cancer in women, its incidence is age related. The disease is rare before age 30. U.S. incidence data from the Surveillance, Epidemiology, End Results Program (SEER), 1973–1977, shows the incidence per 100,000 women to be 0.2 between ages 20 and 24, 1.4 ages 25 to 29, 6.0 ages 30 to 34, and 13.3 between ages 35 and 39. By age 65 to 69, incidence is 102.2 in 100,000 and by more than 85 years old, it is 180.9 in 100,000. The likelihood that any one woman under 45 will have breast cancer is minute; from high school to age 25, it is nearly nonexistent.

5. Of breast lump biopsies done at all ages, somewhere between 1 in 5 and 1 in 8 are malignant. This ratio is less than 1 in 8 in younger age groups because of the low incidence of breast cancer. If all young women were to do BSE, it would become even lower because nearly all lumps found would be benign, therefore false positives. Many lumps are never biopsied; an examining physician,

particularly a breast specialist, is often expert at ruling out malignancy by palpation. Thus, the specificity of BSE is very low. Many lumps found will require a physician's visit followed by referral to a breast specialist. Even if biopsy is not required, these women undergo enormous psychological stress. For those requiring a biopsy to rule out malignancy, the psychological and physical pain are substantial as is the economic cost.

Similar issues are relevant to proposals to teach testicular examination to high school males. Proposals such as those to screen the general population using the hemocult test do not consider the relatively low incidence of colon and rectal cancer, the fact that 95 percent of cases occur in persons over 45 and 75 percent among those over 55, with a median age at diagnosis of 60 to 67 years (Frame & Carlson, 1975). Further, the stool test for occult blood has a very high false positive rate unless a special meat-free, high residue diet is followed and certain medications such as aspirin are avoided. In one mass screening program where test kits were made available to the public through a public radio station, 98,000 kits were distributed. Only twenty-eight percent of these kits were returned. Of these 27,357, 1,024 were positive (3.7 percent). Out of 1,024 positive tests, 695 were seen by a physician. Among these, 21 cancers were detected. All but one of these persons with cancer was over age 60. Median age of individuals with cancer was 67.5 years. Reportedly, 20 of these 21 cancers were in Stage I. A follow-up study will determine whether the survival experience of these screened patients is better than that of colon cancers in the same community diagnosed without screening. Clearly, the screening program's results suggest that such screening should be targeted to the population over 65 years of age. Those with a family history of colon cancer would also be a high-risk group for inclusion. Further, a better rate of diagnostic follow-up on positive tests is required. The psychological and financial cost of follow-ups on 33 persons for every case detected must also be considered.

Clinicians and administrators must continually make decisions about sponsoring public screening programs and whether to use various screening tests in their own practice. Medical supply companies are continually evolving new technologies for screening that they market to clinicians, administrators, and with increasing frequency to the general public. Home screening raises not only concerns about the burdens of following up false positives but also major issues regarding false negatives primarily because there is no control over whether the test proceedure is correctly done. Studies of home pregnancy testing kits found false negative rates as high as 50 percent in consumer use when they were first available (Baker et al., 1976); more recent kits still yielded false negative rates as high as 33 percent (Valanis & Perlman, 1982). Issues that arose included concern that false negative rates might be more frequent among high-risk pregnancies, i.e., teenagers and those of lower socioeconomic status, as a result of poorer compliance to test procedure among these groups. Such negative results might lead these groups to more than their usual delay in seeking prenatal care or those wishing an abortion to seek care too late for a simple first trimester abortion. The news media frequently pick up on such issues and those in clinical practice must be informed about the relevant epidemiological data to speak out on these issues, as they are so often asked to do.

In this era of limited fiscal resources for health, screening programs must be objectively based. Because few programs are systematically evaluated by clinical trial prior to widespread use, available data related to the criteria for screening programs must be reviewed. As new information on disease natural history and changes in treatment become available, reevaluation of existing recommendations may be necessary. Clearly screening procedures are best used in conjunction with a longitudinal program of periodic health assessment, rather than sporatic, one-shot screening programs.

REFERENCES

American Cancer Society. Guidelines for the cancer-related checkup: Recommendations and rationale. *CA: A Cancer Journal for Clinicians,* 1980, *30*(4), 194–230.

Baker, L. D., West, L. W., Chase, M. D., et al. Evaluation of home pregnancy tests. *American Journal of Public Health,* 1976, *66,* 130–132.

Canadian Task Force. Periodic Health Examination. *Canadian Medical Association Journal,* 1979, *121,* 1193–1254.

Elvebach, L. R. How high is high? A proposed alternative to the normal range. *Mayo Clinic Proceedings,* 1972, *47,* 93.

Frame P., & Carlson, S. A critical review of periodic health screening using specific criteria. *Journal Family Practice,* 1975, *2,* 29–36; 123–129; 189–194; 283–288.

Holroyde, J., Valanis, B., & Cameron, B. Life-table analysis of time to next pregnancy of mothers of sickle cell trait infants. Paper presented at Annual Sickle Cell Conference, Hilton Head, S.C., December 1–4, 1981.

National Cancer Institute. *Surveillance, epidemiology, and end results, incidence and mortality data, 1973–77.* DHHS (NIH) publication No. 81-2330, 1981.

National Research Council. *Genetic screening programs, principles and research.* Committee for the Study of Inborn Errors of Metabolism, Division of Medical Science. Washington, D.C.: National Academy of Sciences, 1975.

Schneiderman, L. *The practice of preventive health care,* Menlo Park, Calif.: Addison-Wesley, 1981.

Thiessen, E. V. Breast self-examination in proper perspective. *Cancer,* 1981, *28,* 1537–1545.

Valanis, B., & Perlman, C. Home pregnancy testing kits: Prevalence of use, false-negative rates and compliance with instructions. *American Journal of Public Health,* 1982, *72,* 1034–1036.

Venet, L., Strax, P., Venet, W., & Shapiro, S. Adequacies and inadequacies of breast examinations by physicians in mass screening. *Cancer,* 1971, *28,* 1546–1551.

Clinical Decision-Making

CLINICAL EPIDEMIOLOGY

On a daily basis, clinicians make decisions with respect to individual patient care. These decisions include which tests or assessments should be done to aid in diagnosis, whether or not to treat, and which treatments are likely to be most effective. The ability to deal with these issues by making rational decisions that will lead to optimum therapeutic outcomes is a signal characteristic of an outstanding clinician. How are these clinical decisions reached? Dr. S. J. Roberts in his book, *Epidemiology for Clinicians* (1977), points out that when laboratory investigators make decisions with respect to an experiment, the reasoning behind the decision must be both specified and justified; when clinicians make decisions about individual patient care, they often justify the choices on the basis of an hunch, intuition, or a nebulously defined clinical experience. Perhaps this is one reason that clinical professions like nursing, medicine, and physical therapy are considered at least as much art as they are science. Scientific method, insofar as it consists of observation, classification of phenomena, measurement, hypothesis, and reasoning, has been a part of clinical disciplines largely in the laboratory, where experiments test physiological and biochemical hypotheses about how specific organ systems work. In actual clinical practice, where intervention by the clinician involves procedures to clarify diagnosis or to maintain or improve the patient's well-being, the scientific method is much less often used.

Many clinicians view as alien the idea that any or every action of intervention undertaken in the course of individual patient management should be exposed to the rigors of scientific method. They do not consider the need to collect evidence that will allow others as well as themselves to judge whether or not that action was justified. When a new intervention becomes available, how often do clinicians review the evidence on efficacy prior to adopting it for use with their own patients? How does a clinician decide whether a patient is at high risk for developing a condition and should therefore be screened, or whether a particular intervention will make a difference? On what basis is a judgment made as to what will likely happen to the patient without intervention? These are all questions considered by the science of clinical epidemiology—the application of epidemiological principles and methods to the day-to-day care of patients. Such scientifically-oriented health practice utilizes a systematic, data-based problem solving process to determine if a client has a problem requiring professional intervention, what kind of intervention is needed, and if the intervention has been effective. The rationale for the development of clinical epidemiology as a distinct discipline is presented in Table 14–1.

Clinical epidemiology deals both with the systematic collection and interpretation of clinical data and with the application of findings from these studies in daily clinical decision-making. Prior chapters of this book have addressed the acquisition of epidemiological data and considerations in evaluating such data. This chapter focuses on uses of available epidemiological data in clinical practice, specifically on how epidemiology is used to make decisions regarding care of individual patients.

The clinical issues addressed in this chapter include (1) normality versus abnormality, which involves questions relevant to diagnosis and risk assessment; (2) selection of treatment; and (3) prognosis. These issues and specific related questions are listed in Table 14–2. Questions of cause, although clinically relevant, are discussed in other chapters. While decisions about screening are clearly clinical, this issue also will not be discussed further in this chapter, both because the topic was extensively discussed in Chapter 13 and because screening is usually related to deci-

TABLE 14–1. RATIONALE FOR CLINICAL EPIDEMIOLOGY AS A DISCIPLINE

1. Many clinical decisions are based on information that is uncertain and, therefore, expressed as a probability.
2. That probability is best estimated by means of past experience with similar patients, but a single clinician has a limited range of past experience.
3. Because clinical observations are made on subjects who are free to do as they please, by clinicians with variable skills and prejudices, the observations may be influenced by a variety of systematic errors that can distort the true nature of events and thereby be misleading.
4. To deal with these misleading effects, clinical observations should be based on sound scientific principles, which require understanding the design of scientifically sound human research.
5. Because clinical observations can also be influenced by the play of chance, interpretation of the observations requires an understanding of statistics.
6. Understanding these principles is as important to clinicians who wish to be self-sufficient in judging clinical information as it is to researchers who produce research.

(Adapted from Fletcher, R., Fletcher, S., & Wagner, E. *Clinical epidemiology, the essentials.* Baltimore: Williams and Wilkins, 1982, p. 5.)

sions about groups of persons; this chapter focuses on decisions regarding individual patients. Screening for purposes of case-finding with individual patients is also in Chapter 13.

NORMALITY VERSUS ABNORMALITY

It is rare that patients present with something so grossly different from the usual that it can immediately be recognized as abnormal and categorized by diagnosis. More often, when a patient presents with a complaint, the clinician is immediately faced with the need to determine whether this symptom represents a normal, expected event or a physiological abnormality. If it is abnormal, is it a transient everyday complaint not worth pursuing aggressively or is it a subtle manifestation of disease? For example, is the sore throat a garden variety pharyngitis or a dangerous streptococcal infection? Does the patient with abdominal pain have self-limited gastroenteritis or a more serious intestinal disorder such as peptic ulcer, colitis, or a tumor? Is a 5-foot 6-inch tall woman weighing 160 pounds obese? Does

TABLE 14–2. CLINICAL ISSUES AND QUESTIONS IN THE CARE OF PATIENTS

Issues	Questions
Normality/abnormality	Is a person sick or well?
	What precipitating event led the patient to seek health care?
Risk	What factors are associated with an increased likelihood of disease?
	With likelihood of a specific disease?
	Will altering the factor change the probability of developing disease?
Diagnosis	What are the objective signs, physical findings or laboratory data?
	How accurate are diagnostic tests or strategies used to find a disease?
	What are the costs and risks of diagnostic tests?
	Which of several possible diagnoses is more likely, based on disease frequency distributions?
Prognosis	When should treatment be altered or stopped?
	What is the probable clinical course of this disease?
	What are the consequences of having the disease?
Treatment	What are the ultimate objectives of treatment?
	What treatment options are available?
	How does each change the future course of a disease?
	What are the advantages and risks of treatment compared to no treatment?

her weight post a risk to her health? What are the risks? Is weight alone sufficient justification for a program to reduce her weight? If so, how much should she lose and how fast is it safe to lose the weight? What risks are attached to the use of medication as an aid to lose weight? This first decision as to whether or not an observation reflects illness serves as a precursor to action. If the observation has clinical significance in terms of representing either a risk factor for future illness or probable illness in the present, then intervention is initiated. If it is decided that the observation does not represent illness or abnormality, then no action is taken. The observation is useful in either instance as a yardstick for judging improvement or deterioration. Decisions about normality may also be used as the basis for social and legal decisions, for example, whether compensation is due, or whether someone is mentally competent.

Very few separations of normal from abnormal are based on a clear-cut, dichotomous, yes-or-no measures yielding discrete data. Exceptions are conditions such as cleft lip or cleft palate. Other exceptions are infectious conditions for which there is a laboratory procedure that can grow an organism from the cultured sample only if it is present. A positive culture indicates presence of disease, a negative culture absence of the disease, assuming complete reliability of completing a valid culture procedure. In these instances, decisions about normality are somewhat straightforward.

More often, however, the measures that must be used in assessment are continuous in nature, for example, blood pressure. The likelihood of hypertensive symptoms increases as blood pressure increases. So does the predictive value of blood pressure for occurrence of other conditions such as myocardial infarction or stroke. But the question faced by clinicians is, "when is blood pressure abnormal? When does it require me to do something?" In the case of a blood pressure of 150/90 in a 35-year-old man, for example, the clinical significance can be inferred only from knowledge of the extent to which it is present or absent in other members of the general population, both well and ill, or from measures of the strength of the association between various levels of blood pressure and independent pathological or clinical confirmation of the presence of sickness. The objective is to determine where on the continuum of health to illness this particular patient fits. The natural history of a disease represents this health–illness continuum (see Chapters 3 and 11). Such information on the natural history of each disease is available in the epidemiological literature. Most medical and nursing schools include these data in the content of didactic or clinical courses.

During the prepathogenic phase of the natural history of any disease, the host is healthy. Once a susceptible host becomes exposed to a pathogenic agent, physiological changes begin. Some of these factors represent signs of elevated risk for developing a disease but can also be steps in the development of the disease, although not all individuals go on to develop the illness. At some stages along the health–illness continuum, the only detectable signs of abnormality are subclinical changes that can be detected by laboratory tests. Later, one or several symptoms may appear. As the number or intensity of symptoms increases, the patient will recognize that something is wrong and go to a health care center for diagnosis and treatment. The task of the clinician is to identify where on the natural history continuum the patient currently falls (Table 14–3). This decision serves as the basis for action.

Depending on the particular point along the natural history continuum where the patient's illness lies at the time he or she presents at the health care center, different signs and symptoms will be observed. A physician working in a specialized hypertension clinic will have a very different impression of signs and symptoms associated with hypertension than will a nurse who manages a caseload in a health maintenance clinic. The physician in the specialty clinic sees many patients who were referred because there was something so unusual about their presentation that general practitioners or internists were unable to decide on hypertension as a diagnosis, the patient's hypertension did not respond to usual treatment, or the patient has a complex of chronic diseases requiring a specialist's evaluation of the safest way to treat the newly detected hypertension. Furthermore, once this physician has arrived at a diagnosis and instituted treatment, the patient is usually sent back to the referring source for follow-up. The specialty physician can never really evaluate effectiveness of the treatment. He or she may never see a patient again unless treatment failed, and perhaps not then. Some patients may not comply with the prescribed treatment; some of these will do well and some will do poorly but in neither case will they be a part of the physician's professional frame of reference.

Because health care is often fragmented or specialized, many health clinicians deal with a very limited spectrum of the natural history, health–illness continuum. Thus, clinical expe-

TABLE 14–3. POSSIBLE DECISIONS ABOUT THE NATURAL HISTORY STAGE OF A PATIENT

1. Essentially normal (no risk–no illness)
2. At risk
3. Disease agent present
4. Signs of disease present
5. Symptoms of disease present
6. Disability from disease present
7. Risk of death

rience is often limited. Clinicians are therefore dependent on information derived from epidemiological studies to provide the complete picture, including frequency of symptoms and of the disease, and a description of the natural history. In addition, data from epidemiological studies is needed to answer questions about relative effectiveness of patient treatment or management.

The nurse who manages patients in the health maintenance clinic will see a more representative range of signs and symptoms associated with elevations in blood pressure. He or she will observe patients with a normal range of blood pressures, temporary, stress-related elevations, gradual increases in pressure that may indicate some underlying disease process, patients whose pressure is on the high side but who have been assessed and declared not to require treatment, and patients who may have a sudden increase in blood pressure caused by an underlying disease process. This nurse will observe a wide variety of symptoms associated with hypertension among patients in the clinic. There will be more opportunity to observe long-term compliance with the hypertension treatment regimen and to see both successful and unsuccessful outcomes of treatment. But, even though his or her experience is more representative than that of the speciality physicians, it is limited by little if any experience with the unusual or difficult to manage patient. Furthermore, he or she does not see those persons living in the community who are not receiving regular health care monitoring and follow-up. Thus, the nurse too needs the epidemiological data base to give a complete picture of the disease natural history and frequency of signs and symptoms, and how they are distributed in relation to time of disease onset, severity of disease, and response to therapy.

Epidemiological Criteria for Abnormality

Abnormality can thus be defined through epidemiological data on frequency and on the natural history of the condition. For practical purposes, abnormality is usually defined on the basis of three criteria: (1) it is statistically unusual, (2) it is regularly associated with disease, disability, or death, and (3) treatment leads to a better outcome.

Clinicians generally define normal as whatever occurs often and abnormal as what occurs infrequently. This statistical definition is most often based on frequency of the characteristic in a general population. Often, an arbitrary cutoff point of two standard deviations from the mean is used to separate normal from abnormal, with all values beyond two standard deviations considered to be abnormal. An alternative approach suggested by Elvebach (1972) is the use of percentiles, particularly age- and sex-specific percentiles. This approach has some advantages over the standard deviation approach because it does not assume a normal distribution of values, which is characteristic of few biological measures. Using age- and sex-specific popula- tions as the basis for defining normality increases precision. However, neither of these statistical approaches to normality is adequate in all situations. Fletcher, Fletcher, and Wagner in their book, *Clinical Epidemiology* (1982), list five ways in which the statistical definitions might be ambiguous or misleading:

1. If all values beyond a certain limit (e.g., the 95th percen- tile) are considered abnormal, then the prevalence of all diseases would be the same (5 percent). This is, of course, contrary to our usual way of thinking about disease—few diseases have the same prevalence.
2. There is no general relationship between the statistical definition of how unusual the occurrence of the observed value or symptom is and clinical disease in terms of prognosis for getting worse, developing some other symp- tom or disease condition, or dying. For some diseases, only extreme values are clinically significant and values at the 95th or 98th percentile would mean nothing.
3. Although some extreme values are unusual, they may be preferable to more usual ones. A systolic blood pressure of 90 or 100 is more unusual than one of 160, but is def- initely preferable.
4. Patients may be clearly diseased even though values for laboratory tests diagnostic of their disease are in the usual range for healthy people. For example, some ini- viduals have intraocular pressures within normal range but clearly show retinal damage typical of glaucoma.
5. For many laboratory values, the entire range of values from low to high are associated with risk of disease. For serum cholesterol, for example, risk of coronary heart disease increases throughout the normal range; there is

nearly a threefold increase in risk from "low normal" values to those in the "high normal" range.

For these reasons, statistical definitions of normality must be considered simultaneously with the other two criteria. It is necessary to know which values are regularly associated with disease, disability, or death. Deciding what level of risk is worth preventing is a judgment call based on the data. With blood pressure, for example, 150/90 is used by the National Center for Health Statistics as representing a clinically useful level of risk for treatment. Some physicians would institute treatment at 140/90 in a younger person, however. Others do not feel that treatment is justified unless one or both the values is higher. When some current clinical trials are completed, there may be sufficient evidence to resolve this issue once and for all. It cannot be resolved without systematic collection of data.

The third criterion—what is defined as abnormal should be treatable—is a pragmatic one. Labeling something as abnormal makes little sense if it cannot be treated; the labeling merely causes anxiety for the patient. It is often necessary to reevaluate what is treatable as new data accumulate. Figure 14–1 from Fletcher et al. illustrates beautifully how the definition of treat-

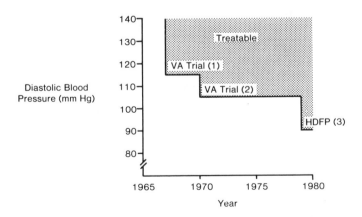

Figure 14–1. The changing definition of treatable disease: accumulative evidence for treating successive lower levels of blood pressure. *(From Fletcher, R., Fletcher, S., & Wagner, E. Clinical epidemiology—The essentials. Baltimore: Williams and Wilkins, 1982, p. 37.)*

able hypertension has changed over time as new evidence from clinical trials accumulated.

DIAGNOSIS

Clinical diagnosis is a process, not a single action. The process is initiated with data collection and analysis, from which an initial diagnostic hypothesis is derived, tested, and refined. Once a diagnostic decision is reached, planning and implementation of appropriate interventions follows. The process ends with evaluation of a client's responses to the interventions.

Carnevali (1984) points out that both tradition and patient well-being require nurses to be sufficiently competent to engage in diagnostic reasoning and to make treatment decisions in at least two disciplines, nursing and medicine. In nursing, nurses hold primary accountability for making judgments regarding the status of the patient and the family's daily life as it affects or is affected by the patient's health. Treatment plans are aimed at helping the individual and the family to manage effectively within the constraints imposed by presenting circumstances, health-related activities, and demands of daily life. In regard to the biomedical domain, in many settings such as industry, home care, private practice, and nurse-managed clinics, nurses hold delegated responsibility for making accurate, appropriate clinical judgments about a patient's pathophysiological health status. On the basis of these judgments, nurses must decide whether to recommend that a patient continue in self-care, continue under nursing management, perhaps seeking consultation from the physician about altering the medical treatment regimen, be referred to a physician for medical diagnosis and treatment, or be retained under the existing medical regimen. Therefore, the following discussion includes illustrations relating both to biomedical and nursing diagnoses.

Deciding whether a laboratory test value or observed symptom represents health or illness is clearly a first step in the process of reaching a diagnosis. The second step is differentiating among the alternative conclusions that can potentially be reached about a patient's condition. This step involves three substeps: (1) reviewing patient characteristics in relation to possible explanatory data, (2) choosing the appropriate clinical measurements for obtaining further information, and (3) reviewing and synthesizing the evidence to determine what diagnostic classification or label best fits the evidence. Once this process is complete, the stage of disease progression can be determined and a treatment can be selected.

Suppose a laboratory value, a symptom, or a cluster of symptoms has been identified as abnormal. What is to be done? Clearly, until the clinical meaning of these observations is established, no action can be taken. Just as epidemiological thinking is useful in deciding initial issues of normality versus abnormality, so it is used in narrowing down the diagnostic options. Epidemiological questions to be considered are:

1. What diseases are prevalent in the community at this time? If, for example, there were a local influenza epidemic at the time a patient presents with fever, headache, weakness, and myalgia and the symptoms were of recent origin, a clinician would be likely to attribute the symptoms to influenza and make recommendations accordingly. At other times, if there were no influenza outbreak, he or she might be more inclined to consider laboratory tests to rule out other explanations.

2. What diseases characterized by these symptoms would fit the characteristics of this patient? As part of the clinical history, information about patient characteristics such as age, race, sex, occupation, habits, and geographical area of residence is gathered. If a middle-aged woman presents with a nonspecific lung lesion, has no history of smoking or hazardous occupational exposure but lives in the Mississippi Valley, histoplasmosis might be immediately expected. If this same woman lived in Arizona and presented with these same symptoms, other diagnoses would need to be explored. No tests may be required when a 38-year-old non-smoking mother who uses little alcohol and has been generally healthy in the past now presents with recent weight loss, fatigue, faintness, forgetfulness, and upset stomach if the screening clinician is aware that she became widowed three months before. These are symptoms frequently associated with the stress of unresolved grief. Thus, many diagnostic decisions can be tentatively reached before examining the patient or doing diagnostic tests, simply by collecting appropriate information and "thinking epidemiologically." In general practice settings (primary

care practice), the probability of finding a serious underlying disease associated with symptoms is much less
than in referral settings. Very often, the action taken
will be to treat the symptom without additional diagnostic tests. Where there is suspicion of underlying disease,
however, additional tests may be required.

Choosing a Diagnostic Procedure

With advances in medical technology come a wide array of new
diagnostic procedures and techniques. When a patient presents
with several symptoms, the physician or nurse clinician, in
order to arrive at a diagnostic classification of the problem that
can be used to plan treatment, must choose from among the
available tests those that are most likely to provide useful, valid
information. Cost of the tests and risks to the patient must also
be considered. In the best of all possible worlds, information on
the relative efficacy of each test or combination of tests, based
on prospective studies, would be available relative to each disease of interest. This is rarely available in practice, however.
More is known about tests that have been in common use for
some time than about many of the newer, less used tests.

The same criteria discussed in relation to screening tests in
Chapter 13 are important in choosing diagnostic tests: reliability; validity as measured by sensitivity, specificity, and predictive values; cost; safety; and acceptability. The most accurate
tests—the gold standards—are often relatively elaborate, expensive, and risky, for example, cardiac catheterization, other
radiological contrast procedures, and tissue biopsies. Usually, in
the initial stages of a diagnostic workup, simpler, less accurate
tests are used. Clearly, when the suspected disease is life threatening but treatable, high sensitivity of the test is essential, e.g.,
childhood leukemia. Sensitive tests are also useful when the
patient's symptoms represent many possible disease conditions
and the objective is to rule out diseases and reduce the number
of viable possibilities that must be considered. For example,
tuberculin skin tests, which are highly sensitive but not highly
specific, can rule out tuberculosis as an explanation for lung
infiltrates; a negative test would direct the diagnostician to look
for alternative explanations. Sensitive tests, in these latter
instances, are thus most helpful when the result is negative.

Because highly specific tests are rarely positive in the

absence of disease, such tests are useful for implicating or confirming diagnoses suggested by other tests. Such tests are necessary before instituting treatment. Thus, one strategy in the use of diagnostic tests is to begin with tests of high sensitivity but reasonable cost and risk. As the number of diagnoses being considered is decreased, then more specific tests are used. Tests with high specificity are also, more often than not, more expensive and pose greater risk to patients, for example, cardiac catheterization. Such tests are also highly sensitive.

Another strategy for maximizing the effectiveness of any diagnostic procedure is to maximize the likely prevalence of the disease by selectively applying the test to those patients at highest risk by history and symptoms for developing the disease. This strategy maximizes the predictive value of the positive test just as screening high-risk populations increases the predictive value of a screening test.

Another strategy is to use multiple tests for the same disease. Because many diagnostic tests have less than 100 percent sensitivity and specificity, use of a single test frequently results in an intermediate probability of disease, for example, 40 or 60 percent. Because treatment cannot be instituted on the basis of a 60 percent certainty that the disease exists, for example, pancreatic cancer, more information or certainty is needed. Multiple tests can be used in parallel (at the same time) or serially (consecutively). With multiple tests, a high degree of certainty is achieved when all tests are positive or negative. Serial testing can be used when rapid assessment is not required, for example, when the suspected disease progresses slowly, is not life threatening, and the patient can be easily followed up, as in an office or ambulatory care clinic. It is also used when some tests are risky or expensive; these risky or expensive tests are used only after the simpler tests are positive. With serial testing, testing is stopped when a negative result is obtained. Serial testing maximizes specificity and positive predictive value but lowers sensitivity and negative predictive value. This approach is useful when no individual test is highly specific. The most specific test should be used first to minimize the number of persons who must be followed up (Fig. 14–2). The possibility of a false negative result must be considered if no alternative diagnostic explanation is confirmed or if additional symptoms that are consistent with the diagnosis develop (Fletcher et al., 1982). It is often the nurse who may be engaged in follow-up care of such patients

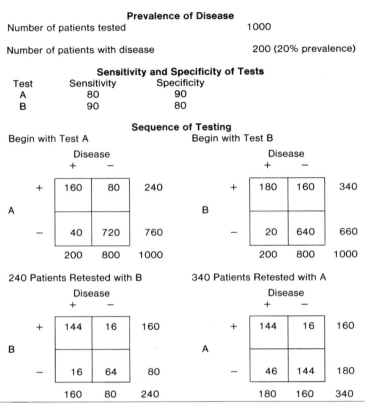

Prevalence of Disease

Number of patients tested	1000
Number of patients with disease	200 (20% prevalence)

Sensitivity and Specificity of Tests

Test	Sensitivity	Specificity
A	80	90
B	90	80

Sequence of Testing

Begin with Test A   Begin with Test B

	Disease +	Disease −	
+	160	80	240
−	40	720	760
	200	800	1000

(A)

	Disease +	Disease −	
+	180	160	340
−	20	640	660
	200	800	1000

(B)

240 Patients Retested with B   340 Patients Retested with A

	Disease +	Disease −	
+	144	16	160
−	16	64	80
	160	80	240

(B)

	Disease +	Disease −	
+	144	16	160
−	46	144	180
	180	160	340

(A)

* Note that in both sequences the same number of patients are identified as diseased (160), and the same number of true positives (144) are identified. But when Test A (with the higher specificity) is used first, fewer patients are retested. The lower sensitivity of Test A does not adversely affect the final result.

Figure 14–2. Effect of sequence in serial testing: A then B versus B then A.* *(From Fletcher, R., Fletcher, S., & Wagner, E. Clinical epidemiology—The essentials. Baltimore: Williams and Wilkens, 1982.)*

and who will be in a position to observe these symptoms and initiate referral to a physician for further testing.

Parallel tests are used when rapid assessment is required—when the suspected disease has a rapid course with high case-fatality rates, when patients are hospitalized, or in cases of emergency. They may also be considered for ambulatory patients who may have difficulty returning for additional visits. This approach increases the sensitivity and negative predictive value of results over those obtained by any individual test. Specificity and positive predictive value are, however, lowered. Although disease is less likely to be missed than with serial testing, a higher rate of false positives requiring additional testing or unnecessary treatment results. For a more complete discussion of these issues, see Fletcher et al., 1982.

Nurses and Biomedical Diagnoses

A nurse faced with the need to make a biomedical diagnosis must do so without access to a sophisticated array of laboratory tests, although in some settings he or she may be able to order or carry out some basic ones, such as a CBC, Pap smear, stool culture, or hemocult test. The nurse's diagnostic task is not to affix a precise diagnostic label but to infer and classify the status of the patient on the basis of present or readily available data. The nurse must determine whether the presenting symptoms represent a mild or self-limiting condition that can be alleviated through nursing intervention or a more serious disease that requires medical diagnosis and treatment.

Suppose that a patient presents with a complaint of watery diarrhea and abdominal cramping. Such symptoms may be acute symptoms of either an infectious process or of exposure to a toxin, or, if chronic, may be a manifestation of a serious disorder. Based on the patient's description of altered fecal output and other history factors such as age, sex, race, occupation, dietary patterns, recent travel experiences, recent stressful incidents, and drug intake, as well as results of a physical examination, the nurse can reach some conclusions about the probable cause of the symptoms. History of an acute onset with no history of psychological, occupational, or pharmaceutical causes, suggests an infectious etiology. Epidemiological evidence suggests that viral infections generally have a short duration of 1 or 2 days and few distinguishing characteristics. Symptoms produced by bacterial organisms that cause diarrhea through production of a toxin rather than infection of the bowel, e.g., staphylococcal food poisoning, while producing severe cramps and diarrhea, are characterized by the suddenness of onset, lack of fever, and self-limited course. Other bacterial and protozoal infections are not apt to be self-limiting, will become more severe with time, and require referral for differential diagnoses to distinguish these inflammatory states from other causes so that appropriate medical treatment can be instituted (Aspinall & Tanner, 1981).

TABLE 14–4. MAJOR CAUSES OF DIARRHEA

Abnormal Initiating Mechanism	Pathophysiology	Clinical State
I. Infection of GI tract	Viral changes in cellular structure of small bowel	Viral enteritis, viral gastroenteritis
	Bacterial invasion of mucosa in colon causing hyperemia and ulceration plus production of enterotoxin causing hypersecretion	Staphylococcal food poisoning, *salmonella, shigella enteritis* (bacillary dysentery), "turista" (traveller's diarrhea), cholera, *clostridium perfringens (C. welchii),* tropical sprue
	Protozoa and parasites produce an inflammatory colitis	Amebic dysentery (Amebiasis), giardiasis, coccidiosis, schistosomiasis, trichinosis
II. Inflammation or irritation of GI tract	Alteration of bacterial flora, overproduction of tissue-lysing enzymes, hypersensitive food reactions, autoimmune reactions, and other less well understood mechanisms initiate an inflammatory reaction, primarily involving mucosa and submucosa of small bowel, with hyperemia, ulceration, and leucocyte infiltration	Ulcerative colitis, Crohn's disease (regional enteritis), diverticulitis, drug-induced colitis (lincomycin, clindamycin, tetracycline, etc.)
III. Malabsorption A. Malabsorption of fats	Deficient production of the pancreatic enzyme lipase	Pancreatitis, carcinoma of pancreas, cystic fibrosis, protein malnutrition (kwashiorkor) pancreatic resection
	Deficient production of bile salts with impaired micille formation and resultant decrease in solubilization of fatty acids	Bile duct obstruction, hepatocellular disease
	Deconjugation of bile	Jejunal diverticulosis,

TABLE 14–4. *(cont.)*

Abnormal Initiating Mechanism	Pathophysiology	Clinical State
	salts by overgrowth of colonic bacteria	scleroderma, diabetic visceral neuropathy, afferent loop obstruction, blind loop syndrome
	Sequestration or precipitation of bile salts	Intake of neomycin, calcium carbonate, cholestyramine, liquid paraffin
B. Alteration of intestinal mucosa absorptive surface	Defective assimilation pathways due to deficiency of enzymes, damage to intestinal mucosa, infiltration of intestinal mucosa by other cells or matter, etc.	Celiac disease, nontropical sprue (gluten-induced enteropathy), Whipple's disease, lymphosarcoma infiltration, radiation enteritis, amyloidosis, pernicious anemia, hypogammaglobulinemia, mastocytosis
	Loss of absorptive area by surgical resection	Short bowel syndrome, gastrocolic fistula, gastroileostomy
C. Metabolic abnormality	Genetic or acquired deficiency of disaccharidases, with impaired hydrolysis of disaccharides	Lactase deficiency, lactose interolance, sucrase deficiency, glucose–galactose malabsorption
	Genetic defect in amino acid transport in intestinal mucosa and renal tubules	Cystinuria, Hartnup disease
	Release of potent bioactive humoral agents:	
	serotonin	Carcinoid syndrome
	gastrin	Pancreatic tumors (Zollinger–Ellison syndrome)
	Dysfunction of endocrine glands, with resultant alteration in neuromuscular function and malabsorptive disorders	Thyrotoxicosis, adrenal insufficiency, hypoparathyroidism

(continued)

TABLE 14–4. (cont.)

Abnormal Initiating Mechanism	Pathophysiology	Clinical State
D. Altered vascular supply	Congestion and edema of the mucosa, abnormality of mucosal lymphatics, or ischemia from altered blood supply	Mesentery artery insufficiency/occlusion, vasculitis, constrictive pericarditis, congestive heart failure
IV. Altered neurologic function	Surgical interruption of parasympathetic nerve supply results in poor emptying of gallbladder and inadequate stimulation with malabsorptive states	Postvagotomy
	Psychogenic initiation of sympathoadrenal response	Irritable colon syndrome, anxiety states
V. Mechanical factors	Partial obstruction of the bowel causing colonic distention with frequent expulsion of liquid stool around lesion	Neoplasms, adhesions, fecal impaction, stenosis
	Osmotic effects of nonabsorbable matter with movement of fluid into bowel lumen	Laxatives (sorbitol, magnesium), heavy metals, dumping syndrome

(From Aspinall, M. J., & Tanner, C. A. *Decision making for patient care: Applying the nursing process.* New York: Appleton-Century-Crofts, 1981, pp. 200–201.)

Parameters for assessing diarrhea lasting longer than 3 days include: (1) frequency and urgency, which can provide clues to the site of the lesion, (2) amount and character of stools, (3) relationship of abdominal pain to defecation and eating, (4) presence or absence of blood in stools, unrelated to dietary intake, (5) presence or absence of mucus, and (6) weight loss. Diagnostic tests that might be done by the physician include stool testing for occult blood; microscopic examination for pus, ova, or parasites; a stool culture; other laboratory analyses of the stool; protoscopy and/or sigmoidoscopy; roentgenologic examination; serum carotene levels (for steatorrhea); and tests for electrolyte losses (Aspinall & Tanner, 1981). Major causes of diarrhea that need to be considered are shown in Table 14–4.

Nursing Diagnoses

The following case in an acute care setting was presented by Aspinall and Tanner in their book, *Decision-Making for Patient Care: Applying the Nursing Process* (1981) and serves to illustrate epidemiological thinking in nursing diagnosis.

> Mrs. L. is a 63-year-old diabetic who has been in coronary care for five days with the diagnosis of acute MI complicated with recurrent premature ventricular contractions. She has been receiving lidocaine IV drip at 2 to 4 mg/minute, currently at 2 mg/minute. She has an abrasion over the left eye, sustained in a fall prior to admission. Her history indicates one prior hospitalization for cataract removal. When the afternoon nurse comes on duty, Mrs. L. is disoriented as to time and place. She is out of bed, brushing her teeth, and is quite agitated about the monitor wires restricting her freedom. When told that she is in the hospital, she comments that she has given enough time to the "equipment check" referring to all the people coming in the room to check the monitor. There is no record of her having been confused before.

The question is what is the cause of Mrs. L's confusion? Based on knowledge of the epidemiology of diabetes, heart disease, and head trauma, the nurse must consider as probable diagnoses hypoglycemia, reduced cerebral perfusion caused by low cardiac output, and increased intracranial pressure from the head trauma. Sensory deprivation caused by not having her glasses and having no visitors or diversions is another possibility. The nurse must gather information to confirm or rule out one or all of these possibilities.

Available data indicates that the patient's skin is warm and dry, pulse is 72 and full, blood pressure is stable at 128/60. The patient last received 40 units of NPH insulin 8 hours ago. NPH generally peaks in 8 to 12 hours. The last S and A was done at 11:30 A.M. and was 2+/neg. Further assessment indicates that the IV is patent with lidocaine at 30 cc/hour. There is no evidence of tremors, sinus rhythm is normal with no dysrythmias, urinary output has been stable for the past 8 hours (800 cc), peripheral circulation is good, pulse is stable at 72 beats per minute, and skin color is good. The nurse concludes there is no evidence of low cardiac output that could produce disorientation. Head trauma seems unlikely as a cause because pupils are equal and react to light, the patient denies headache, and early admission data indicate no evidence of substantial head trauma sustained in the preadmission fall. Based on this data, the nurse concludes that hypoglycemia or sensory deprivation are the two most likely causes.

Administration of orange juice should lead to some improvement if hypoglycemia is the cause. Meanwhile, the nurse has blood drawn for glucose tests and can continue to monitor the patient and request her eyeglasses from home, increase frequency of visitors, and provide for other diversions to reduce sensory deprivation. In a sense, this nurse has used the approach of multiple tests for each competing diagnosis. All tests were negative for the hypothesized diagnosis of reduced cerebral perfusion caused by low cardiac output and increased intracranial pressure from head trauma. The tests for hypoglycemia were not highly sensitive but were specific in the sense that they ruled out elevated blood sugar, leaving low blood sugar as a possibility. The blood glucose test is a more sensitive test. Meanwhile, the intervention of administering orange juice may help. If not, no harm is done.

Another kind of diagnostic challenge facing the nurse clinician is the diagnosis of abnormal health status resulting from a prescribed medical treatment regimen. Epidemiological studies provide data on likely complications of various treatments. Awareness of common complications or side effects enables the nurse to diagnose such problems promptly. An epidemiologically oriented nurse caring for a patient on high-dose, short-term steriod therapy would be alert to the potential for alteration in glucose metabolism. Because this patient is at higher risk for such outcomes, the nurse should routinely monitor the patient's urine for glucose and acetone a.c. and h.s., monitor results of serum glucose tests, and observe the patient for signs and symptoms of steroid-induced diabetes, such as polydypsia, polyuria, and polyphagia. Positive results on these measures will likely lead the nurse to a diagnosis of steroid-induced alteration in glucose metabolism. This diagnosis then offers several alternatives for intervention, including teaching the patient to limit his or her intake of high carbohydrate foods and alerting the physician who may wish to alter the steriod therapy or institute additional treatment for diabetes. In this same patient, if the nurse detects a temperature elevation accompanied by cough, skin lesions, dysuria, redness, swelling, heat or pain in eyes, ears, throat, abdomen, joints, genital, or rectal areas, flushed appearance, or malaise, lethargy, myalgia, he or she will probably diagnose an infection and alert the physician.

Health Risk Appraisal

Health risk appraisal is a way of estimating personal risk. It provides a basis for offering practical advice on how to reduce that risk by changing life style.

Risk is the probability that an untoward event will occur, e.g., the probability of becoming ill or dying within a stated period of time or by a specific age. The term risk factor is variously used by epidemiological authors to mean any of the following (Last, 1983):

1. An attribute or exposure associated with an increased probability of a specified outcome, such as occurrence of a disease. Also called a risk marker, it need not be a causal agent.
2. An attribute or exposure that increases the probability of occurrence of a disease or specified outcome, i.e., a determinant.
3. A determinant that can be modified by intervention, thereby reducing the probability of occurrence of a disease or other specified outcomes. May be referred to as a modifiable risk factor.

As used in the following discussion, risk factor refers to modifiable risk factors as in definition 3.

Many life style factors are known risk factors for specific diseases. Examples were discussed in Chapters 7 through 10 in relation to stages of the life cycle. In Chapter 11, risk factors were discussed in relation to onset and progression of disease. Identification of individuals at risk of specific diseases was discussed in relation to disease prevention and control in Chapters 3, 5, 6, and 12. The following brief discussion centers on a currently popular approach to health risk appraisal in clinical practice.

Evidence that life style is associated with health status comes from a study of 7000 California residents by Belloc and Breslow (1972) that showed that health status and longevity varied by living pattern. Habits associated with good health included eating breakfast daily, eating moderate regular meals and no snacks, maintaining weight, avoiding smoking, limiting alcoholic beverages to 7 per week and sleeping 7 to 8 hours per night. There was a positive association between the number of these habits followed and both health status and life span. A follow-up study 9 years later showed an inverse relationship between these good habits and mortality (Breslow & Enstrom, 1980). Evidence suggesting the positive effects of good health practices on physical health status comes from a recent study by Reed (1983).

Risk for individual patients can be estimated from tables identifying mortality rates for the leading causes of death in ensuing 10-year periods (Geller–Gelsner tables). Such tables, based on the top ten causes of death, are available for each 10-year age group from 5 to 75 years of age. Because the top ten causes of death account for two-thirds of deaths in each age group, with the rest scattered among more than 1000 causes, the incidence for these other causes is extremely low.

Based on the natural history of each cause, specific precursor risk factors can be identified for each cause of death. For example, risk of heart attack caused by atherosclerotic heart disease is associated with sedentary life style, smoking, overweight, hypertension, diabetes, and triglyceride levels. These risk factors can be combined to give a composite risk using either a mathematical formula or probability tables. The mathematical formula method uses information on the individual level of risk on each factor relative to the average population risk, which is set at 1.0. The individuals risk is then expressed as greater or less than 1.0. The calculation multiplies together factors with risk of less than 1.0 and adds to that result factors greater than 1.0. This composite risk factor is multiplied by the known average number of deaths from that specific cause for individuals of the same age, sex, and race. The resulting value represents a risk for the individual that can be compared to the average person's risk. This appears to be a meaningful measure for patients and serves as motivation to change behavior.

Calculations can be done by hand as illustrated by Robbins and Hall (1979) or by computer using a form with a brief medical history and physical examination data* (Ross, 1981). Such

---

*Some sources are: Life Extension Institute, Control Data Corp., Minneapolis, MN; U. of Wisconsin, Stevens Point, WI; Medical Datamation, Belleville, OH; St. Louis County Health Dept., Duluth, MN; Div. of Health Educ., Centers for Disease Control, Atlanta, GA; Project Well Aware, U. of Arizona, Tuscon, AZ.

computer risk assessments are being done with increasing frequency as part of health fairs and occupational health programs. Some physicians use this assessment in the office setting. The patient receives a printout of health strengths and weaknesses and suggested ways to reduce risk, accompanied by counseling and planning of specific measures, such as the specific changes that may be made in diet or exercise in view of the patient's general health status. Such programs can be a useful means of promoting health.

It is, of course, not necessary to quantify risk so precisely. A major advantage of quantification is that it seems to express risk in terms that are easy for both the clinician and the patient to understand. Also, it provides a baseline against which progress can be measured subsequent to life-style changes (Table 14–5) and provides a data base with both baseline and follow-up data that could be used to study the effects of life-style changes as long as adequate information is recorded about these behavioral changes. Without quantification, a clinician can still identify for individual patients the risk factors for the specific major causes of death as long as the clinician is well informed about the natural history of these conditions. Monitoring of biological and behavioral risk factors can be used to assess whether health behaviors have improved and whether concurrent changes in the biological risk factors have occurred. Using the example in Table 14–5 of arterosclerotic heart disease, cholesterol, triglycerides, blood pressure, and weight could be monitored concurrently with patient reports of changes in smoking, exercise, and so on.

Another aspect of risk assessment concerns the identification of factors that place patients at higher risk of particular complications from medical interventions. These are discussed further in the following sections on prognosis and treatment.

PROGNOSIS

The disease prognosis represents the expected clinical course and outcome for the patient, that is, the relative probabilities that a patient will develop each of the alternative outcomes of the natural history of the disease. In the absence of intervention, prognosis is a function of the general progressive nature of the disease itself, the pathogenicity and virility of the disease

TABLE 14–5. RISK PROFILE FOR ARTERIOSCLEROTIC HEART DISEASE (HEART ATTACK) FOR JANE DOE

Average risk	1,260	
Your current risk	2,898	(2.3 × Avg)
Your achievable risk	491	(.4 × Avg)

Contributing Factors	Risk Factor	Risk-Reducing Factors	Risk Factor
BP—144/80	.08	BP—120/80 or less	.6
Cholesterol—200 mg%	.7	Cholesterol—180 or less	.6
Diabetes—No	1.0		1.0
Exercise—Sedentary	1.4	Supervised exercise	1.0
FH ASHD No Early Deaths	.9		.9
Smoker—1 pack/day	1.9	Not smoking	.9
Weight—166 lbs	1.2	Weight—134 lbs or less	1.0
No Hx of Abnormal ECG	1.0		1.0
Trig—231 mg%	1.6	Triglycerides—<151 mg%	1.3
Excessive stress may increase risk—exact risk factor not yet available			

Factors That May Offer the Greatest Reduction in Risk	Achievable Benefit with Change of These Factors
Not smoking	2.7 years
Not drinking	1.1 years
Exercise	.9 years
Weight reduction	.9 years
Blood pressure reduction	.3 years
Cholesterol reduction	.1 years
Other	1.5 years
Total reduction in risk	7.0 years

(Adapted from Ross, C. M. Health hazard appraisal. In Schneideman (Ed.). *The practice of preventive health care*. Menlo Park, Calif.: Addison-Wesley, 1981, p. 32.)

agent, and characteristics of the host. Influenza, for example, is usually an acute, self-limiting condition, producing unpleasant symptoms in the host, but not threatening life. Certain variants of the influenza virus may be more virulent than others. These occasional virulent strains may be characterized by a much higher attack rate and by higher case-fatality than for the more common less virulent strains. Certain subgroups of the population—the elderly, the very young, and the poor—may be more susceptible to infection and more likely to have clinically apparent disease with complications that may lead to death.

Thus knowledge of prognosis guides decisions about the

need for intervention. What we tell the patient about his or her illness is based on knowing the prognosis. Should we reassure the patient that the illness is trivial or prepare him or her for major changes in health status or even death in the future? Is there anything the patient can do after the prognosis, for example, changes in lifestyle after myocardial infarction? Prognosis also influences what we do for the patient, whether we merely follow for observation or initiate treatment.

Medical intervention in the form of treatment is intended to change the disease prognosis and lead to a more favorable outcome for the patient. Each time a physician prescribes a medicine or performs an operation, he or she must weigh the potential for benefit against the potential for harm. Similarly, nursing interventions are intended to change patient outcome and must be weighed in terms of potential for benefit versus harm. Many therapeutic interventions offer potential for harm as well as benefit. Drugs have undesirable side effects; even the ubiquitous aspirin tablet presents a risk to certain individuals. Surgical procedures carry risk of infection, organ failure, and death. Extended bed rest may be as undesirable as excessive exertion. Bladder catheterization of a postoperative patient with a severely distended bladder may be helpful in preventing refluxing of urine to the kidneys, rupture of the bladder, or other complications but also poses the threat of introducing infectious organisms into a patient whose resistance may be low. Although this risk may be low in the average patient, in an immunosuppressed patient this risk must be weighed against the risks to the patient of waiting too long to void.

CHOOSING A TREATMENT

Choosing between two or more possible choices of action requires that choices be clearly identified and that a method be available to assess the overall value of the outcome for each choice. Data from epidemiological and clinical studies provide information as to the probable effects of an action on the prognosis for the disease, both generally and for particular subgroups of patients. Even where adequate data are available, two additional elements influence the decision-making process: (1) uncertainty about the future outcome and (2) the value or worth assigned to the various possible outcomes. These conditions apply to physicians who must decide, for example, whether to prescribe or not to prescribe a particular drug or whether or not to operate. Nurses must make decisions such as whether to administer morphine to a postoperative patient complaining of pain, but who appears to be suffering signs of respiratory distress.

Today, even patients are faced with treatment decisions; they are required to give informed consent for medical procedures such as surgery. In other instances, they may need to decide among alternative treatments; for example, a woman may have one physician recommend a modified mastectomy for treatment of breast cancer whereas another physician may have recommended a lumpectomy with subsequent radium implant. A nurse is often asked to help such patients think through their decisions.

Sound clinical judgments in any of the above situations require a command of a sufficient body of facts and the skill to combine facts appropriately. Such skills are rarely taught; rather it is assumed that with acquisition of sufficient experience, the clinician will somehow acquire clinical judgment. But the essence of clinical judgment resides in the ability to weigh advantages and disadvantages of a diagnostic or therapeutic procedure and to choose a course of action for a particular patient based on estimates of costs and benefits.

Sackett et al. (1985) have identified three principal decisions inherent in determining the rational treatment of any patient:

1. Deciding the ultimate objective of treatment, whether cure, palliation, symptomatic relief, limitation of structural or functional deterioration, preventing later complication or recurrence.
2. Selecting the most efficacious specific treatment.
3. Specifying an identifiable (measurable) treatment target as a guide for when to stop or alter treatment. Poor progress towards the target suggests a need to change the intensity or form of treatment.

Making and recording these decisions provides a basis for coherent patient management, even by a treatment team. Without such decisions, chaos can ensue. For example, unless a decision to provide only palliative care and to maintain comfort and dignity for a terminally ill patient is recorded, personnel covering when the primary physician is off duty might order x-rays, blood counts, and antibiotics if the patient spikes a temperature.

Treatment decisions must be based on the best available evidence on risks and benefits of treatment. Ideally, evidence is available from studies on patients with characteristics similar to the one being treated. Critical assessment of the validity and applicability of the evidence is essential. The other elements to be considered are the patient's social, psychological, and economic circumstances.

Clinical decisions about treatment should be made only after a patient's need is determined. The issue becomes one of choosing from among several potential interventions the one that will have the highest probability of achieving the most valued or desirable outcome. The four components to be considered are: (1) a set of possible actions, (2) potential outcomes associated with those actions, (3) the probability that a particular outcome will occur if a given action is taken, and (4) the value of the outcome to the decision-maker. It is assumed that the patient's values are an element in determining relative values of particular outcomes to the decision-maker. Certainly the value of an outcome to a patient will affect his or her compliance with the treatment. In general, clinical decision-making takes place in an open system, that is, complete knowledge of factors affecting the outcomes is usually unknown. These unknowns lessen the complete rationality of the decision-making process. Even so, nursing and medical decisions can be made more objective and systematic if outcomes are consciously and deliberately narrowed to a limited number that are then ordered by their values and if the relative potential of available nursing actions to achieve these outcomes is weighed. Practical strategies for such decisions are found in decision analysis.

Decision Analysis

The necessity of making treatment decisions in the face of uncertainty about outcome is an integral part of the life of a clinician. Confronting uncertainty is never easy. Uncertainty is minimized, however, when all available information enters into the process of decision-making in a logical manner. Imagine a surgeon faced with a 59-year-old male patient, married, with two children, one a college sophomore, the other a third year law student. The patient owns and runs a small hardware store. The patient, who has a family history of heart disease, has recently recovered from a heart attack and complains of severe chest pains almost daily. Coronary angiography shows partial blockage of all three major arteries feeding the heart and a probable developing clot in one artery. The surgeon is aware that bypass surgery is one treatment option. Another is treatment with one of the newer drugs for dissolving the clot. The drugs may have side effects and there is the possibility that another clot may form at a later time. The only group for whom bypass surgery has clearly been shown to prolong life is the group of patients with obstruction of the left main coronary artery. For patients with prior heart attacks, partial obstructions, or developing infarction, no improved survival has been demonstrated (NIH, 1981). Although bypass surgery has been thought to relieve chest pain and numerous studies find an enhanced "quality of life" among patients with bypass surgery, other evidence suggests this could be a placebo effect—a group of over 100 patients whose vein grafts had ceased to function after their surgery reported such amelioration of symptoms just prior to finding out that their bypasses were blocked (Preston, 1977).

The surgeon is faced with a difficult decision in regard to what treatment to recommend. The bypass surgery carries a 2 percent risk of death, a 5 percent risk of heart attack on the table, and a 5 to 10 percent risk of a serious complication such as stroke, weakening of the heart muscle, or infection. The final decision is the patient's; therefore the physician's recommendation will probably include a discussion of the pros and cons of the alternatives. But, as the expert, the surgeon must choose and support the option that is likely to have the best outcome. Although bypass surgery remains an option if drug treatment fails, there is some risk of another fatal heart attack in the interim or weakening of the heart muscle, which will make surgery more dangerous at a later time. In the face of such decisions, many clinicians are turning to decision analysis as a way of arriving at the best possible logical decision.

Decision analysis involves application of analytical and mathematical tools to assist in making the "best" choice. Decision analysis assumes that (1) decision makers wish to maximize some measure of value for outcomes of the decision and (2) people are generally limited in the amount of information they can process at any one time about complex decisions. Thus, the goal of decision analysis is to break complex decisions into smaller, more easily assimilated pieces that human decision makers can handle well, and then to use mathematical techniques to put all the pieces together to solve the larger, more complex decision (Fryback, 1981). This process is operationalized through the decision tree, a diagram showing the interrelationships of three pieces of the problem: (1) possible actions, (2) possible outcomes associated with each possible action, and (3) probability of each outcome occurring if a given action is taken. The values of the outcome to the decision maker and to the patient also need to be considered and may be included in the decision tree.

Figure 14–3 shows relationships between possible actions and outcomes in a simple decision tree format. The root of the tree is the initial available decision alternatives. Branches of the tree move away from the root showing these alternatives. The point of branching is called a decision node. Each alternative leads to several potential, mutually exclusive outcomes, one of which must occur. These represent additional branches coming out from the appropriate initial branch. The ordering of branches from the root represents information in the order in which it becomes available to the decision maker and therefore the order in which the decisions must be made. For example, in Figure 14–3, if Treatment A is done first, the three possible outcomes are a successful outcome, (the patient recovers), an equivocal outcome (the patient is improved, but not recovered), and a negative outcome (no improvement or condition worsens). Imagine for the surgeon's decision discussed earlier that Treatment A is drug treatment, that Treatment B is single bypass surgery, and that Treatment C is double bypass surgery. If the surgeon considers bypass surgery, he or she knows that the probability of a negative outcome is 12 to 17 percent (death 2 percent, heart attack on table 5 percent, stroke or other complication 5 to 10 percent). In regard to successful outcomes, probability of prolonging life, based on the NIH study (1981), is 0 percent. Probability of reducing pain is high, however, probably 80 percent. There is a 20 percent probability of little or no change. In the event of an equivocal (no change) outcome, he or she can still try Treatment A or C. In the event of the negative outcomes,

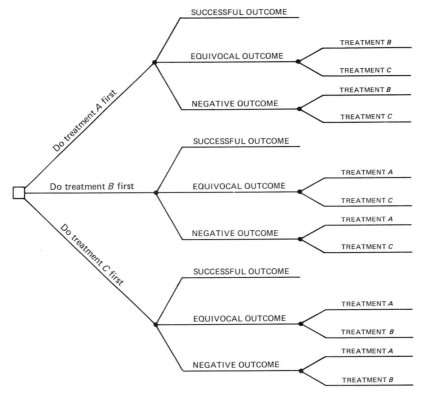

Figure 14–3. Hypothetical decision tree where three potential treatments are available.

except death, the surgeon could also try the other treatments, but the damage cannot be corrected. The surgeon would work through similar probabilities for outcomes if Treatment A or C were tried first.

In order to assign values to the various outcomes, the physician needs to consider how each outcome would affect the patient's ability to support the family, maintain self-esteem or whatever else might be important in that patient. Numerical values to represent these patient values can be assigned to each outcome if the surgeon wishes to do a mathematical analysis of the decision tree. These numerical values, called utilities, would be multiplied by the probabilities of the occurrence for each alternative decision. Scores for the alternatives can then be compared. The physician could choose to restrict the analysis to a qualitative analysis. For more detailed discussion of quantitative decision analysis, see Aspinall (1979), Parker and Kassier (1980), or Weinstein and Feinberg (1980).

The decision tree does not indicate a single best decision, only options and possible consequences. The best decision is based on a variety of factors that can be assigned to one of two categories: (1) probabilities of the various outcomes (obtainable from epidemiological data combined with judgment of the clinician) and (2) values of the various outcomes to the patient and the decision maker. Both the probabilities and the values of particular outcomes are a function of the condition or circumstances of the patient in question. For example, potential options and outcomes remain the same for virtually all patients for whom arteriography is considered, but probabilities of particular prognostic outcomes and the associated values differ from patient to patient; the decision is influenced accordingly. The probabilities and assigned values of a particular outcome can be added to the branches of the decision tree and either a formal, quantitive analysis or a qualitative analysis of the tree can be done. To simplify either analysis, probabilities and the values of various outcomes can be used to "prune" the tree. Pruning involves removing branches that are relatively unimportant (e.g., of low probability for this particular patient) and consolidating others to reduce the problem to manageable proportions.

In many clinical situations, a thought process similar to constructing and pruning a decision tree occurs instinctively and informally without the clinician describing or being able to describe the process. Such behavior would be expected of the experienced clinician whose knowledge and experiential base of probabilities and knowledge of probable utilities of potential outcomes lead to an instinctive best decision. For the younger, less experienced clinicians, however, conscious use of a decision tree can develop the sound patterns of decision-making that will eventually lead to such intuitive decisions in the future.

Probabilities are derived from empirical and clinical studies. Many of these probabilities are part of the knowledge base acquired by clinicians during their professional education and may be a subconscious factor utilized in making clinical decisions. Grier, in a study of nurses' decision-making about patient care, demonstrated that when nurses were asked to rank alternative actions, the preferred actions were generally consistent with the nurses' knowledge of the probabilities of the various outcomes and with the nurses' values for the outcomes. Values of the outcomes varied by whether the nurses worked in an inpatient or community setting (Grier, 1976). This variation in values assigned to outcomes probably results because judgments about the value or utility of an outcome are necessarily more subjective than are probabilities of an outcome occurring. Assessment of probabilities is exclusively the responsibility of the clinician and requires up-to-date knowledge of the most recent research. Because different individuals assess the value of outcomes differently, assessment of values must be done in cooperation with the patient and the family. For example, a 45-year-old patient with hypertension may prefer to take antihypertensive medications for an indefinite period than to face the risks and discomforts involved in a diagnostic evaluation and surgical correction of hypertension of probable renovascular origin. Another patient of similar age, cardiovascular status, and other characteristics may prefer the risks of the diagnostic and operative maneuvers to the prolonged need of drug therapy.

In a more nursing-oriented example, a 78-year-old widowed blind woman with diabetes may prefer the option of sharing her home with a stranger in need of a place to live who would help with shopping, cooking, and her insulin injections to the option of moving in with a relative. Another woman in similar straits may prefer giving up the independence of her own home and living with relatives to the option of dealing with a stranger.

Let us consider the following example of how a decision tree approach can be used by a nurse. The example uses a qualitative approach rather than quantitative analysis. The visiting nurse visits the home of the Jacksons, an elderly couple in their mid 70s. Mr. Jackson, the patient, is recovering from a stroke and is paralyzed on his right side. His wife, who has been caring for him since his return home from the hospital appears to have an upper respiratory infection. She is slightly flushed and appears tired, which is unusual. Although she claims to have a slight cold that doesn't amount to anything, she continues to carry out her busy schedule of caring for her husband, keeping their home clean and neat, baking treats for her husband, and making dolls for a church bazaar. Her oral temperature is 101.2 and other vital signs are somewhat elevated. Her throat is red, she has considerable nasal congestion and some shortness of breath. The nurse must decide what activity recommendation would be best for Mrs. Jackson—continue ambulating, sitting, or staying in bed. Outcomes that need to be considered are effects on (1) circulation/ventilation, (2) fatigue/overexertion, (3) GI/urinary elimination, (4) image of self, (5) muscle/joint mobility, (6) sensory stimulation, (7) skin integrity, and (8) resistance to infection. Figure 14–4 shows a decision tree for decisions in relation to effects on fatigue/overexertion and resistance to infection. The tree has been pruned to show resistance to infection outcomes for only those mobility outcomes that favor maintaining present mobility. The probability of each outcome is strictly hypothetical. Based on these probabilities, however, bed rest would appear to be the best decision because short-term bed rest carries a minimal risk of decrease in mobility and a high probability of preventing worsening infection caused by fatigue. When patient values are also considered, however, sitting may be a preferred choice because Mrs. Jackson can still keep her husband company and work on her dolls. The problem is that

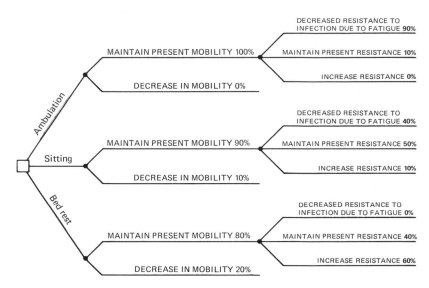

Figure 14–4. Decision tree for Mrs. Jackson (example described in text). At the square node, the choice is in the hands of the decision-maker and at the circular nodes, the outcome is dictated by probability. The probabilities of each outcome as estimated by the author are shown on each branch. The tree has been pruned to remove outcomes relating to resistance to infection for the decreased mobility outcomes.

she may still tend to overdo and become more ill as a result of a decrease in resistance to infection. Because Mrs. Jackson values her activities, she must be helped to weigh the relative impact on her long-term function of submitting to a short period of bed rest or limiting her activities to those that can be done while sitting. If the latter is preferred, then she must be made aware of the risks of overdoing, namely that if her respiratory infection worsens, she may need to spend a longer period in bed to recover. Placement of a temporary home health aide to assist in care of her husband or exploration of family resources to help out (e.g., an adult child living nearby) could ameliorate her concerns for her husband's care, thus reducing the value of ambulation to Mrs. Jackson and assuring that Mr. Jackson's needs would also be met.

A similar analytical process would be applied to each of the three choices in regard to the other seven outcomes and the choice that leads to optimal status on the most outcomes would be selected.

Decision theory could be considered a way of formalizing common sense. Although it provides no magical formulas for correct decisions, it provides a logical framework for analyzing clinical decision problems, from the simplest to the most complex, based on clinical preferences and knowledge. As medical and nursing care becomes more complex, such a framework for organizing available knowledge for the purpose of reaching optimally effective decisions becomes necessary. It also provides a framework that clinicians can use to help patients understand the various treatment options available to them.

Similar thinking processes are useful in deciding whether an observed side effect is caused by the drug used to treat the presenting condition. Like decisions about what treatment to use, decisions about whether an observed side effect is caused by drug treatment and what action should be taken rely on epidemiological evidence and the value of alternatives. In this instance, it is necessary to know with certainty that this drug does cause the observed side effects in some patients and also that it causes these particular side effects in patients with characteristics similar to this one. If the answers to these two questions are yes, then consequences of alternative courses of action need to be considered in a systematic fashion as was illustrated in choosing the initial treatment.

READING THE CLINICAL LITERATURE

It should be clear by now that clinicians rely heavily on epidemiology for building the knowledge base necessary for clinical decision-making. In Chapter 2, suggestions were provided in regard to how to read critically epidemiological articles investigating disease etiology. A few hints on what to look for in articles introducing new therapies and modifications or evaluations of previous therapies may be helpful. As previously stated, the best way to investigate efficacy of therapies is through randomized, controlled trials. Table 14–6 lists important points to consider. Each of these points is briefly discussed.

Random assignment to treatment is intended to assure that every subject has an equal probability of receiving one or the other treatment. The method of random assignment should be described in the article. Usually random assignment is based on use of a table of random numbers. Evidence that random assignment accomplished its task and produced comparable groups of experimental and control patients should be provided. This usually takes the form of a table comparing entry characteristics for the two groups and a statement about their similarity.

Characteristics of study patients are an important factor in determining whether the study results can be generalized. Thus, criteria for cases entered into the study should be clearly stated. Many studies use only patients with advanced illness. Results of

TABLE 14–6. QUESTIONS FOR EVALUATING NEW THERAPIES

1. Were patients randomly assigned to treatment groups?
2. What are the characteristics of patients in the study?
   a. Are study patients representative of patients with the condition, i.e., do they represent a spectrum of disease severity, age, race, and so on?
   b. Are they similar to my patients?
3. Were all clinically relevant outcomes included?
4. Were treatments administered according to protocol?
5. Is the therapeutic intervention feasible in my practice?
6. How was significance of findings determined?
   a. Were both statistical and clinical significance assessed?
   b. If study findings were negative, was the trial large enough to show a clinically important effect if it occurred?
7. Were all patients entering the study accounted for at its conclusion?

such studies provide little or no information about effectiveness of the treatment for patients at other stages of the disease. When a representative cross-section of patients is studied, results should be compared for various subgroups, e.g., different age groups, in order to establish that treatment efficacy is equivalent for all types of patients. This information also provides a basis for each clinician to evaluate the relevance for his or her own practice. The importance of a clear statement of case definition and that all cases met these criteria cannot be overemphasized.

In caring for your patients, what outcomes, good or bad, are you concerned about? Outcomes related to quality of life may be as relevant as 5-year survival rates, infection rates, or other purely physiological criteria. Differences in frequency of clinical disease are probably more important than frequencies or levels of risk factors. All of the relevant outcomes should be examined by the study.

Treatment protocols for all treatment groups should be described. Ideally, neither the investigators nor the patients should know which patients are receiving which treatment. This is called blinding. In a single blind trial the patients are unaware of what treatment they are receiving. In double blind trials, the investigator is also unaware of treatment assignment. In triple blind trials, the individuals analyzing the data are also blind as to which group received which treatment. Blinding is intended to reduce bias. Blinding can be effected with relative ease in studies where the treatment involves administration of medication because placebos can be given to those not receiving the treatment. In contrast, when the treatments under study involve clearly different approaches, e.g., surgery versus medical treatment or audiovisual versus written patient teaching programs, blinding cannot be done.

The description of study methods should include safeguards assuring that treatment was given as intended. With many people involved in the care of a single patient, there are numerous opportunities for interference with the prescribed protocol. In a study of infection rates associated with different frequencies of changing dressings, for example, a temporary nurse on a unit might change a dressing that appeared soiled or loose unless she had been notified about the study protocol and instructed to leave it alone. When trials involve outpatients, patient compliance becomes an operative factor.

In addition, some patients may be intolerant to an assigned treatment and may be getting worse or having life-threatening complications. The design should specify how such cases are to be handled. One large trial, the University Group Diabetes Programs (1970), designed to determine whether better control of elevated blood sugar could reduce or retard the incidence of vascular complications in maturity onset, nonketosis prone diabetics, has received major criticism for the way in which this issue was handled. Patients who stopped or switched their treatments during the study were counted in their original group for the analysis. This study has also been criticized because not all patients met the entry criteria for diabetes and because of poor randomization; more high-risk subjects ended up in the treatment group receiving tolbutamide than in the two groups receiving insulin treatments (Seltzer, 1972; Kilo, 1980). A clear, easy to follow analysis of this study is presented in Chapter 12 of *Clinical Epidemiology* (Fletcher et al., 1982).

Specific interferences with study protocols have been termed contamination and cointervention (Sackett et al., 1985). Contamination occurs when control patients accidentally receive the experimental treatment. Cointervention is the performance of additional diagnostic or therapeutic acts on experimental, but not control, patients. The likelihood of such interferences occuring in a systematic manner is reduced when blinding can be used. Whenever possible such interferences should be recorded so their effect can be assessed in analysis.

The question of whether all patients entering the study were accounted for at the conclusion of the study is related to the previous issue, in that final status of each subject must be accounted for, whether they changed treatments, dropped out of the study, died, or were lost to follow-up. If 142 patients began the study, then 142 should be accounted for at the end. Be suspicious when the final analysis is based on a smaller sample than began the study, particularly when no explanation is given. More often than not, loss of subjects is related in some way to poor outcomes ranging from inability to tolerate a treatment or unwillingness to comply to severe effects such as death. Particularly when such losses occur from the group receiving a new, experimental treatment, results should be viewed cautiously.

Two measures of outcome may be used in clinical trials: statistical significance of results and clinical significance. Statistical significance deals with whether the findings are real, i.e., whether differences in outcome between treatment groups are likely chance phenomena or can be attributed to treatment. A p value of .05 means that the risk of concluding erroneously that that treatment A is better than treatment B is only 5 in 100. Ninety-five times in 100, a conclusion that treatment A is better, would be correct. Statistically significant effects, however, may be too small from a clinical viewpoint to justify changing clinical practice. Suppose that a randomized, controlled trial of the effects on infant birthweight of high protein food supplements for pregnant women found an increase of 15 g in birthweight in the supplemented group compared with the nonsupplemented and that this difference was statistically significant at $p = .01$. Is this statistically significant difference clinically important? Should pregnant women be given protein supplements on the basis of these findings? Obstetricians and clinical nurse specialists in maternal–child health might argue that at least a 50 to 100 g change in birthweight is needed to have any impact on infant morbidity or mortality. Thus, 15 g would not be considered clinically important and resources would not be diverted to supplementation programs for pregnant women. A related question, however, is whether the sample size in the trial was sufficiently large to show a clinically significant difference if it had occurred. A well-designed study will set in advance what is considered to represent a clinically significant effect. The power of this study to detect such an effect should be stated.

Finally, if the study design is deemed adequate and conclusions valid, clinicians must judge whether the new therapeutic intervention is feasible for their practice. Feasibility may depend on the nature of the therapeutic maneuver and availability of personnel and technological resources. For example, individualized self-hypnosis relaxation training has recently been demonstrated in a randomized, controlled trial to be an effective form of antiemetic therapy in children (Cotanch et al., 1985). Training the children in the procedure requires a trained nurse-therapist and 30 to 40 minutes per child as well as a quiet setting. Such an intervention is probably not feasible in a busy outpatient pediatric chemotherapy clinic with a single nurse, because of both environmental and personnel limitations.

Literature in the health care field in general, and nursing in particular, is growing rapidly as new information becomes available and new treatments are tested. Critical assessment of the literature is necessary if nurses are to do more good than harm to patients and to aid in containing health care costs. Knowledge of the natural history of diseases and principles for applying epidemiological thinking to planning patient care can contribute to quality care for patients.

REFERENCES

Aspinall, M. J. & Tanner, C. *Decision making for patient care: Applying the nursing process.* New York: Appleton-Century-Crofts, 1981.

Aspinall, M. J. Use of a decision tree to improve accuracy of diagnosis, *Nursing Research,* 1979, *28*; 182–185.

Belloc, N. & Breslow, L. Relationship of physical health status and health practices. *Preventive Medicine,* 1972, *1*, 409–421.

Breslow, L. & Enstrom, J. D. Persistence of health habits and their relationship to mortality. *Preventive Medicine,* 1980, *9*, 469–483.

Carnevali, D. *Nursing care planning: Diagnosis and management* (3rd ed.). Philadelphia: J. B. Lippencott, 1983.

Cotanch, P., Hockenberry, M. & Herman, S. Self-hypnosis as antiemetic therapy in children receiving chemotherapy. *Oncology Nursing Forum,* 1985, *12*(4), 41–46.

Elvebach, L. R. How high is high? A proposed alternative to the normal range. *Mayo Clinic Proceedings,* 1972, *47;* 93–97.

Fletcher, R. H., Fletcher, S. W., & Wagner, E. H. *Clinical epidemiology: The essentials.* Baltimore: Williams and Wilkins, 1982.

Fryback, D. G. A note about decision trees. In M. J. Aspinall & C. Tanner (Eds.). *Decision making for patient care: Applying the nursing process.* New York: Appleton-Century-Crofts, 1981.

Grier, M. R. Decision-making about patient care. *Nursing Research,* 1976, *25*(2), 105–110.

Kilo, C., Miller, J. P., & Williamson, J. R. The Achilles heel of the University Group Diabetes Program. *JAMA,* 1980, 243; 450–457.

Last, J. M. (Ed.). *A dictionary of epidemiology.* New York: Oxford University Press, 1983.

McIntosh, H. P. *Overview of aortocoronary bypass grafting for the treatment of coronary artery disease: An internist's perspective.* Rockville, Md.: National Center for Health Care Technology Monograph Series, DHHS, 1981.

Parker, S. G., & Kassier, J. P. Clinical application of decision analysis: A detailed illustration. *Seminars in Nuclear Medicine,* 1980, *302;* 1109.

Preston, T. A. *Coronary artery surgery: A critical review.* New York: Raven Press, 1977.

Robbins, L. C., & Hall, J. H. *How to practice prospective medicine.* Indianapolis, Slaymaker Enterprises (Rev. ed. 1979). Indianapolis: Methodist Hospital Press.

Ross, C. M. Health hazard appraisal. In Schneideman (Ed.). *The practice of preventive health care.* Menlo Park, Calif.: Addison-Wesley, 1981.

Sackett, D. L., Haynes, R. B., & Tugwell, P. *Clinical epidemiology: A basic science for clinical medicine.* Boston: Little, Brown, 1985.

Schneideman, L. *The practice of preventive health care.* Menlo Park, Calif.: Addison-Wesley, 1981.

Seltzer, H. S. A summary of criticisms of the findings and conclusions of the University Group Diabetes Program (UGDP). *Diabetes,* 1972; *21;* 976–979.

Weinstein, M., & Feinberg, H. *Clinical decision analysis.* Toronto: Saunders, 1980.

15

Health Planning and Evaluation

This chapter focuses on epidemiological considerations for the planning and evaluation of health activities, services, or programs. In the planning and ealuation of health activities, excess or unusual morbidity and mortality may be viewed as problems. A clinic nurse may be concerned about the problem of noncompliance with prescribed therapy among hypertensives. A staff nurse may be concerned about the problem of an increase in nosocomial infections in the unit. A hospital administrator may be concerned about an unusual suicide rate among hospital staff. A public health nurse may be faced with the problems of unusually high rates of alcohol-related fatalities or of an increase in childhood infectious diseases. Such excesses or increases, when viewed as problems, may be addressed by a problem-solving approach. This approach allows for a thorough assessment of the problem, its causes, likely solutions, and determination of the best method to address the problem. At the same time, the problem-solving approach lends itself to integrating evaluation into the process of planning health care activities. This chapter provides a discussion of the cyclic nature of planning and evaluation, a brief overview of the planning and evaluation process, followed by a more thorough discussion of community assessment, the problem-solving process, and other aspects of planning and evaluation that should incorporate epidemiological principles and methods.

CYCLIC AND CONTINUOUS NATURE OF PLANNING AND EVALUATION

Planning and evaluation, along with the implementation and performance of an activity are all part of a dynamic, cyclic, continuous process. In a new program, planning is the first step, then activities are implemented. These activities then occur routinely for some period of time, after which evaluation is done. This process of planning, action, and evaluation may be considered one cycle of the total process of eliminating a health problem (Fig. 15–1A). Several aspects of the process may occur simultaneously in an existing program, but emphasis on any one aspect of the process will vary from week to week, month to month, and year to year.

As one planning/evaluation cycle is completed, a second planning effort should occur. Planning at this stage considers any problems from the previous cycle that were identified during the evaluation. New information that becomes available during evaluation may lead to major or minor program changes. In some instances, it may be necessary to do additional research to verify or determine the causes of any new problems that become apparent as a result of evaluation.

During the first planning/evaluation cycle, the planner will have only a limited amount of information about the problem. Choices must be made in this atmosphere of uncertainty and many unanswered questions will still exist as the program begins. As the program or activity is implemented and evaluation is carried out, the planner learns more and is able to reduce his or her level of uncertainty, thereby making better choices and refining the plan on the basis of indications derived from the new information. This, then, starts a new cycle. Modifications of the original plan reflect the needed changes in activities. New data are collected as the modified activities are initiated so that the modified activities can subsequently be evaluated. Such planning and evaluation becomes a process that may be likened to an upward spiral, where each cycle is one level on the spiral (Fig. 15–1B). Each time the cycle is completed, the planner continues moving up the spiral until all goals are met.

Cervical cancer serves as an example of this process. This example is being simplified in the interest of brevity. It is not meant to imply that the decisions made or the evaluation methods used were the best or ideal. The example is for illustrative

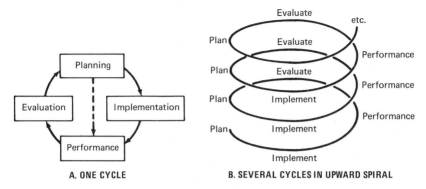

Figure 15–1. Relationship of planning and evaluation.

purposes only. For this example, we move back in time to the approximate beginning of the spiral. Pathologists have just demonstrated that cervical cancer mortality can (theoretically) be reduced by Pap smear screening. Following a community assessment in which both cervical cancer mortality patterns in the community and current Pap smear rates were measured and described, the nurse planner develops a public education program to encourage women to see their physician for a Pap smear. The first public education effort is made through newspaper and television ads and articles. The nurse implements that program. After a year, as called for in the evaluation plan, he or she reviews pathology reports to determine how many women have been screened and how many cases of cervical cancer have been found. Although the nurse routinely collects data on cervical cancer mortality rates so he or she will be able to monitor them, the formal evaluation of mortality patterns is delayed because it will be some time before screenng efforts are likely to impact on mortality rates (3 to 5 years). Logically, an objective of reduced mortality will be met only if women are being screened. Therefore, the evaluation plan does call for consideration of Pap smear screening rates and the rate at which cervical cancers are being identified among screened women. In this program, Pap smear screening rates were found to be within those specified in program objectives. Cycle 1 is now complete.

Before proceeding with this discussion, it is important to point out that public education is only one of several possible actions that might have been taken to address this problem. Public screening programs could have been set up rather than relying on private physicians to do screening. A law could have been passed to require that all women entering hospitals be screened for cervical cancer or that all women examined by a physician must be screened. Workplace screening programs might also have been set up. The planner, however, made the choice to implement the public education program as the best approach. Because the Pap smear was a new procedure, the nurse planner felt that this choice would produce a substantial public response at a lower cost than other action alternatives.

Continuing with the example, several cycles of planning, action, and evaluation subsequently occur. Evaluation finds substantial increases in screening participation and reduced mortality. These changes are in line with program objectives (cycles 2 to 8). Now, however, the most recent evaluation suggests that current actions are no longer effective in meeting program objectives. The planner suspects that some modifications are needed in the public education effort. A descriptive study is done to identify those women not being screened. It is found that many of these women did not know about Pap smears because they do not read newspapers or watch television. These women say they would be willing to have a Pap smear. The planner decides to continue previous efforts but also to send information to mothers through schools, to put informational posters around in the community, and to do lectures in churches, work sites, shopping centers, and women's clubs. These efforts produce some further increase in Pap smear rates but program objectives are not being met (completion of cycle 9). It is not apparent from program evaluation that public education, by itself, is insufficient to meet program goals. The evaluation has shown that most of those not screened are less educated and lower income women who cannot afford preventive screening. As a result, a public screening program is planned and implemented. Cycle 10 begins and so the process continues.

PLANNING AND EVALUATION ACTIVITIES: AN OVERVIEW

As used here, planning includes the whole sequence of activities necessary to develop a sound, data-based program to meet a community's need. The sequence includes a community assessment, identification and description of the problem, determination of the problem's causes, identification of possible methods for solving the problem, establishing goals and objectives, determination of costs for the various methods, estimating the likely feasibility and effectiveness of each potential method, documenting likely risks versus benefits for each method. Next, after comparing, for each method, the costs, effectiveness, risks, time requirements, and feasibility, methods should be prioritized. Finally, an evaluation plan must be developed. Other activities of planning are preparation of budget, formulation of detailed time plans, allocation of resources (personnel, financial, and materials) and obtaining approval and funding.

Evaluation includes all the activities designed to determine the value of efforts that have been made to reach the stated objective of a program. The two criteria most often considered in health care evaluation are the effectiveness and the efficiency of the program. Effectiveness is defined as "the extent to which a specific intervention procedure, regimen, or service, when deployed in the field, does what it is intended to do for a defined population" (Last, 1983). In simpler terms, the effectiveness represents the proportion of the program objective that was met. For instance, if the objective is that 80 percent of adult recipients of Aid to Dependent Children will receive educational materials and 60 percent did receive such materials, then the program has been 75 percent effective in meeting its objective (60/80). Because a change in the quantitative value of the objective affects the value of the effectiveness, such measures of effectiveness must be interpreted with caution. If the objective for the previous example had been 65 percent and 60 percent had been reached, the program would have been 92 percent effective.

Efficiency is defined as "the effects or end results that are achieved in relation to the effort expended in terms of money, resources, and time" (Last, 1983). Maximum efficiency obtains the most effectiveness for the least possible cost in resources. Efficiency is usually reported as the planned dollar cost per case (the objective) divided by the dollars actually expended per case. In a screening program, for example, this might be evaluated in two ways: (1) as cost per patient screened and (2) as cost per case identified. If the objective is 30 dollars per patient screened and the project spent 28 dollars then the program is 107 percent efficient. If, on the other hand, 50 dollars was spent per patient screened, then the program was only 60 percent efficient. Efficiency, when calculated by this method, is dependent upon the cost specified in the project objective. The closer that a program efficiency approaches 100 percent, the better it is. An efficiency over 100 percent represents savings per case over what was projected as the cost per case.

Evaluation plans include the objectives to be evaluated, a prioritization of evaluation activities, the identification of target subjects and of activities to be evaluated, the measures of evaluation to be utilized, the data collection instrument(s), and the data analyses that are planned. The process of evaluation includes carrying out the evaluation plan by collecting and analyzing data, reviewing findings, and stating conclusions. The result of evaluation should be plans for additional research, if needed and/or a plan to vary or change the program activities to more effectively meet goals and objectives. This chapter addresses only epidemiological considerations of planning and evaluation. The reader should refer to health administration references for a thorough discussion of all aspects of planning and evaluation (Deniston, 1968, 1970; Fink, 1978; Fitz-Gibbon, 1978; Franklin, 1976; Guttentag, 1975; Hilleboe, 1978; Morris, 1978; Suchman, 1967).

Community Assessment

Community assessment is the process of describing a community, its patterns of morbidity and mortality, and identifying those patterns that are clearly in excess. Since this step provides the data for defining the problem, it is preparatory to the utilization of the problem solving process. *The purpose of doing community assessment is to identify problems that need to be addressed and to identify those factors that may contribute to or cause the problems that have been identified.* The steps in community assessment are listed in Table 15–1 and discussed below.

Population Characteristics. A community assessment in the health care field focuses principally on the health of the community or lack thereof. A community assessment is in large part a description of the community and its health/illness patterns. The first part of a community assessment is to describe the characteristics of the population in the community. For the hospital practitioner, the population encompasses the patients, the staff,

TABLE 15–1. STEPS IN COMMUNITY ASSESSMENT

1. Describe the population in the community.
2. Describe the epidemiological characteristics of morbidity and mortality patterns in the community.
3. Describe the environmental characteristics of the community.
4. Collect information on other similar communities, if necessary.
5. Determine which of the accidents, diseases, defects, or other pathologies may be defined as a problem.
6. If desired, rank the priority for addressing each of the identified problems.

and the wider population from which the patient population is drawn. For the practitioner associated with a clinic, the community encompasses the clinic staff, the clinic patients, and the population from which the clinic patients are derived. For the public health nurse, the community is the entire population of the city, county, or state, depending upon the practice area (e.g., city nurse versus county nurse versus state nurse). In other words, the population to be considered in community assessment is much broader than the patients who are served over a short period of time. This information on the broader population allows for the computation of incidence and prevalence rates and it allows for consideration of whether any differences of etiological significance (i.e., bias or confounding factors) exist between the patient population and the population as a whole.

A description of the population in the community should include total population census and subcategorizations by age, sex, race, and neighborhood. The socioeconomic status of each neighborhood should also be characterized in some way. Options include average income, percentage below federal poverty guideline, percentage on welfare, and other relevant factors. Most of this information is generally available in publications from local government or the U.S. Bureau of the Census.

Although health care providers may be considered a subcategory of the population as a whole, they should be described separately, because this information is necessary to formulate a list of potential etiological factors and to formulate methods to attack the problem. The professional health care staff in hospitals, clinics, and other facilities should be characterized by professional degree (R.N., M.D., R.D.), by speciality (cardiovascular, gastroenterology, oncology, and so on) and by where they

practice. Within a hospital, the location of practice would be a
unit. Within a city, the location of practice would be the hospital
and/or clinic. This information is necessary in formulating an
etiological hypothesis, because professional staff plays a role in
disease transmission or in availability of services. Staff may
spread infectious diseases; various specialities may obtain better
or less compliance with treatment regimens; location of practice
may make it prohibitive for many medical needs of the poor to
be met; and, inadequate numbers of some specialists may lead
to unnecessary deaths. Each of these examples are of major
importance in understanding some of the health care problems
facing various communities today.

Community Health. The next part of a community assessment
is to describe the epidemiological characteristics of community
morbidity and mortality. Morbidity and mortality is used here
in the broad sense to include birth defects, low birth weight,
mental illness, accidental injury, alcohol- and drug-related pathologies, lack of compliance with treatment regimens, pain, or ill
health of any variety. The frequency count and the incidence
and prevalence rates for each condition are determined. These
rates are then given by age, sex, race, and unit of hospital or
neighborhood in the community. The amount of detail and the
degree to which subdivisions or subcategorization are done is
dependent upon the practice setting and the amount of information available. Frequency counts and rates should be generated for several years to allow for comparison of the present and
the past. In some situations, such as infectious diseases, daily,
weekly or monthly rates will be necessary. Other epidemiological characteristics that may be included are length and/or quality of survival by type of condition, level of function by condition, level of compliance by treatment regimen and condition,
rates of side effects by condition, and rates of psychological
effects by condition. Although survival rates are usually available, it is less likely that data are available on these other characteristics. Occasionally, the clinic or hospital practioner may be
able to determine these rates for their practice unit. The planner is cautioned in generalizing to other populations from data
limited to one institution as it is subject to small numbers and
possible biases related to who utilizes the facility. For instance,
a university hospital may only see the worst cases of myocardial
infarction (MI) and there may be personality differences between

the worst cases and those who have less severe cases of MI. Therefore, conclusions about compliance with treatment regimens may differ between the two groups. The practitioner who serves only an inpatient population may find such information helpful if conclusions and programming are directed only to inpatients of their institution.

Institutional nosocomial infection and accident rates should be reported per unit within the hospital. The entire patient population is used as the denominator for hospitalized patients in studying nosocomial conditions. Where the number of cases is sufficient to do so, rates should also be reported by primary condition, age, and sex.

Ordinarily, community assessment encompasses all the major health problems of the community and is not limited to one or two specific problems. Although in some circumstances, only one type of problem may be considered, for example, a mental health nurse considering only mental illnesses in the community or the infection control nurse considering only infectious diseases, it is preferable to start with a broad community assessment, because it is frequently difficult, if not impossible, to understand the dynamic etiological factors involved if information is available on only one aspect of health. For instance, should a marked increase in the suicide rate be found during a study of mental illness in the community, it probably would not be recognized that a high rate of incurable cancers may be a partial explanation of excess suicides, unless data on cancer in that community were simultaneously available. An infection control nurse who does not assess overall diagnostic patterns of patients in that institution might not recognize the role that an increase in leukemic cases plays in any increase in nosocomial infections. Thus, because one of the purposes of community assessment is to identify factors that contribute to or cause the problem, it is normally necessary to include in any community assessment all diseases that may occur in the particular practice setting. If a limitation on the diseases to be considered is necessary, it may be better to limit the degree to which diseases are subdivided. For example, total birth defects may be reported rather than each type of birth defect, if birth defects are not the condition of primary interest. Diabetes and heart disease could be given as general categories rather than obtaining rates for all diabetic and heart pathologies such as diabetic retinopathy or mitral valve prolapse. The degree to which subdivisions are made depends on the practice setting. A nurse caring for infants with birth defects will definitely want to consider the various types of defects. The nurse working in the mental health area will need to know about birth defect and cancer rates in the community, but may not need to know the rates for each type of birth defect and for all types of cancer. This nurse, however, will be concerned with all specific psychiatric diagnoses.

Environment. In addition to the population characteristics of the community and the patterns of health/illness in the community, a community assessment includes a description of the community environment. Environment includes pollution, weather, geographical characteristics, industries, institutions, sanitation, food, transportation, laws and rules, and the attitudes, customs, and beliefs that prevail in the community. Of course, in any one community assessment all of these factors will not necessarily be considered. Which environmental factors will be considered depends upon the focus of the practitioner, that is, the type of practice setting dictates the relative importance of the different environmental aspects. For instance, the environment for a hospital population encompasses the types of units within the hospital: the physical layout, including furniture arrangements within the units, arrangements of patient rooms in relation to other specialized areas (treatment rooms, surgical suite, cafeteria, and so on), lighting, heating, and ventilation systems; food; clothing; housekeeping practices; safety rules and other hospital procedures; and patient and staff attitudes.

The community health nurse considers environment at a broader level. This broader level encompasses geographical and neighborhood characteristics, weather patterns, transportation, commerce and industry, local, state, and federal laws, health care facilities, community economics, and religious affiliations. In short, the environment encompasses all aspects of the community that may affect health either directly or indirectly. Individuals may not follow their prescribed drug treatment program because the nearest drug store is too far to walk to, no one will deliver, private cars are rare, and no public transportation is available. Unemployment may be so high that suicide, violence, depression, malnutrition, and alcoholism are all increased. Teenage pregnancy rates may be high due to lack of contraceptive availability to teenagers as a result of community religious mores. For the hospital practitioner, it may be that nosocomial infections have increased because of a change in housekeeping or cooking procedures. Spontaneous abortions may be above normal in staff working in operating rooms because of inadequate ventilation of waste anesthetic gases. In all these cases, knowledge of the environment is necessary to formulate the possible causes of any identified problems.

Determining Which Conditions May Be Problems. In epidemiology, an epidemic, defined as a significant excess or unusual increase in the rate of a particular condition, is normally the criterion for a situation to be considered a problem. But health planners may define a problem more generally, as "any deviation from a standard, desired, or expected state of affairs" (Bales, 1983). The comparison rate for identifying deviations can be derived in two ways: (1) in comparison with previous rates for the setting or community of interest or (2) by comparing disease rates for various settings or communities. The important issue is choosing an appropriate comparison population. An annual cervical cancer mortality rate of 1 per 10,000 would not be seen as a problem if it were compared with a national rate of 4 per 10,000 (NCI, 1981). If, however, the rate of 1 per 10,000 were compared with that of a similar community with a rate of 0.02 per 10,000, it may be considered a problem. Some administrators may view any cervical cancer mortality as a problem. In this later case, a comparison community is unnecessary. When an external comparison population is needed, the community should be compared to similar communities in order to draw valid inferences. National or state rates tends to be relatively insensitive for comparison purposes.

Caution should be used in interpreting comparisons of rates for present and past conditions in a single community when substantial changes in the population composition or in the community structure and services available have occurred. A hospital that hires a recognized specialist in heart disease may begin seeing more of the worst cases of MI and may show a increase in MI mortality rates. Such an increase may appear to be an epidemic if the change in case severity is not recognized. This mortality rate may be undesirable and may be a problem, but it is not an epidemic of MI deaths and therefore approaches to dealing with the change will be different from those needed if this represented an epidemic. A change in diagnostic or treatment practices may also falsely suggest the presence of an epidemic. If more infants under 500 grams were born alive as a result of improved prenatal and delivery practices but if these infants die within a year after birth, the local community may see a sudden increase in infant mortality rates. Again, this mortality pattern is undesirable, but it is not an epidemic. It actually represents a shift of when these infants are dying. Previously, the infants died before delivery, now they die after delivery. The endemic infant mortality rate has not, in reality, changed. In general health care, many situations that are endemic may be considered undesirable and thus a problem. Lack of utilization of available services may be unexpected and as a result may be considered a problem.

The individual practitioner must decide during a particular community assessment whether to use the all encompassing definition of a problem as any deviation from a standard, desired, or expected state of affairs, or whether to consider only epidemics and significant upward trends as problems. Scarcity of staff and financial resources often limits the definition of a problem to the presence of an epidemic or a significant upward trend in the incidence or prevalence rates.

An additional step may be added during community assessment when a practitioner has general responsibilities or concerns as opposed to a focus on a single disease area such as infection control or childhood problems. Such individuals as the supervisory nurse responsible for all the units in the hospital, the public health nurse administrator, and other practitioners faced with multiple problems will find it necessary to assign a priority to each of the identified problems. Efforts to solve the problems are then directed by this priority ranking. Problems with high mortality rates or substantial effects on quality of life are usually addressed first. Criteria that might be utilized to rank problems could include severity of health effect (e.g., death, disability, defect and illness, and so on), number or rate of those suffering from the problem, cost to the individual and society, and ability of the health care practitioner to impact on the problem.

Problem Solving

Preparation of Problem Definition. Table 15–2 provides a summary of steps for effective problem solving. The first step in

TABLE 15–2. SUMMARY OF STEPS TO EFFECTIVE PROBLEM SOLVING

Identify and describe problem

List potential causes of the problem

Determine or verify causes

Rank causes of problem (relative to how much of the problem has been caused by each causative factor)

Depict problem hierarchy and interrelationships of causative factors

Determine target group(s)

Determine potential methods and activities to attack each cause

Determine feasibility of each method and probability of success for each method

Determine resources needed for each method

Prioritize methods based on target group characteristics, target group accessibility, feasibility, probability of success, potential impact on the overall problem, and required resources

Choose or recommend a program (which may include several methods or activities) to attack the problem

the problem solving approach is to describe and define the problem (Bales, 1983). A simple way to define a problem statement is to describe the who, what, when, how much, where, relative importance of the problem to all other problems, and the cost to individuals and society. A problem definition includes:

The specific type of problem

The extent of the problem

The time period covered by the problem

The trend for the problem over time

The standards by which the situation is judged to be a problem

Evidence that is available illustrating a deviation from the standard

The effect of the problem if it continues or the problem becomes worse

The relationship or relative rank of this problem to other problems for your area of practice

The costs associated with the problem

If the community assessment has been completed, all of the information needed for this problem statement will be in the assessment.

The description of the problem incorporates several aspects of epidemiology. The problem is usually a disease state or a less than optimal state of health. The problem statement must be specific in identifying the type or nature of the problem, the extensiveness of the problem, and the probable effects if the problem continues or worsens. The specific type of problem might be identified as hypertension, cervical cancer deaths, birth defects, or diabetic acidosis. Extensiveness of the problem is stated in terms of the overall incidence, prevalence, and attack rate and the age-, sex-, and race-specific rates for this problem. Whether a choice was made to use prevalence or incidence rates or both would depend on the specific problem being addressed. Incidence rates, for instance, would more often be used for infectious diseases since each case is usually of short duration and quick elimination of the problem is desirable and possible. For chronic diseases of noninfectious origin like hypertension, prevalence rates would, perhaps, be the most useful. Whether the condition has decreased, increased, or remained the same over time is described by daily, weekly, monthly, or annual rates (the trend over time).

It is usually desirable to review rates for a period of 2 to 30 years, depending upon the condition or the problem of interest. Cancers and other chronic health problems require observation of rates over the longest periods. Acute health problems may be assessed over a shorter time frame, but a minimum of 3 to 5 years is usually necessary because many acute diseases are cyclic or seasonal and because some fluctuation of rates may always be present.

The problem statement must include a definition of the word "problem" for the specific problem statement being prepared. As previously discussed, this definition may be based on deviation from a standard or an undesirable situation or an unexpected situation. The definition within the problem statement might be:

> In this document, a problem is defined as a deviation from a standard state of affairs

or,

> In this document, a problem is defined as a deviation from a desired state of affairs

This may sound silly, but it greatly simplifies and clarifies things for readers of the document. Once it is clear how the author defines a problem, data consistent with that problem definition should be presented in the problem description as evidence of the problem. If this problem is an epidemic then data are presented to support the contention that it is an epidemic. Endemic rates generated from previous data from the same community or by a comparison to a similar community would be provided for comparison. Graphs frequently represent the most efficient way of demonstrating an epidemic when the comparison is previous data from the same community. The term epidemic may not be appropriate in some comparisons of one community to another. Significant differences may be present between communities without the presence of an epidemic. Such differences will, however, provide sufficient evidence for the existence of a problem. If any efforts were made to rule out changes in reporting habits, screening, diagnostic, or treatment practices as the cause of this problem, appropriate data should be reported as evidence supporting that this is a real problem rather than an artifact of such changes.

The problem statement should also include an analysis of effects, should the problem continue or become worse. This analysis could include projection of future disease rates or costs, for example. Table 15–3 lists examples of categories of costs associated with ill health: costs to individuals, costs to society, and costs to employers. The relationship of this problem to other problems within the practice setting or the community should be described; ranking where this problem falls relative to the other problems may be useful. Any criteria used to rank the problems should be clearly described. Current costs associated with the problem should also be reported in the problem statement.

Potential Causes of the Problem. The next step after preparation of the problem statement is to determine the likely causes of the problem. Determination of causes includes reviewing the literature for previously identified factors associated with the problem, listing of all possible causes, and research or study of whether the suspected causes have been documented as causes. Causes may be of four different types: predisposing factors, enabling factors, precipitating factors, and reinforcing factors. *Predisposing factors,* such as age, sex, race, state of suscep-

TABLE 15–3. TYPES OF COSTS ASSOCIATED WITH ILL HEALTH

Costs to the Individual

Lost work time
Out-of-pocket expense
Health insurance cost
Cost associated with number of years of lost
Survival time, a theoretical value usually
   based on earning power if the individual had lived life the average length of time
Value associated with diminished quality of life

Costs to Society

Public health programs
Institutional care
Welfare
Disability
Unpaid medical bills
Excess insurance costs that are absorbed by the community as a whole (e.g.,
   nonsmokers' health insurance rates reflect the cost of treating the health
   problems of smokers)

Costs to the Employer

Health insurance
Training of replacement employees
Decreased productivity
Equipment down time
Workmen's compensation (for occupation-related problems)
Possible government fines (for violation of occupational health laws)

tibility, or attitudes toward health services, in some way condition, prepare, or sensitize the individual so that the individual reacts in a specific way to a disease agent. *Enabling factors* are such things as climate, personal support systems, income, nutrition, health insurance coverage, housing, and availability of medical care. *The Dictionary of Epidemiology* (Last, 1983) defines enabling factors as "those that facilitate the manifestation of disease disability, ill health, or the use of services, or conversely, those that facilitate recovery from illness maintenance or enhancement of health status or more appropriate use of health services." *Precipitating factors* are the types of causes that are "associated with the definitive onset of a disease, illness, accident, behavioral response or course of action" (Last, 1983). Examples of precipating factors are exposure to a drug, a noxious agent, a specific disease, an occupational stimulus, a physical trauma, or a new knowledge or information. The last type of cause is *reinforcing factors,* such as repeated exposure to the same noxious agent, presence of financial incentive or disincentive, and deprivation of personal satisfaction. Reinforcing factors tend to aggravate or perpetuate the presence of the particular health problem. They tend to be persistent, recurrent, and repetitive. Such factors may or may not be the same as the precipitating, enabling, and predisposing factors.

Determination of Causative Factors and Ranking of Causes. When reviewing the literature on causality of any disease condition, the concepts presented in Chapter 2 in the section Criteria for Evaluating Causality in the Literature should be used. A list of all possible causes should be formulated using the information gained both from the literature and from the community assessment. Attention should be paid to all the different types of causes that may play a role in the development, presence, or continuation of the problem under consideration. It should be recognized that it is not necessary to understand the specific cause of a disease to be able to solve or reduce the problem. For instance, although it is still not known what causes cervical cancer, the problem has been greatly reduced in recent years. Lack of a Pap smear may contribute to a fatal case of cervical cancer, but its lack did not cause the disease. A consideration of all of the different types of factors that may cause or contribute to onset of or death from cervical cancer would include: exposure to a precipitating agent (currently not known), sex (female) age (more than 15 years old, usually), multiple sexual partners, multiple pregnancies, lack of efficiacy of Pap smear, lack of knowledge about need for Pap smears, interval between smears too great, no health insurance, low income, no or inadequate transportation, gynecological services inaccessible or insufficient, gynecological service hours inadequate, fear, failure to follow-up on suspicious smears (by physician or the woman), laboratory error (false negatives), physician attitude (complacent or apathetic), treatment failure, failure to follow recommended treatment, or time delays in reporting suspicious laboratory reports or in receiving treatment. This list is a list of *possible* causes of the problem. Although, in forming the list it is not necessary to provide supporting evidence when adding an item to the list of possible causes, the practitioner should have some reason for adding an item to the list.

The next step, documentation of a causal role for each of the potential causal factors, is critical. Lack of such documentation is the major reason why many planners go wrong and why many problems have not been solved. *Never, ever assume causation.* Many activities and programs have failed merely because someone assumed what the cause of the problem was. For example, suppose the overall problem is the need to reduce mortality from cervical cancer. Most individuals today view the cause of this problem as a lack of a Pap smears. *This is an assumption.* It is possible that all or a major portion of the women who died from cervical cancer have had Pap smears. They may be dying not because they did not have a Pap smear, but because they did not have enough money for treatment, or the laboratory report of the test was a false negative. In other cases, their doctor may not have followed up on a positive report. Any one or a combination of factors may have contributed to the death, even though the women had had a Pap smear.

The point is, unless research is available on this factor for the community of interest, it is totally inappropriate to assume that if women are dying from cervical cancer it is because of the lack of Pap smears. The role of each of the potential causative agents in contributing to the problem should be documented. Existing research from other settings may suggest a role for many agents but assessment of whether they are operating in the current setting must be assessed. The planner must, however, be careful that the findings are timely. Prior data from this community may not be applicable. When a screening test is new on the market, the major reason that it is not used is lack of public and professional knowledge. Five to ten years later, cost, fear, or accessibility may play the largest role. Addition of an income-adjusted fee type of clinic in a local neighborhood could change the subsequent relationship of income to the problem. In other words, the factors that contribute to the problem vary in their relative magnitude to each other at different points in time.

The relative rank of a cause also varies by area of the community. Income may play no role in failure to obtain Pap smears in an affluent neighborhood, whereas it may play a major role in a upper lower class neighborhood (above eligibility for government support but insufficient to cover the additional cost). Because of these differences in relative rank of the causative factors in time and place, the planner must be extra careful not to assume that today's problem is the same as yesterday's problem and that the problem in neighborhood A is the same as that in neighborhood B. Although the same factors may be involved, a difference in the relative rank of a contributing factor could make the difference of whether or not a problem solving effort is successful as program efforts go forward in time.

The Pap smear in relation to cervical cancer mortality is an excellent example of the problem discussed above. Originally, lack of knowledge about test availability was a major factor in not preventing deaths from cervical cancer. Although *assuming* that lack of knowledge continues to be a major factor, public health administrators have added to their list of causative factors fear, income, accessibility and transportation. In many instances, these are assumptions! They may or may not be correct assumptions of why women do not get Pap smears in a particular community. Are they correct assumptions for why women are still dying of cervical cancer? Answering this question requires an epidemiological study of women who have died. Such a study was done for cervical cancer. It was found that 82 percent of the women who had invasive cervical cancer had had Pap smears. Forty-two percent had received annual tests. In this study, it was found that laboratory error, failure to follow up on suspicious Pap smears, lost reports, and personal choices not to follow up on suspicious smears were the major factors that probably led to these deaths. An additional group appeared to have had rapidly proliferating tumors that were not identified early enough with annual smears (Martin, 1972). The planner must be able to have some estimate of the current relative rank of each of the contributing factors to attack the problem with any efficiency. A substantial amount of time, cost, and effort has probably gone into programs that are unlikely to have much impact on the problem because they did not assess these factors. Cervical cancer is one example of inefficient and inadequate problem solving.

Although causes or contributing factors have been classified as predisposing, enabling, precipitating, and reinforcing factors, another classification system that has been used is perhaps easier for planning purposes. This classification is useful because it assists in identifying the types of activities that are useful in solving the problem. Examples for each category in this classification include:

Biological
   age, sex, susceptibility to infectious agent, allergies

Screening and/or Treatment
    screening test; drug, surgical, radiation, or other
    treatment modality
Environmental
    Exposures: sanitation, air, water, soil contamination
    work, food additives, infectious agent
    Sociological: family support, number of people living
    in same space, influence of peers, etc.
    Physical stressors: lifting, heavy labor, etc
    Economic: income, insurance
    Community: access to medical services, adequacy of
    medical services, location of services, transportation
Educational/Counseling
    Habits: smoking drinking, nutrition, sedentary life-
    style
    Education: lack of knowledge, lack of awareness
    Psychological: motivation, fear, belief patterns
Administrative
    lack of quality control, lack of follow-up, inadequate
    or insufficient staff, untrained staff, insufficient funds,
    poor quality of provided services, service hours, location
    of services

Causes or contributing factors, in addition to varying in their relative rank in time, are frequently interdependent. Seldom do each of these potential causative factors exist in isolation. Usually causes are interdependent. As a result of this interdependence, a plan directed at one cause may not be sufficient to reduce the problem significantly. In some cases, if activities and methods are directed at a minor cause or if the only cause or factor under attack is highly interdependent upon another factor, no impact on the problem will be observed. For example, distance to medical services (access) may be a risk factor associated with not having a periodic Pap smear. In a particular hispanic community distances to such services are long. In addition, peer group pressure against having a Pap smear may be strong in a hispanic community. In such a case, it is unlikely that a program utilizing a mobile screening unit (attacking the access problem) will have much impact. It is therefore important that the planner recognize the interrelationship or the interdependence of the various contributing factors.

Problem Hierarchy. As the potential causes are studied, it becomes apparent that each cause is a problem with its own causes. The original problem can be depicted as a problem hierarchy. Cervical cancer may, again, serve as an example. Suppose that an epidemiological study of women who died of cervical cancer (compared to women who did not die of cervical cancer) has been done as part of the problem solving process and suppose that, as in the study previously mentioned, a large proportion of the women who were dying from cervical cancer had had a Pap smear. The overall problem is unnecessary cervical cancer mortality. But there are now two problems: (1) a lack of Pap smears (demonstrated by women who die without having had Pap smears) and (2) ineffective Pap smear programs (demonstrated by women who have died despite having had Pap smears. We shall assume for this example that Pap smear screening is efficacious (an assumption that could be questioned). Each of these problems has causes. Lack of knowledge may be one cause of failure to have a Pap smear. Lack of knowledge then becomes a problem with its own causes. Lack of public education on the subject may be one cause for this lack of knowledge. Lack of public education becomes a problem. Lack of funds may be a cause of the lack of public education. The same cause or contributing factor may exist for several problems. Lack of funds, lack of education, and lack of services are frequently contributing to several different problems. Attitudes and fears are also contributing factors at the root of many problems. Although the contributing factors may be interrelated and interdependent in some cases, they may be unrelated in other cases. For instance, if lack of quality control is the major cause of laboratory error, then a quality control program may significantly impact on the problem of laboratory error. But a laboratory quality control program will have no impact on why a physician does not choose to follow up on a suspicious smear (when the report is accurate). The causation/problem hierarchy should be graphically illustrated with appropriate patterns of interrelationships. This problem hierarchy should be limited to significant contributing factors. An example is given in Figure 15–2 for cervical cancer.

Determination of Target Groups. At this point, the planner should have completed a problem statement, have listed potential causes of the problem, determined or verified the role of the

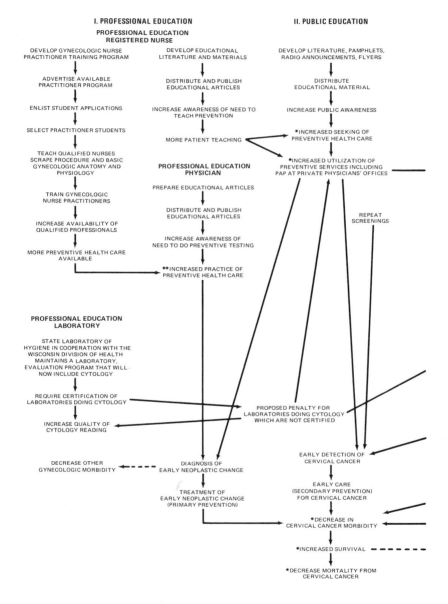

I. PROFESSIONAL EDUCATION

II. PUBLIC EDUCATION

PROFESSIONAL EDUCATION
REGISTERED NURSE

DEVELOP GYNECOLOGIC NURSE
PRACTITIONER TRAINING PROGRAM

DEVELOP EDUCATIONAL
LITERATURE AND MATERIALS

DEVELOP LITERATURE, PAMPHLETS,
RADIO ANNOUNCEMENTS, FLYERS

ADVERTISE AVAILABLE
PRACTITIONER PROGRAM

DISTRIBUTE AND PUBLISH
EDUCATIONAL ARTICLES

DISTRIBUTE
EDUCATIONAL MATERIAL

ENLIST STUDENT APPLICATIONS

INCREASE AWARENESS OF NEED TO
TEACH PREVENTION

INCREASE PUBLIC AWARENESS

SELECT PRACTITIONER STUDENTS

MORE PATIENT TEACHING

*INCREASED SEEKING OF
PREVENTIVE HEALTH CARE

TEACH QUALIFIED NURSES
SCRAPE PROCEDURE AND BASIC
GYNECOLOGIC ANATOMY AND
PHYSIOLOGY

PROFESSIONAL EDUCATION
PHYSICIAN

*INCREASED UTILIZATION OF
PREVENTIVE SERVICES INCLUDING
PAP AT PRIVATE PHYSICIANS' OFFICES

TRAIN GYNECOLOGIC
NURSE PRACTITIONERS

PREPARE EDUCATIONAL ARTICLES

INCREASE AVAILABILITY OF
QUALIFIED PROFESSIONALS

DISTRIBUTE AND PUBLISH
EDUCATIONAL ARTICLES

REPEAT
SCREENINGS

MORE PREVENTIVE HEALTH CARE
AVAILABLE

INCREASE AWARENESS OF
NEED TO DO PREVENTIVE TESTING

**INCREASED PRACTICE OF
PREVENTIVE HEALTH CARE

PROFESSIONAL EDUCATION
LABORATORY

STATE LABORATORY OF
HYGIENE IN COOPERATION WITH THE
WISCONSIN DIVISION OF HEALTH
MAINTAINS A LABORATORY,
EVALUATION PROGRAM THAT WILL
NOW INCLUDE CYTOLOGY

REQUIRE CERTIFICATION OF
LABORATORIES DOING CYTOLOGY

PROPOSED PENALTY FOR
LABORATORIES DOING CYTOLOGY
WHICH ARE NOT CERTIFIED

INCREASE QUALITY OF
CYTOLOGY READING

DECREASE OTHER
GYNECOLOGIC MORBIDITY

DIAGNOSIS OF
EARLY NEOPLASTIC CHANGE

EARLY DETECTION OF
CERVICAL CANCER

TREATMENT OF
EARLY NEOPLASTIC CHANGE
(PRIMARY PREVENTION)

EARLY CARE
(SECONDARY PREVENTION)
FOR CERVICAL CANCER

*DECREASE IN
CERVICAL CANCER MORBIDITY

*INCREASED SURVIVAL

*DECREASE MORTALITY FROM
CERVICAL CANCER

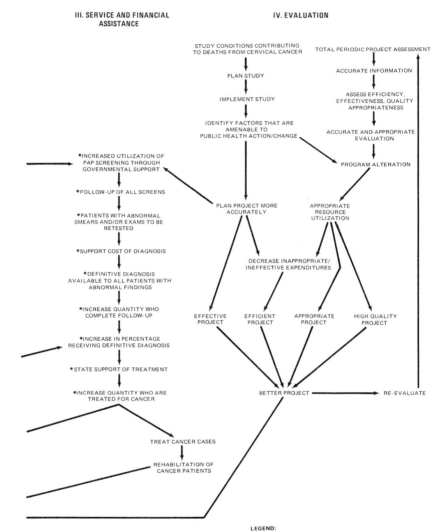

III. SERVICE AND FINANCIAL
ASSISTANCE

IV. EVALUATION

STUDY CONDITIONS CONTRIBUTING
TO DEATHS FROM CERVICAL CANCER

TOTAL PERIODIC PROJECT ASSESSMENT

PLAN STUDY

ACCURATE INFORMATION

IMPLEMENT STUDY

ASSESS EFFICIENCY,
EFFECTIVENESS, QUALITY
APPROPRIATENESS

IDENTIFY FACTORS THAT ARE
AMENABLE TO
PUBLIC HEALTH ACTION/CHANGE

ACCURATE AND APPROPRIATE
EVALUATION

*INCREASED UTILIZATION OF
PAP SCREENING THROUGH
GOVERNMENTAL SUPPORT

PROGRAM ALTERATION

*FOLLOW-UP OF ALL SCREENS

*PATIENTS WITH ABNORMAL
SMEARS AND/OR EXAMS TO BE
RETESTED

PLAN PROJECT MORE
ACCURATELY

APPROPRIATE
RESOURCE
UTILIZATION

*SUPPORT COST OF DIAGNOSIS

*DEFINITIVE DIAGNOSIS
AVAILABLE TO ALL PATIENTS WITH
ABNORMAL FINDINGS

DECREASE INAPPROPRIATE/
INEFFECTIVE EXPENDITURES

*INCREASE QUANTITY WHO
COMPLETE FOLLOW-UP

*INCREASE IN PERCENTAGE
RECEIVING DEFINITIVE DIAGNOSIS

EFFECTIVE
PROJECT

EFFICIENT
PROJECT

APPROPRIATE
PROJECT

HIGH QUALITY
PROJECT

*STATE SUPPORT OF TREATMENT

*INCREASE QUANTITY WHO ARE
TREATED FOR CANCER

BETTER PROJECT

RE-EVALUATE

TREAT CANCER CASES

REHABILITATION OF
CANCER PATIENTS

INCREASE MOTIVATION THROUGH
KNOWLEDGE IF INCREASED
SURVIVAL

LEGEND:
* PORTION OF PROJECT TO BE EVALUATED
** PREVENTIVE HEALTH CARE IS DEFINED AS ANNUAL
PHYSICAL EXAMINATIONS, INCLUDING PELVIC, PAP
AND BREAST

Figure 15–2. Wisconsin Division of Health Cervical Cancer
Detection Program Flow Chart.

contributing factors, determined or verified the role of the contributing factors, determined the rank of the contributing factors relative to each other in contributing to the problem, and depicted the problem hierarchy and the interrelationships of the contributing factors. The next step is to determine who are the potential target groups for the activities that will be planned. The target group is dependent upon which part of the problem hierarchy is to be addressed. For laboratory errors, the target would be those laboratories without a quality control program or with an inadequate quality control program. For women who have not had a Pap smear, the target group should be those women who have not had a Pap smear and who are at high risk of developing the disease, i.e., low income, multiple sexual partners, early age at first intercourse, multiple pregnancies, and of low educational attainment. Such women might be found through venereal disease or government family planning programs or through particular neighborhoods. When the target group is the group of individuals most at risk of developing the disease, the scientific literature is the best place to obtain informaton on the characterisitcs of the individuals most likely to get the disease. The target group should be described in terms of their age, sex, race, socioeconomic, and neighborhood (or unit) characteristics. Frequency counts on the size of the target group as a whole and for the particular units or neighborhoods should be stated.

Selecting Methods to Resolve the Problem. The information on the causation/problem hierarchy and on the target groups is then used to identify potential methods for attacking or resolving each level of causation. A thorough understanding of the causation/problem hierarchy frequently makes these methods quite obvious. Methods frequently used are education, counseling, quality control program, behavioral modification, isolation, immunization, screening, drug or surgical therapy, and rehabilitation.

Probability of success must then be estimated for each method relative to each identified contributing factor. Probability of success is dependent on the method to be used and the target group. A simple, quick, nonthreatening, low risk, low cost method that is easy to explain and easy to arrange in terms of patient access is more likely to meet with success. Well educated, upper socioeconomic, health conscious adults are the easiest target group. Health professionals, however, may be greatly resistant to change. The probability of success does not have to be expressed in quantitative terms. Rather, the different methods can be ranked for probability of success. For instance, a new screening tool of proven efficacy will often achieve the largest rate of response through public and professional education programs. After a tool has been available for several years, the best method for resolving the problem may change.

Probability of success is determined for each problem within the problem hierarchy. There may only be one activity or method for attacking some problems, whereas other problems within the hierarchy may be attacked in several ways. For example, Pap smear screening could be made available through a stationary clinic within a high-risk neighborhood, through private physicians, through hospitals, through mobile screening vans, through screening set up in various neighborhood locations (schools, shopping centers, and so on), or through provision of self-test Pap kits. In ranking the probability of success, the planner should rank activities for each problem within the hierarchy.

The cost in resources and the feasibility of each method is then considered for each problem within the problem hierarchy. The methods are then prioritized by the following criteria: target group characteristics, target group accessibility, feasibility, probability of success, potential impact on the overall problem, and required resources to carry out the activity. Ideally, the method with the lowest cost, the largest impact, and the highest probability of success should be chosen. This results in a list of preferred methods for attacking each of the problems within the problem hierarchy. The total problem hierarchy is then reviewed. This review must again include a prioritization of which methods out of the methods selected for each part of the problem will most likely meet with success and which methods will have the largest impact on the overall problem. This is necessary because it is usually not possible to implement a program that will attack all of the contributing factors for the overall program. With the cervical cancer example, this is exemplified by the findings that a major reason why women are still dying is problems associated with screening. When the majority of the women that will respond to a screening program have already been screened, it is extremely expensive in terms of resources to significantly increase the number of screenees any further. If only 20 percent of those dying are nonscreenees, a program aimed at the problems associated with women who have been screened may be more successful. That is, the cost per life saved and the number of lives saved may be far greater with methods that attack a major portion of the problem and that have greater chance of success. In many cases, a problem must be approached sequentially. If laboratories do not know how to do a test or if the laboratory does not have the equipment necessary to do a test, public education programs will be of little benefit until that problem has been resolved.

Program Plan

At this point the planner is ready to put together the program plan. The program plan contains a summary of all the items previously discussed; the problem statement, the program goals and objectives, a list of major contributing factors that have been verified as contributors, a ranking of the contributing factors, the potential methods for attacking the problems within the problem hierarchy, the rank of each method in terms of likely success and feasibility, the estimates of the cost for each method (rough estimates for those methods that were not selected), the potential impact for the chosen methods, and the rationale for the choices made. This serves as a background and supporting rationale for the plan that is developed. The plan consists of a description of the recommended program, including goals and objectives, activities, a time plan for implementation of the plan, and a budget. (A complete list of inclusions for the Program Plan is given in Table 15–4). If staff for the program have already been determined, then the plan should include their names and qualifications. Letters of support from any individuals or groups that volunteer to support the program in any way should also be included. If portions of the program must be subcontracted, then it is advisable to demonstrate the availability of subcontractors and their willingness to subcontract. Sample contracts may also be necessary. Anytime the program is dependent upon other groups or individuals a demonstration of their willingness to cooperate is necessary. Any

TABLE 15–4. PROGRAM PLAN INCLUSIONS

Problem statement
Program goals and objectives
List of major contributing factors with evidence supporting their role as contributing
  factors
Rank of contributing factors
Illustration of the problem hierarchy and interrelationships
List of potential methods of attacking each of the problems in the problem
  hierarchy
Rank of each method in terms of likelihood of success and feasibility for each
  objective
Cost estimates for each method (rough estimates of methods not selected for
  utilization in final program plan)
Potential impact on the problem for the chosen methods
Rationale for recommended program
Time plan for implementation of each activity associated with each objective
Statement of what effect the lack of any program would have
Time plan for implementation of each objective
Statement of program limitations and potential risks
Indication of protection of human subjects requirements and how the requirements
  will be met
Informed consent statements, if needed
Professional staff and their credentials
Data collection instruments or program forms
Sample subcontracts, if needed
Letters of support
Budget
Evaluation plan

record-keeping forms for the program should be specified and example forms should be developed whenever possible. The program plan must also include an evaluation plan.

The program plan should also clearly state the limitations of the plan and any potential negative consequences of the program. The parts of the problem or the contributing causes that are not addressed should be clearly stated in the program plan. The consequences or the potential consequences of not addressing these problems or contributing causes should be stated. For example such a statement might read, "It is estimated that approximately 20 percent of the problem will remain at the completion of this program. The prevalence rate for this problem is projected to be approximately 2 per 100,000 women in the state in 1990." As in this example, the estimates should be as specific as possible in projecting the rate and time frame and in identifying the community for which the forecast is being made. Any potential negative consequences of program activities should also be stated. Private physicians may resent a public screening program and sabotage its efforts. Drugs may have significant side effects. A screening or diagnostic device may cause health problems, for example, a proctoscope perforating the colon or repetitive mammography causing a breast cancer. The risk of such negative effects should be stated. This statement of risk should specify the degree of risk and who is at risk. Such a statement of risk might read, "It is estimated that a perforated colon will occur once in every 10,000 proctoscopic examinations of the target group."

A program plan should also reflect that the program has passed all requirements of the law, the institution or agency, the community, the government, and the funding agency. Informed consent may be required for participation in the program. If informed consent is necessary, an informed consent form should be included with the program plan.

In some institutions, the planner may have to develop several different program plans to submit to administration for consideration. The shorter, clearer, and more concise the recommendation(s), the more likely they are to get serious and thorough consideration by administration.

Developing Goals and Objectives. Goals and objectives serve as a framework for the design of the program plan and evaluation. A goal is usually stated in rather global terms, for example:

1. Cervical cancer mortality will be reduced, or
2. Nosocomial infections will be reduced, or
3. Compliance with prescripted treatment will be improved

Notice that these goals are not specific, do not quantitate the degree to which the probem will be reduced, do not include a time frame for accomplishment of the goal. This overall goal usually reflects the original problem that was in need of resolution.

Objectives specify for each of the problems within the problem hierarchy to be addressed, the outcomes to be achieved. No objectives are necessary for parts of the problem that will not be addressed. Objectives should be specific to the activities to be carried out. An objective must specify the outcome to be expected, a time period for accomplishing the objective, a quantitated measure of success, the target group, the location of the activity or the target group, and any qualitative aspects necessary to the objective. One way to do this is to approach the objective in a segmented way—first, a general statement of the specific objective may be made, then a sentence relative to qualitative aspects of the objective may be stated, then a quantitative sentence is provided. The activities associated with each objective should be stated. An example of objectives handled in this way is provided in Table 15–5. A one sentence objective for each of the problems within the problem hierarchy, which will be attacked, may be used if it is specific as to the expected outcome, the time period for accomplishing it, the quantitated measure of success, and the target group. The objectives must be this specific if an adequate evaluation plan is to be developed.

Program outcomes that are specified in the objectives may be of several types, including patient outcomes, process outcomes, administrative outcomes, and economic outcomes. The main focus of interest for health professionals is one or more health outcomes. These outcomes may be at the primary, secondary, or tertiary levels of prevention (see Chapter 2). Examples of *patient outcomes* are length and quality of survival, death rates, level of function, rates of psychological or physical illness, birth defects, and birth weight. Patient satisfaction, disease understanding, medical regimen compliance, and alteration of risk are *process outcomes*. Alteration of risk is usually accomplished through life-style changes or changes in exposure such as smoking cessation, exercise, nutrition, and use of protective equipment in the workplace. Service utilization, waiting time for service, length of time to notification of test results, and distance to services are *administrative* types of *outcomes*. Ordinarily, meeting objectives for patient outcomes is dependent upon meeting process, administrative, and economic outcomes. The type of outcome for a given objective depends on which contributing factor is being addressed by the activities of the program. That is, different problems within the problem hierarchy have different types of outcomes associated with their objectives.

TABLE 15-5. CERVICAL CANCER PROGRAM OBJECTIVES

Ultimate goal: To reduce morbidity and, thereby, mortality from invasive cervical cancer.

Primary objective: To reach, screen and diagnose those most at risk for cancer in situ of the uterine cervix (5 to 10 years).

Secondary objective: To reach, screen and diagnose those most at risk for invasive cervical cancer (5 to 10 years).

Rationale: Future morbidity and mortality will be most affected by preventing the occurrence of invasive stages. At the same time, alteration in the present mortality may be brought about by screening directed to those now at high risk for invasive cervical cancer.

Service and Financial Assistance: All women presenting themselves for screening who are at high risk of cervical cancer will receive quality screening and follow-up (3-year).

Subobjectives	Qualitative	Quantitative (year 1)	Activities
1. Medically indigent women will have been screened for cervical cancer.	Medically indigent women over age 20 will have had a Pap smear. Emphasis on 25 to 55-year-olds.	There will have been a 15% increase in the number of medically indigent women who will have received a Pap smear in the last 12 months.	Screening will be carried out at Milwaukee County Hospital, Family Planning, Planned Parenthood Clinics, VD Clinics, and selected industries.
2. The screened population represented a group of women at high risk.	Screened women were 25 to 55, low socioeconomic, early 1st coitus, and poor Pap history.	80% of those screened were at high risk.	Screenee enumeration by age, socioeconomic, 1st coitus, and Pap history.
3. The services were sufficient to serve the needs of the target population.	Women who are at high risk were able to get a screening appointment.	90% of high-risk women calling for an appointment were able to get a screening appointment.	Record of women who did not get appointments who were at high risk.
4. The services were available to and accepted by the target population.	The high-risk population did report for screening.	15% of the population in need in areas served reported for screening.	Need level will be compared against those responding to screening.
5. The services were acceptable to the target population.	Women screened felt that services were acceptable.	90% of women screened felt that services were acceptable.	Random sample of those served. Test instrument to be developed. Including: reasonable wait time, courteous staff, questions answered, etc.
6. The screening test as administered provided results that were acceptable.	Screening test were acceptable in terms of sensitivity, specificity, underreferral, and overreferral.	Sensitivity plus .75 Specificity plus .99 Underreferral – 1/1000 screened Overreferral – 10/1000 screened	Screening test results to be measured.

EVALUATION

Evaluation Plan

The evaluation plan is developed during program planning and preferably is part of the program plan. It is utilized as a plan for the actual evaluation and incorporated into the final evaluation report. Such a plan must always be developed *before* doing any evaluation. If an evaluation plan was not developed during program planning it will be necessary to develop one before beginning any evaluation. A complete list of the items that should be included in an evaluation plan is given in Table 15–6.

An evaluation plan should be based on objectives of the program. If the specific objectives do not include the expected outcome, a quantitative measure of success, a time frame, and the specification of the target group for programs or activities, a major problem in evaluation arises. Until objectives can be stated in this fashion, an evaluation cannot be done. If the desired outcome is unknown, it cannot be determined if the outcome has been produced. This demonstrates the importance of clear objectives during the planning process.

For each program objective a method of evaluation must be described. This description should specify which activities contribute to a given objective (a single activity may contribute to more than one objective). It should also specify what data will be collected and how they will be collected for the evaluation of each objective, sources for any data that are not generated internally by the program (e.g., mortality rates), the frequency of evaluation, and the analyses planned to evaluate each objective. The criteria for a judgment of acceptability or of nonacceptability for meeting each objective should be stated. For example, if the objective is to have 250 adult women participate in a coun-

TABLE 15–6. EVALUATION PLAN INCLUSIONS

Program plan or a reconstruction of the program plan and its objectives (if no plan exists for a program already in existence)

Identification of evaluative measures, methods, and acceptability criteria

Ordering and prioritization of objectives for evaluation

Data collection forms and mechanisms

Analysis plan, time frame, and frequency

seling program for one year, then has the objective been met if
175, or 70 percent, of the adult women have participated? A specific cutoff of acceptability may be specified or the program planner may choose to grade or rank the program's effectiveness in
meeting its objective. One such scheme might be:

90 to 100 percent	Very good
70 to 89 percent	Good
50 to 69 percent	Questionnably acceptable
49 percent or less	Unacceptable

Criteria for judging the acceptability of costs or efficiency should
also be stated for each objective that is to be evaluated for efficiency. If an activity affects more than one objective, then the
efficiency estimates should reflect only the costs of the proportion of the activity that were related to the particular objective
being evaluated. As previously stated the quantification of the
effectiveness of a program is dependent upon the value given in
the objectives. For the new program, the quantity or value
stated in an objective may be little more than a guess. Frequently, it will represent a value that the planner thinks will
look good for the projected costs and looks realistic for the size
and nature of the group. Obviously, a program planner can
make the program look quite good if an underestimate is made
of its ability to impact on the problem. The smart planner will
choose an intermediate to low estimate. Too high or too much of
an overestimate could make a program look pretty bad. With an
ongoing program, it is possible to make more realistic estimates
of impact. When revising objectives it is advisable to utilize
findings of the data generated during evaluation and to try to
project the highest goals that seem reasonable for the resources
going into the activities associated with the objective.

The order for evaluating objectives should be stated in the
evaluation plan and reflect a prioritization of the objectives. An
evaluation time schedule should be developed which reflects this
prioritization. If for some reason, a total evaluation cannot be
completed, evaluation should be done on the most important
objectives referring back to the ranking of the problems within
the problem hierarchy for assistance in prioritization of objectives.

Data Collection Forms and Mechanisms. All of the program
forms that provide data for evaluation should be included in the

evaluation plan. The evaluation plan for each objective should specify all of the data items and all of the forms on which the item is found. The easiest way to do this is for each form to have a unique identification number and for each item within the form to have a unique identifier. Such specification of the sources of the data for evaluating each objective assures that when it comes time for evaluation, the necessary data are available.

A lack of appropriate data is a major problem in evaluating an existing program that does not have a plan or objectives. The evaluator must make a concerted effort to evaluate the reconstructed objectives to the best extent possible. Existing data may be useful; if data are available, the plan should provide copies of forms that will be used to obtain the information and state which data items on which forms are to be used for evaluating each objective. In some cases the evaluator may be in a position to collect new information as part of an evaluation effort. A survey of people served by the program may be done. Or, data may be collected retrospectively for the situation before and after the program was initiated. For instance, pathology laboratories could be surveyed to determine how many Pap smears were done annually before March 1975 (which is when the program began) and how many Pap smears were done annually from March 1975 until the present. Pap smear rates can then be determined for each period of time, that is, before and after the program began. If the program consisted of a public education effort, it will not be possible to conclude that any change in Pap smear rates occurred because of the program's public education effort. Other factors on which no information is available may have caused this change. This example illustrates some of the problems that occur as a result of failure to build evaluation into the program design.

Analysis Plan, Time Frame, and Frequency. The evaluation plan should specify the analyses that are planned for evaluating each objective. A profile of the target group (information available in the plan) for each objective should be provided and descriptive data should be provided to illustrate how the actual participants compare to the target group. In one cervical cancer screening program it was found that most of the participants were middle to upper class, well educated white women with few pregnancies who had had Pap smears within 6 months prior to being screened by the program. The target group was lower socioeconomic, poorly educated minority women with multiple pregnancies who had not had a Pap smear in the last 3 years. The evaluator should make sure that the time frame utilized in analysis is the same as the time frame specified in the objective. In other words, do not evaluate 6 months worth of daa for a 12-month objective. The formulas that are to be used for determination of effectiveness, efficiency, adequacy, or other measures of program accomplishments should be included in the plan. (Although only one formula was given in this chapter for effectiveness and efficiency, there are several methods of calculating them.) Sensitivity, specificity, and predictive value should be calculated when evaluating any screening or diagnostic procedures (see Chapter 13).

A time frame for evaluation should be included in the evaluation plan. When evaluation will begin and when it is projected to end should be stated. The frequency of evaluation activities should be stated also. If different objectives require evaluation at different intervals at different points in time, the intervals and the length of time for the evaluation for each objective should be stated or illustrated.

Potential Biases and Limitations of Evaluation Plan. The last item to be included in the evaluation plan is a statement of any biases or limitations of the evaluation. This is always important but it is extremely important for programs that have never had a program plan or specific objectives.

Program or Method Efficacy. The question of program efficacy is sometimes raised during program evaluation. Efficacy is defined in the *Dictionary of Epidemiology* as "The extent to which a specific intervention, procedure, regimen, or service produces a beneficial result under ideal conditions. Ideally the determination of efficacy is based on the results of a randomized controlled trial" (Last, 1983). It is this author's opinion that an activity should not be implemented as part of an ongoing program until efficacy has been demonstrated. It may, however, be of value to periodically reassess efficacy when a program is using a method of proven efficacy. A method of efficacy proven under ideal conditions may not be efficacious under everyday field conditions. Testing of efficacy in existing programs usually will be very difficult. Because randomized controlled trial is not usually possible (for ethical reasons) in an existing program, other methods would need to be used. Retrospective or prospective studies may be carried out for this purpose. These types of studies are not as definitive as a randomized controlled trial and they do require substantial time and resource efforts. The result is that it is rare to find a study of efficacy as part of an existing program. Problems related to measuring efficacy for screening or diagnostic tools purporting to impact on the natural history of a disease are discussed in Chapters 11 and 13. If the only methods available that may be of value in resolving a problem have never been tested for efficacy, then it is advisable to do a randomized controlled trial before beginning the program. Subjects would be randomly assigned to several treatment modalities and then followed over time. Such trials may be rather complicated to design. Multiple references are available on the subject. This is one situation where an expert consultant should be utilized.

The Evaluation Report

The actual evaluation leads to the preparation of an evaluation report. This report must describe the problem, the program objectives, the problem hierarchy, the methods of evaluation, the measures of evaluation used, the findings, criteria used for judging the acceptbility of the findings, the potential biases and limitations, conclusions, recommendations for program modifications or for research that is needed, and the rationale for any recommendations. Findings include all of the pertinent data that are generated during analysis. The findings that are reported reflect the items chosen for analysis in the analysis plan previously discussed under the section on the evaluation plan.

Conclusions and inferences should be limited to those areas where evaluation has been done. If a topic has not been evaluated, it should not be discussed in the conclusions unless findings related to several objectives, when taken together, point in a particular direction. If the findings related to several objectives together appear to point to a particular conclusion, then the stated conclusion should include a discussion of which findings when taken together support the conclusion. How the findings support the conclusion should also be discussed. Pertinent literature references may be utilized in drawing these conclusions or in supporting the findings from the evaluation.

Recommendations should be included in the evaluation report. A program that is meeting its objectives within acceptable limits will most likely receive a recommendation to continue as is. Objectives with evaluation findings that are outside of acceptable limits should be submitted for problem solving and then a recommended plan of action developed. Failure to meet the overall goal even though program objectives are being met, should lead to a reassessment of the problem. An example of reassessment was discussed at the beginning of this chapter under the discussion of the cyclic nature of planning and evaluation.

Sometimes the findings of evaluation lead to a recognition of an unrecognized problem or factor that may contribute to the original problem. Evidence supporting the existence of such a problem should be included in the reporting of any such problem. If it is a significant problem or factor that has a significant impact on the overall problem and if there is evidence substantiating the existence of this contributing factor, then it should be incorporated into the problem hierarchy. It should also be ranked with the other contributing factors. In short, it requires a complete revision of the problem statement. If this problem prevents a program from meeting its overall goal, then a complete revision of the program plan is necessary. If a contributing factor is not significantly interfering with meeting of program objectives, then it should not be added to the problem hierarchy and should not result in revisions of the program plan.

The findings of a program evaluation may point to the need for a study of efficacy or it may point to the need to do a study of the risk associated with the suspected causes of the problem. This was the situation with cervical cancer, which was described under the cyclic nature of planning and evaluation. That is, research was needed to determine what factors were largely responsible for the deaths now occurring from cervical cancer. Any research of this type must utilize epidemiological methods of study. The focus of such studies, however, is on causative factors that are subject to disease control methods. Factors that are subject to disease control methods are Pap smear status, time since last Pap smear, knowledge about Pap smears, socioeconomic status, laboratory error, and so forth.

CLOSING COMMENT

It must be emphasized that although cervical cancer has served as an example in most of this chapter, the described approach to planning and evaluation can and should be used for all types of health-related problems. The described approach is not as complicated as it may sound. The process of planning and evaluation is not difficult as long as the steps are followed as specified. Most of the required information is available from government sources, scientific literature, or institution and agency records. Locating the information may take some effort. The bulk of the effort for using this approach is mental effort. Real thought is required to generate a problem hierarchy and to understand how all the problems within the hierarchy interrelate. And, real thought is required to consider all of the factors and issues involved in making a good decision as to which methods or activities are the best choices for a given problem. It also takes some real thought to decide the best way to collect the data necessary for evaluation. Hard thinking can be enjoyable and growth producing. It will also lead to effective problem solving and the effective and efficient resolution of today's health care problems.

REFERENCES

Bales, V. S. *Problem solving for managers.* Unpublished manuscript, U.S. Centers for Disease Control, 1983.

Deniston, O. L., Rosenstock, W. W., & Getting, V. A. Evaluation of Program Efficiency. *Public Health Reports,* 1968, *83*(7); 603.

Deniston, O. L., Rosenstock, I. M. Evaluating health programs. *Public Health Reports,* 1970, *85*(9); 835.

Fink, A., & Kosecoff, A. *An evaluation primer.* Washington, D.C.: Capitol Publications, 1978.

Fitz-Gibbon, C. T., & Morris, L. L. *How to design a program evaluation.* Beverly Hills: Sage Publications, 1978.

Franklin, J. L., & Thrasher, J. H. *An introduction to program evaluation.* New York: John Wiley & Sons, 1976.

Guttentag, M., & Streuning, E. L. (Eds.). *Handbook of evaluation research* (vol. 1 & 2). Beverly Hills: Sage Publications, 1975.

Hilleboe, H. E., & Schaefer, M. Evaluation in community health: Relating results to goals. *Bulletin of the New York Academy of Medicine,* 1968, *44*(2), 140.

Last, J. M. (Ed.). *A dictionary of epidemiology,* New York: Oxford University Press, 1983.

Martin, P. L. How preventable is invasive cervical cancer? A community study of preventable factors, *American Journal of Obstetrics and Gynecology,* 1972, *113*, 541–548.

Morris, L. L., & Fitz-Gibbon, C. T. *Evaluators handbook.* Beverly Hills: Sage Publications, 1978.

Morris, L. L., & Fitz-Gibbon, C. T. *How to calculate statistics.* Beverly Hills: Sage Publications, 1978.

Morris, L. L., & Fitz-Gibbon, C. T. *How to deal with goals and objectives.* Beverly Hills: Sage Publications, 1978.

Morris, L. L., & Fitz-Gibbon, C. T. *How to measure achievement.* Beverly Hills: Sage Publications, 1978.

Morris, L. L., & Fitz-Gibbon, C. T. *How to measure attitudes.* Beverly Hills: Sage Publications, 1978.

Morris, L. L., & Fitz-Gibbon, C. T. *How to measure program implementation.* Beverly Hills: Sage Publications, 1978.

Morris, L. L., & Fitz-Gibbon, C. T. *How to present an evaluation report.* Beverly Hills: Sage Publications, 1978.

National Cancer Institute. *Surveillance, epidemiology & end results: Incidence and mortality data, 1973–1977.* NIH Publication No. 81-2330, June, 1981.

Suchman, E. A. *Evaluative research: Principles and practice in public service and social action programs.* New York: Russell Sage Foundation, 1967.

Glossary

accuracy: the degree to which a measurement represents the true value of the attribute being measured.

agent: a factor whose presence, excessive presence, or relative absence is essential for the occurrence of a disease.

association: a relationship between two factors or events, usually expressed as the degree of statistical dependence. Factors or events are said to be associated when they occur more frequently together than one would expect by chance alone.

attributable risk: *See* risk.

biological plausibility: a reasonable physiological mechanism to explain how a casual factor could operate to bring about a particular disease.

carrier: a person or animal that harbors a specific infectious agent in the absence of clinical disease, thus serving as a potential source of infection to others.

    chronic carrier: a person or animal who harbors a specific infectious agent for an indefinite period of time.

    convalescent carrier: a person or animal who no longer has an acute infectious disease, but remains infectious to others because of continued shedding of the viable organism.

    inapparent carrier: a person or animal who is infected with an infectious organism and never develops clinical disease, but is a source of infection to others.

    incubating carrier: a person or animal who is infectious to others while incubating an infectious disease prior to development of clinical symptoms.

case: any person identified as having a particular disease based on presence of defined criteria.

case-control study: a study that begins with the identification of persons with the disease (or other outcome variable of interest) and a suitable comparison (control) group of persons without the disease, then compares the diseased and nondiseased with regard to the frequency or level of presence of the hypothesized causal (or associated) attribute.

case-finding: a concerted effort to search for previously unidentified cases of a disease.

causality: the relating of causes to the effects they produce.

cause: a stimulus that brings about an effect; usually defined operationally by determining that changing the amount or frequency of a suspected cause changes the amount or frequency of the related effect.

necessary cause: a factor that must always be present before an event.

sufficient cause: a factor that inevitably initiates or produces the effect.

chronic disease: all impairments or deviations from normal with one or more of the following characteristics: permanent, leaves residual disability, is caused by non-reversible pathological alterations, requires special training of the patient for rehabilitation, or may be expected to require long periods of supervision, observation, or care.

clinical disease: the stage in the natural history that begins when sufficient anatomic or functional changes have occurred to produce observable signs and symptoms of disease.

clinical epidemiology: the application of epidemiological principles and methods to the day-to-day care of patients.

clinical horizon: a point in the natural history when clinical disease becomes evident.

cluster: a closely grouped series of events or cases of a disease or other health-related phenomena with well-defined time and/or place distribution patterns.

cohort: any designated group of persons who are followed or traced over a period of time.

cohort anaylsis: the following of a component of the population born during a particular period and identified by period of birth so that its characteristics (e.g., causes of death) can be ascertained for each successive period of time and age.

cohort study: a study in which subsets of a defined population can be identified as exposed, not exposed, or exposed in varying degrees to a factor or factors hypothesized to cause a disease or other outcome. Subjects are then followed over time, and frequency of disease occurrence is determined.

comparison group: any group with which the index group is compared; a control group.

community assessment: the process of describing a community, its patterns of morbidity and mortality, and identifying those patterns which are clearly in excess of normal.

cost–benefit: the ratio of the economic benefit of preventing an additional case to the economic cost of preventing an additional case. When the ratio is greater than 1, the benefits outweigh the costs.

critical point: a theoretical time representing a point in disease natural history that is crucial in determining whether there will be major or severe consequences of the disease. Intervention prior to this point can change the subsequent course and prognosis of the disease. Intervention after this point does not alter the course of the disease.

cross-sectional study: a study that determines for each member of a study population or a representative sample of a population the presence or absence of hypothetical causal factors and disease at a single point in time.

decision analysis: application of probability theory to assist in making "best-choice" clinical decisions by breaking such decisions into smaller, more easily assimilated series of decisions; often expressed graphically in the form of a decision tree diagram which indicates alternative decision choices and eventualities in the order they are likely to occur and which assigns quantitative values to each outcome.

detection point: the point at which a disease is detectable by technological methods.

ecological fallacy: an error in inference caused by failure to distinguish between different levels of organization, e.g., assuming that relationships between factors and diseases observed for groups can be equally applied to individuals.

ecological study: a study that looks for relationships between factors or events and disease frequency or level, based on aggregate data for entire populations; joint presence or absence of disease and the etiological factor for individuals is not established.

efficacy: the extent to which a specific intervention, regimen, procedure, or service produces a beneficial result under ideal conditions.

efficiency: the effects or end results achieved in relation to the effort expended in terms of money, resources, and time.

endemic disease: the habitual presence of a disease or infectious agent in a defined geographical area or population.

environment: all external conditions and influences affecting the life of living things.

epidemic: rates of a disease clearly in excess of normal or expected frequency in a defined geographical area.

common source epidemic: an epidemic caused by exposure of a group of persons to the same source of an agent, e.g., the same water supply.

epidemic curve: a graphic plotting of the distribution of cases by time of onset.

propagated epidemic: an epidemic caused by person-to-person transmission of a disease agent.

epidemiology: the study of the distribution of states of health and of the determinants of deviations from health in populations.

analytical epidemiology: use of epidemiological methods to test hypotheses about causality; the second phase of epidemiological investigations.

descriptive epidemiology: the first phase of epidemiological investigation; applying epidemiological methods to generate descriptions of the time, place, and person characteristics of disease distribution.

experimental epidemiology: use of experimental studies to establish disease causality.

substantive epidemiology: the collection of epidemiological knowledge about diseases.

etiology: postulated causes that initiate the pathogenic process; *see also* cause.

evaluation: an objective, systematic process for determining the relevance, effectiveness, and impact of program activities in relation to program objectives.

experiment: a study in which subjects are randomly assigned to each experimental condition and the conditions of the study are under the control of the investigator; also called a randomized, controlled trial.

factor: one of the elements, circumstances, or influences that contribute to produce a result.

false negative: a negative test result in a subject who possesses the attribute for which the test is conducted.

false positive: a positive test result in a subject who does not possess the attribute for which the test is conducted.

health: complete physical, mental, and social well-being.

health risk appraisal: a method of estimating an individual's risk of developing a disease or other outcome.

host: a person or living animal that affords subsistence or lodgement to an infection.

hypothesis: a supposition provisionally adopted to explain observations and to guide investigation.

immunity: the resistance of an individual to a specific infectious agent or its products.

> *active immunity:* resistance developed in response to stimulus by an antigen (infective agent or vaccine) and usually characterized by the presence of antibody produced by the host.

> *natural immunity:* species-determined inherent resistance to a disease agent.

> *passive immunity:* immunity conferred by an antibody produced in another host and acquired naturally by an infant from its mother or artificially by administration of an antibody-containing preparation.

immunization: administration of a living modified agent, a suspension of killed organisms, or an inactivated toxin to protect susceptible individuals from infectious disease.

incidence: the frequency of newly occurring cases of a disease in a specified population during a given time period.

incubation period: a time interval beginning with invasion by an infectious agent and continuing until the organism multiplies to sufficient numbers to produce a host reaction and clinical symptoms.

index case: the first case in a defined population unit to come to the attention of the investigator.

induction period: the period of time from causal action of a factor (exposure) to initiation of the disease.

infection: the entry and establishment of an infectious agent in a host.

subclinical infection: an infection detectable through anti-body tests but not manifest in clinical signs or symptoms.

infectivity: the property of being able to lodge and multiply in a host, thus the ability to infect a host.

isolation: separation, for the period of communicability, of infected individuals from those who are susceptible or who may spread the agent to others.

lead time: the time gained in the natural progression of a disease through earlier diagnoses.

lead time bias: a systematic error arising when follow-up of two groups does not begin at strictly comparable times, e.g., a group diagnosed early in the natural history through screening is compared with cases detected because of symptoms.

natural history: stages in the process of development and progression of a disease without intervention by man.

nosocomial: relating to a hospital; arising while a patient is in a hospital or as a result of being in a hospital.

outcomes: all possible results that may arise from exposure to a factor or an intervention.

pandemic: epidemics that involve populations in widespread geographical areas of the world.

parallel testing: the simultaneous application of multiple diagnostic tests.

pathogenesis: the postulated mechanisms by which an etiological agent produces disease.

pathogenicity: the ability of an organism to produce overt disease.
  pathogenicity rate: a measure of the pathogenicity of an organism in a population; the percentage of all infected persons who have clinical disease.

person–year: a statistical measure representing one person at risk of developing a disease for one year.

potential years of life lost: a measure of the loss to society due to youthful or early deaths, calculated as the sum, over all persons dying from that cause, of the years these individuals would have lived had they experienced a normal life expectation.

precision: accuracy of a test or measure.

predictive values: in screening and diagnostic tests, the probability with which test results represent correct identification of disease status.

positive predictive value: the probability that a person with a positive test has the disease.

negative predictive value: the probability that a person with a negative test does not have the disease.

presymptomatic disease: an early stage in the natural history of disease when physiological changes have begun but no clinical signs or symptoms are present.

prevention: the act of hindering or forestalling development or progression of disease.

primary prevention: actions directed toward intervening in the natural history of disease during the stage of susceptibility, before any pathological changes occur in a host. These actions seek to keep the agent away from the host or to increase host resistance.

secondary prevention: actions directed toward early detection and treatment of disease.

tertiary prevention: actions directed toward limiting disability from disease or restoring function.

proportion: a specific type of ratio in which the numerator is included in the denominator and the resultant value is expressed as a percentage.

prospective study: *See* cohort study.

quarantine: limitation of freedom of movement of well persons exposed to a communicable disease for a period of time no longer than the usual incubation period of the disease. The purpose of quarantine is to prevent contact with persons not exposed during the time the exposed individuals are infectious to others.

rate: a special form of proportion that includes specification of time. *See also* proportion; *see text for specific rates.*

ratio: the relationship between two numbers expressed as a fraction; the value obtained by dividing the numerator of the fraction by the denominator.

register, registry: the file of data concerning all cases of a particular disease or other health-relevant condition in a defined population, so that cases can be related to a population base and incidence calculated. Regular, ongoing follow-up of cases to monitor remissions, exacerbations, prevalence, and survival is often done. The register is the actual document, the registry is the system of ongoing registration.

relational study: a study that uses information on presence or level of both the hypothesized causal factor or event and the health-related outcome or disease in each individual in order to examine relationships between the factor or event and the health-related outcome or disease.

relationship: See association.

reliability: the degree of stability exhibited when a measurement is repeated under identical conditions, i.e., the repeatability or replicability.

reporting system: See registry.

reservoir of infection: the habitat in which a living organism lives and multiplies.

retrospective study: See case-control study.

risk: the probability that an unfavorable event will occur.

risk appraisal, risk assessment: an estimation of an individual's risk for developing an outcome, e.g., a specific disease or death.

risk factor: this term is used in three ways:
1. an attribute or exposure associated with an increased probability of a specified outcome; a risk marker.
2. an attribute or exposure that increases the probability of occurrence of disease or other specified outcome; a determinant.
3. a determinant that can be modified by intervention, thus reducing the probability of occurence of a disease or other specified outcome; a modifiable risk factor.

screening: the presumptive identification of unrecognized disease or defect by tests, examinations, or other procedures that can be applied rapidly.
mass screening: application of screening tests unselectively to entire populations or selectively to high-risk groups.
multiphasic screening: simultaneous application of screening tests for a variety of diseases or conditions, e.g., multiple tests on single blood sample.

sensitivity: the proportion of persons with a disease who test positive on a screening test.

serial testing: the application of diagnostic tests consecutively, one at a time. The decision to use each subsequent test is dependent upon results of the previous test.

specificity: the proportion of persons without a disease who have negative results on a screening test.

stage-specific risk factor: A risk factor associated with only one stage in the natural history of a disease.

statistical power: the relative frequency with which a true difference of specified size between populations would be detected by the proposed experiment or test.

statistical relationship: See association.

surveillance of disease: the system of keeping watch over all aspects of occurrence and spread of a disease that are relevant to effective control.

susceptibility: state or quality of lacking resistance to an agent and therefore being likely to develop effects if exposed.

toxoid: a toxin, treated to destroy its toxicity but still able, upon injection, to stimulate antibody formation in a host.

transmission of infection: any mechanism by which an infectious agent is spread through the environment or to another person.

    direct transmission: transfer of an infectious agent from the reservoir to a receptive portal of entry through which human infection can take place.

    indirect transmission: transport of an organism by means of air, vehicles, or vectors from a reservoir to a receptive portal of entry through which human infection can take place.

true negative: a negative test result for a subject who does not have the disease.

true positive: a positive test result for a subject who has the disease.

vaccine: immunobiological substance used for active immunization. By introducing into the body a live modified, attenuated, or killed infectious organism or its toxin an immune response is stimulated in the host, who is thus rendered resistant to infection.

validity of measurement: an expression of the degree to which a measure represents what it purports to measure.

validity of a study: the degree to which generalization of study results beyond the study sample is warranted when account is taken of study methods, representativeness of the study sample, and the nature of the population from which it is drawn.

variable: any attribute, phenomenon, or event that can have different values.

    confounding variable: a factor that causes change in the frequency of a disease and also varies systematically with a third, potentially causal factor being studied. When uncontrolled, a confounding variable masks or distorts the effect of the study variable.

vector: an insect or other living carrier that transports an infectious agent from an infected individual or its wastes to a susceptible individual or its food or immediate surroundings.

vehicle: an inanimate substance that transports an infectious agent to a susceptible host, e.g., food or water.

virulence: the disease-provoking power of a microorganism, measured as a ratio of the number of cases of overt clinical infection to the total number of individuals infected, as determined by immunoassay.

web of causation: the interrelationship among multiple factors that contributes to the occurrence of a disease.

Index